LITHIUM EFFECTS ON GRANULOPOIESIS AND IMMUNE FUNCTION

ADVANCES IN EXPERIMENTAL MEDICINE AND BIOLOGY

Recent Volumes in this Series

LITHIUM EFFECTS ON GRANULOPOIESIS AND IMMUNE FUNCTION

Edited by

Arthur H. Rossof
Rush Medical College
Chicago, Illinois

and

William A. Robinson
University of Colorado Medical Center
Denver, Colorado

PLENUM PRESS • NEW YORK AND LONDON

Library of Congress Cataloging in Publication Data

Workshop on Effects of Lithium on Granulopoiesis and Immune Function, Rush University, 1979.
Lithium effects on granulopoiesis and immune function.

(Advances in experimental medicine and biology; v. 127)
"Proceedings of the Workshop on Effects of Lithium on Granulopoiesis and Immune Function, held at the John L. and Beatrice Keeshin International Biomedical Systems Planning Center of Rush University, Eagle River, Wisconsin, June 6-9, 1979."
Includes index.
1. Lithium – Physiological effect – Congresses. 2. Granulocytes – Congresses. 3. Immune response – Regulation – Congresses. 4. Lithium – Therapeutic use – Congresses. I. Rossof, Arthur H. II. Robinson, William A. III. Title. IV. Series.
QP535.L5W67 1979 615'.718 80-116

DOI 10.1007/978-1-4757-0259-0

Proceedings of the Workshop on Effects of Lithium on Granulopoiesis and Immune Function, held at the John L. and Beatrice Keeshin International Biomedical Systems Planning Center of Rush University, Eagle River, Wisconsin, June 6–9, 1979.

MyCopy version of the original edition 1980
A Division of Plenum Publishing Corporation
227 West 17th Street, New York, N.Y. 10011

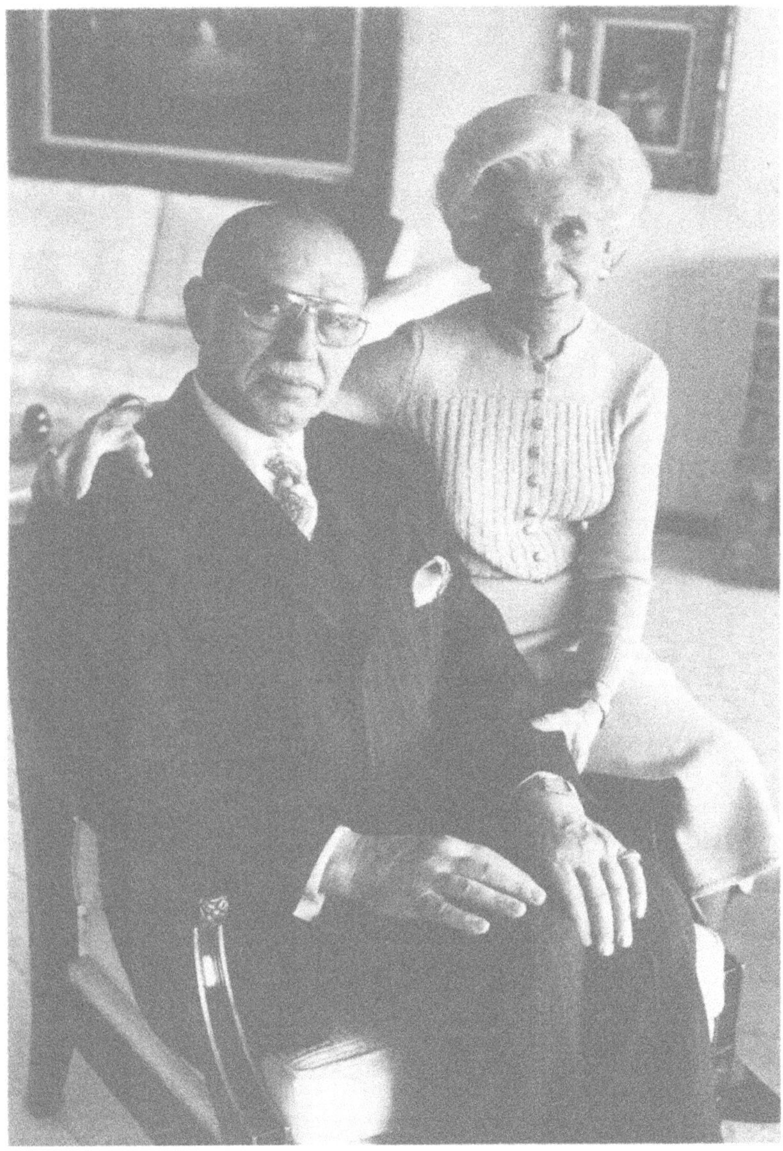

In 1978, Mr. and Mrs. John L. Keeshin donated their summer home, near Eagle River, Wisconsin, to Rush University of Chicago, Illinois. In so doing, the John L. and Beatrice Keeshin International Biomedical Systems Planning Center was born, dedicated to functioning as a biomedical think tank and providing a spacious and idyllic northwoods environment to foster the exchange of promising ideas and experiences in biomedical research. The facility consists of nearly 5000 square feet of meeting, dining, and residential space located on the shore of Catfish Lake.

Rush University is pleased to have been the recipient of this most generous gift. The June 6–9, 1979 Workshop on the Effects of Lithium on Granulopoiesis and Immune Function was the first formal international meeting held at the Keeshin Center and it was a great success. We thank Mr. and Mrs. Keeshin for providing this excellent meeting facility and for the continuing interest in the dissemination of biomedical knowledge.

FOREWORD

This monograph contains papers which resulted from an international workshop on the effects of lithium on the hematopoietic and immunologic systems. The meeting was held at the John L. and Beatrice Keeshin International Biomedical Systems Planning Center of Rush University in Eagle River, Wisconsin from June 6 through June 9, 1979. The object of this conference was to bring together scientists from around the world with an interest in the effects of lithium and its potential use in human disease to bolster and stimulate the hematologic and immune systems. These topics seemed to us to be important and the time seemed right for bringing together the workers in these fields to exchange ideas and recent research results. We sought to bring together basic research scientists trying to uncover the mechanism of action of lithium in the stimulation of granulopoiesis and in its immunologic effects, together with those involved in clinical care and the use of lithium as a therapeutic tool in neoplastic and non-neoplastic disorders. This was the first use of the Keeshin Center for such a program. The sessions were conducted in a relaxed atmosphere with a good deal of give-and-take by all the participants. The editors of this book hope that it will be useful as the first volume completely devoted to these applications of lithium in these new and, as yet, incompletely developed fields.

After editing by each of us, each paper was laboriously and carefully recomposed on a Xerox 850 Typing Display word processor. We are deeply grateful to Ms. DeLois A. Simmons and Mrs. Felice E. Witmer for their accuracy and speed in retyping these manuscripts. Any residual typographical errors are the responsibility of the editors. We hope that the authors and the readers of this monograph will overlook any minor typographical errors which may remain. They have resulted from our zeal for rapid publication.

The workshop was supported by funds provided in part by the International Cancer Research Data Bank, program of the National Cancer Institute, National Institutes of Health (US), under Contract No. N01-CO-65341, (International Cancer Research Workshops - ICREW) with the International Union Against Cancer, Geneva, Switzerland and by Smith Kline and French Laboratories, Philadelphia, Pennsylvania.

This monograph is dedicated to our patients. Their needs have fostered the research discussed in the following pages.

A.H.R. Chicago, Illinois
W.A.R. Denver, Colorado

November, 1979

CONTENTS

Section I: INTRODUCTION

Section II: MECHANISMS OF LITHIUM-INDUCED GRANULOCYTOSIS

Section IV: LITHIUM ATTENUATION OF ANTI-CANCER CHEMOTHERAPY

Section VI: NEUTROPHIL FUNCTION IN THE PRESENCE OF LITHIUM

LITHIUM CARBONATE IN MEDICINE AND PSYCHIATRY

Jan Fawcett

Department of Psychiatry
Rush-Presbyterian-St. Luke's Medical Center
Chicago, Illinois 60612

The history of lithium carbonate is a striking example of the fundamental unity of psychiatry and medicine. The medical use of lithium began in the mid-1800's somewhat after it was discovered in 1817 by Arfvedson while working in the laboratory of Berzelius (Jefferson and Griest, 1977). Isolated from the mineral petalite and named lithium after the Greek word for stone, it was used ineffectively in the treatment of urinary calculi and gout based on the *in vitro* observation that uric acid bladder stones dissolved in the lithium salt of uric acid. Lithium became popular as a medical panacea and waters from "lithia" springs were bottled and widely used well into the 1900's in the unsubstantiated hope that a wide range of medical ills could be cured or prevented. In the early twentieth century, the lithium salt of bromide was used both as a hypnotic and an anti-epileptic agent but this use faded as the use of bromides fell into disfavor.

In 1949 contrasting events were taking place in the United States and Australia, which had opposite effects on the use of lithium in medicine. Corcoran *et al*. (1949) reported in the American medical literature the coma and subsequent death of a patient presenting initially with symptoms of giddiness, nausea, confusion, apathy and gross tremor who was found to represent an example of fatal lithium intoxication secondary to its unrestricted use as a salt substitute (Corcoran et al., 1949). All medical uses of lithium salts were abruptly discontinued in the United States following this report. In the same year, in the Australian literature, Dr. John Cade (1949) reported the successful treatment with lithium salts of 10 patients suffering from mania. He further observed that one of his patients experienced relapse of the mania when the lithium was discontinued. Among his cases, he reported a 51 year old male patient who had been a particularly difficult patient manifesting regression and hostility during a five year hospitalization with chronic manic excitement, who, when treated with lithium, improved sufficiently to be discharged from the hospital and return to work. The use of lithium salts spread to the European continent where it was used in England and Scandinavia in the treatment of affective disorders. The efficacy of lithium in the treatment of mania was first reported in the American literature by Gershon and Yuwiler (1960) and it was rapidly put into use by research oriented psychiatrists and psychopharmacologists by the middle 1960's. It was officially approved for use in acute mania by the Food and Drug Administration in 1970. Subsequently, lithium was approved for use by the FDA in the prevention of recurrences of mania in 1974. The delay in official sanction of the use of lithium carbonate in America is related to the fact that the drug had caused fatalities when used in unrestricted amounts before its toxic potential was recognized, as well as the fact that blood levels were necessary to monitor safe usage of the drug. The fact that this simple salt of lithium could not be patented by any one pharmaceutical company and, therefore, was not commercially worth investing the large sums necessary for double blind trials to achieve official FDA approval, probably also delayed its official acceptance and earlier wide-spread use in psychiatry in this country. Since the introduction of lithium, it has gained acceptance as an effective agent for the treatment and prevention of mania and has to a significant extent replaced the use of neuroleptic drugs such as chlorpromazine and the use of electroconvulsive therapy in the treatment of manic depressive illness (Baastrup et al., 1970; Davis, 1976).

A review of double blind studies of the use of lithium in acute mania has not definitely shown it to be superior to chlorpromazine in resolving an acute manic state (Prien et al., 1974). However, the fact that lithium carbonate normalizes thought, mood, and behavior in the manic patient without sedation and tends to prevent recurrences, whereas chlorpromazine masks the manic state at the price of significant sedation without any basic change in the manic thought disorder, has made lithium the primary choice of therapy except in situations where the severity of a manic excitement requires more immediate control, in which case neuroleptic drugs are still used at least early in the course of treatment.

Mania is most precisely defined by the interim DSM-III Operational Criteria as one or more distinct periods with a predominantly elevated expansive or irritable mood which may not be related to alcohol or drug intoxication (DSM III Draft, 1978). In addition, at least three of the following symptom categories must be present to a significant degree:

1. More active than usual - either socially, at work, sexually or physically restless.
2. More talkative than usual - often associated with a pressure to continue talking.
3. Flight of ideas or the subjective experience that thoughts are racing.
4. Inflated self-esteem and/or grandiosity.
5. Decreased need for sleep.
6. Distractability.
7. Excessive involvement with activities without recognizing the high potential for painful consequences.

In addition, the period of illness must be clearly distinguished from usual functioning and sustained for at least one week, and the patient may not manifest symptom criteria which suggest schizophrenia.

The introduction of lithium carbonate in psychiatry has resulted in increased emphasis in research into the biochemical aspects of psychiatric disorders as well as dramatically emphasizing the importance of differential diagnosis in psychiatry. Specific treatment for specific conditions has replaced the notion that diagnosis was less important than individual psychodynamics.

The efficacy of lithium in the treatment of depression is a matter of continuing controversy. While reviews by Mendels (1976) and studies by others (Goodwin et al., 1972; Friedel, 1976) have shown that lithium does in fact exert a positive effect in depression, especially in manic depressive patients, clinical experience with the use of lithium in depression often shows that the degree of improvement is adequate in only a relatively low percentage of cases (Goodwin, et al, 1972; Friedel, 1976; Mendels, 1976). The September, 1975 conclusions of the American Psychiatric Association Task Force on Lithium Therapy found that experimental results were not sufficiently conclusive to define clearly the value of lithium in acute depression, but did find it effective in the prophylaxis against recurrent depression, especially in cases of manic depressive illness, more recently termed bipolar affective illness (Task Force on Lithium Therapy, 1975). Lithium has not yet been approved by the FDA for the treatment of acute depression or for prevention of the recurrence of depressive episodes in the absence of mania, although there is now ample evidence that lithium has prophylactic effects against recurrent depression.

Claims have been made for the efficacy of lithium in other psychiatric disorders where its therapeutic value is still a matter of controversy. Schizoaffective disorders (a combination of symptoms of mania and symptoms of schizophrenia) may sometimes benefit from treatment with lithium salts (Procci, 1976). Several studies done in prison populations have shown that lithium carbonate may be effective in reducing the occurrence of aggressive and violent behavior (Sheard, 1971; Sheard, 1975). Studies of the possible efficacy of lithium in improving the prognosis in alcoholism have suggested, particularly in patients with depressive mood associated with alcoholism, that lithium therapy may reduce recidivism and morbidity from this disease (Kline et al., 1974; Merry et al., 1976). There is also evidence in both animal and human studies to suggest that lithium may produce taste aversion to alcohol (Sinclair, 1974). More carefully controlled studies are necessary to evaluate the possible therapeutic uses of lithium in the treatment of alcoholism and to specify what particular subtypes of alcoholics might benefit from this treatment. Studies of lithium in the treatment of emotionally unstable character disorders, catatonia, drug abuse, obsessive-compulsive disorders, phobic disorders, paranoid states, and premenstrual tension have been inconclusive.

Lithium carbonate is ordinarily given in doses ranging from 900 to 1800 mgs. daily, attaining a serum lithium level of 1.0 to 1.4 meq/L for maximum therapeutic effect. The use of the drug is generally avoided or it is given with great care in patients with significant cardiovascular or renal disease and the substance must be given carefully, especially in the first week or two of treatment because of possible wide variations in the renal excretion of lithium. Before administering lithium, one should establish that renal function is normal which can usually adequately be determined with a serum creatinine level. Baseline thyroid studies are also a good idea since it has been shown that lithium may compromise thyroid function. A serum lithium level should be obtained five days after the beginning of a course of lithium therapy and levels should be obtained at weekly intervals for the next three or four weeks until a stable level has been obtained on a given dose. Thereafter, blood levels at monthly intervals and, eventually, three month intervals, are generally adequate. Side effects and toxic symptoms of lithium carbonate are quite consistent. The most common side effect is that of a fine intention tremor of the hands which is intensified by social stress. This symptom will often develop when the patient is drinking coffee in front of friends or affixing a signature while others are watching. The symptom is of little medical consequence, but since tremors are very upsetting socially, suggesting the possibility of drug addiction, withdrawal reactions (such as shakes in the alcoholic), and the fear of an impending seizure or fit, this symptom frequently interferes with the use of lithium. When the tremor cannot be removed by decreasing the dosage of lithium, the use of benzodiazepines such as diazepam, or the use of propranolol will often suppress the tremor. Loose stools and cramps may also occur but these can frequently be avoided by giving the medication with meals.

Loss of appetite, aversion to food, nausea and vomiting are common early signs of lithium toxicity. They usually develop before more serious toxic symptoms develop. For this reason, the symptoms should be taught to any patient using this substance. Symptoms of extreme lethargy, forgetfulness and confusion, and neuromuscular twitching herald the danger of coma and possible death from lithium toxicity. Early toxic symptoms may occur when the blood level exceeds 1.5 meq/L or less, but usually do not develop until the blood concentration has reached about 2.0 meq/L. Toxicity intensifies with confusion, lethargy and neuromuscular twitching proceeding to stupor as the blood level approaches 4.0 meq/L. Plasma lithium levels of 4.0 meq/L or over may be fatal. Occasionally, the loss of memory and confusion seen in the middle stages of lithium toxicity can occur in the elderly patient or the individual with chronic brain damage who is receiving lithium in normal dosage and with blood levels in the normal therapeutic range.

Lithium toxicity can occur in patients who have been stabilized at a therapeutic blood level if conditions change decreasing the dietary intake of sodium to a significant degree, or increasing the loss of sodium to a significant degree. A patient of mine, who was stabilized at a plasma level of 1.5 meq/L of lithium developed a severe gastrointestinal illness with severe diarrhea while traveling in Central America. He returned to the United States early because of profound fatigue and lethargy which accompanied these symptoms. He was evaluated for an intestinal infection and treated with anti-diarrheal medications but his condition persisted and his weakness increased. After his condition failed to respond to treatment, the patient presented himself in the emergency room with profound weakness, mild neuromuscular twitching, and, as observed by the medical resident, "a difficulty in connecting his thoughts." A plasma lithium level obtained at this point revealed a level of 4.1 meq/L with markedly elevated serum creatinine and blood urea nitrogen levels. This young man was admitted to the hospital and treated with fluids, sodium and potassium, as well as diuretics and showed a progressive decrease in his lithium levels and, subsequently, his creatinine levels. His mania recurred dramatically, resulting in the need to control him with very high doses of neuroleptic drugs until his lithium toxicity had been fully treated and it could be demonstrated that his renal function had returned to normal as measured by creatinine clearance studies.

Until mid-1977, lithium carbonate, though recognized as a potentially toxic drug, was considered essentially a benign substance if its administration was carefully controlled and monitored. Since that time Hestbech _et al._ (1979) and others have published several small series of patients who, after being maintained on chronic lithium carbonate, had renal biopsies - sometimes after evidence of repeated lithium toxicity but in later studies on a more random basis - which raised the question of chronic renal toxicity associated with lithium carbonate maintenance therapy (Hestbech _et al._, 1977). Over the past year and a half, various investigators, principally from Europe but also from the United States, have reported renal changes in the biopsies of approximately 150 patients who were receiving lithium carbonate for varying periods of time. The changes described are those of a glomerular sclerosis described as an interstitial fibrosis with damage to the proximal or distal tubule (Burrows _et al._, 1978). This picture was unlike that of glomerular nephritis in its most traditional forms. It has been associated by several of the investigators with patients showing evidence of lithium toxicity with normal blood lithium levels, whereas others have associated the findings with patients maintaining blood levels over 1.4 meq/L experiencing prominent polyuria and polydipsia. These findings have raised increasing concerns among psychopharmacologists concerning the possibility that lithium carbonate may cause chronic renal damage that may only be demonstrated after years of administration of the salt. Most recently, Raphaelson (1979) reported renal damage of a severe degree in four of fifty cases of chronic lithium carbonate therapy while fifteen cases showed evidence of moderate damage (Raphaelson, 1979). The degree of damage was related to the chronicity of lithium usage. For these reasons the criteria for selection of patients receiving lithium carbonate are becoming more carefully scrutinized, and the patients are being monitored more often with repeat creatinine levels and creatinine clearance tests as well as plasma lithium levels. Whether or not this potential for renal damage is related to lithium effect alone, interactions with other drugs, related to high blood lithium levels, associated with some inherent sensitivity or vulnerability to this effect, or is being seen in patients with some unrecognized renal disease unrelated to lithium, is not known. While the number of patients showing clinical manifestations of renal toxicity is, at this time, extremely small relative to the number of patients receiving chronic lithium carbonate therapy, these findings must be evaluated carefully by psychopharmacologists. Since manic depressive illness has a life time mortality from suicide alone of 15%, not to mention its severe morbidity and the ruination of careers and families, there is thus far a reluctance to conclude that the dangers of lithium carbonate outweigh the benefits in a large number of cases (Pitts and Winokur, 1964). Questions raised by these findings with regard to the indications for the use of lithium carbonate are unanswered at this time pending the further analysis of data concerning the possible renal toxicity of lithium carbonate.

Drug interactions are another area of interest in the medical use of lithium salts. In general, lithium carbonate is not highly interactive with other medications with a few notable exceptioins. Diuretics, in particular thiazides, with sites of action distal to the proximal tubule have been shown to *decrease* lithium clearance and *increase* serum lithium levels, sometimes to the point of toxicity. Chlorthiazide has been shown to cause a 26% increase in plasma lithium concentration both in normals and in manic depressive patients (Petersen et al., 1974). Himmelhoch et al. (1977) have suggested that this combination may even have some enhanced therapeutic value in obtaining effective intracellular lithium levels (Himmelhoch et al., 1977). It is believed that diuretics acting distal to the proximal tubule are likely to cause lithium retention whereas those agents that act at the proximal tubule such as mannitol and urea, as well as carbonic anhydrase inhibitors, have been shown to increase lithium excretion (Himmelhoch et al., 1977; Jefferson and Griest, 1977). In general, it is believed that lithium dosage should be decreased during the concurrent administration of most diuretics in order to maintain plasma levels in a therapeutic range.

The question has been raised in the literature whether a combination of lithium and the neuroleptic drug haloperidol may produce neurotoxicity in some patients. At present this contention is considered unproven although the 1975 American Psychiatric Association Task Force on Lithium recommends that high simultaneous dosages of these drugs be avoided if possible (Task Force on Lithium Therapy, 1975). Amongst a number of other contentions concerning the interaction of lithium with other medications, which to this point are unsubstantiated, the possible effect of lithium in prolonging the action of neuromuscular blocking agents seems to be receiving continual support in both studies of clinical cases and animal studies (Hill et al., 1976). This interaction may represent a potential hazard to patients undergoing surgical procedures or electroconvulsive therapy (ECT) modified with succinyl choline and suggest that lithium should be discontinued prior to the use of ECT or of surgery.

As in the case of any relatively new and effective drug, lithium carbonate has been claimed to be useful in a large number of medical conditions, and to date there is little substantiation of its value, except, possibly, in few of these disorders. Lithium has not been demonstrated as effective, despite some positive claims, in epilepsy, Huntington's Chorea, Parkinson's disease, spasmodic torticollis, or Tourette's syndrome, but has been found of possible usefulness in the treatment of thyrotoxicosis through its effect of causing a fall in serum thyroxin and iodine levels in thyrotoxic patients (Tempel et al., 1972; Berens and Wolfe, 1975; Poust et al., 1976; Jefferson and Griest, 1977). Lithium apparently rapidly and effectively blocks iodine release from the thyroid gland and therefore it may be of value in the reduction of circulating thyroid hormone levels. Based on the observation that one side effect of lithium, that of polyuria from inhibition of ADH-sensitive renal adenyl cyclase, lithium carbonate was successful in causing a water diuresis and a correction of hyponatremia in a patient with inappropriate ADH secretion syndrome (White and Fetner, 1975). Subsequent cases have been reported that were unresponsive to lithium. Lithium carbonate has been reported as helpful in treating the painful shoulder syndrome and has tentatively been reported as helpful in treating the symptoms of Meniere's disease (Tyber, 1974; Thomsen et al., 1974). At present the best results are suggested by one open study in which 70% of the patients with Meniere's disease, who could tolerate lithium therapy, obtained at least temporary remissions (Thomsen et al., 1974).

The effect of lithium on the hematopoietic system, which is the subject of this conference, was first observed as a benign reversible side effect in manic depressive patients receiving lithium in 1970 by O'Connell, with subsequent reports by others. White counts were reported frequently to reach 14,000 to 15,000/mm^3 and were found to remain elevated during the course of lithium therapy, returning to normal if the drug was discontinued (O'Connell, 1970). In other patients, the total white blood count remained normal with a relative increase in granulocytes. The leukocytosis appeared to be unrelated to lithium dose, serum lithium level, or psychiatric diagnosis. Tisman et al. (1973) suggested that this change was due to a true increase in the body granulocyte pool. It was speculated that the drug may have a role in the treatment of granulocytopenic conditions. More recently Rossof and Coltman (1976) showed that lithium at therapeutic or toxic levels did not interfere with one aspect of polymorphonuclear neutrophil function. This effect on hematopoietic elements, first noted in psychiatric patients, has generated great interest in the potential value of lithium as a treatment for granulocytopenia of various etiologies, as well as stimulating interest in its mechanism of action regarding the hematopoietic system. The series of studies in this symposium attests to the new potentials for the use of lithium in medical hematology and oncology -- another new facet of this unusual substance.

REFERENCES

Baastrup, P.C., Poulsen, J.C., Schou, M., Thomsen, K., and Amdisen, A., 1970, Prophylactic lithium: double blind discontinuation in manic depressive and recurrent depressive disorders, Lancet 2:236.

Berens, S.C. and Wolfe, J., 1975, The endocrine effects of lithium in "Lithium research and therapy," (Johnson, F.N., ed.) London, New York, Academic Press.

Burrows, G.D., Davies, D., and Smith, P.K., 1978, Unique tubular lesions after lithium, Lancet 6:1310.

Cade, J.F.J., 1949, Lithium salts in the treatment of psychotic excitement, Med. J. Aust. 2:349.

Corcoran, A.C., Taylor, R.D., and Page, I., 1949, Lithium poisoning from the use of salt substitutes, JAMA 139:685.

Davis, J.M., 1976, Overview: Maintenance therapy in psychiatry: II. Affective disorders, Am. J. Psychiatry 133:1.

Friedel, R.O., 1976, Lithium and depression, Am. J. Psychiatry 133:976.

Gershon, S. and Yuwiler, A., 1960, A specific pharmacological approach to the treatment of mania, J. Neuropsychiatry 1:229.

Goodwin, F.K., Murphy, D.L., and Dunner, D.L., 1972, Lithium response in unipolar versus bipolar depression, Am. J. Psychiatry 129:44.

Hestbech, J., Hansen, H.S., Amdisen, A., and Olsen, S., 1977, Chronic renal lesions following long-term treatment with lithium, Kidn. Intern. 12:205.

Hill, G.E., Wong, R.C., and Hodges, M.R., 1976, Potentiation of succinylcholine neuromuscular blockade by lithium carbonate, Anesthesiology 44:432.

Himmelhoch, J.M., Forrest, J., Neil, J.R., and Detre, T.P., 1977, Thiazide-lithium synergy in refractory mood swings, Am. J. Psychiatry 134:149.

Jefferson, J.W. and Griest, J.H., 1977, "Primer of lithium therapy," The Williams and Wilkins Company, Baltimore, Md.

Kline, N.S., Wren, J.C., Cooper, T.B., Varga, E., and Canal, O., 1974, Evaluation of lithium therapy in chronic and periodic alcoholism, Am. J. Med. Sci. 261:15.

Mendels, J., 1976, Lithium in the treatment of depression, Am. J. Psychiatry 133:373.

Merry, J., Reynolds, C.M., Bailey, J., and Coppen, A., 1976, Prophylactic treatment of alcoholism by lithium carbonate, Lancet 2:481.

O'Connell, R.A., 1970, Leukocytosis during lithium carbonate treatment, Int. Pharmacopsychiatry 4:30.

Petersen, V., Hvidt, S., Thomsen, K., and Schou, M., 1974, Effect of prolonged thiazide treatment on renal lithium clearance, Br. Med. J. 3:143.

Pitts, F.N., Jr. and Winokur, G., 1964, Affective disorders II. Diagnostic correlates and incidence of suicide, J. Nerv. Ment. Dis. 139:176.

Prien, R.F., Klett, C.J., and Caffey, E.M., 1974, Lithium prophylaxis in recurrent affective illness, Am. J. Psychiatry 131:198.

Procci, W.R., 1976, Schizo-affective illness, fact or fiction? Arch. Gen. Psychiatry 33:1167.

Poust, R.I., Mallinger, A.G., Mallinger, J., Himmelhoch, J.M., Neil, J.F., and Hanin, I., 1976, Effect of chlorothiazide on the pharmacokinetics of lithium in plasma and erythrocytes, Psychopharmacol. Comm. 2:273.

Raphaelson, O., 1979, Ayd medical communications, in "Lithium and the Kidney," (F.J. Ayd, ed.), International Drug Therapy News Letter 14:25.

Rossof, A.H. and Coltman, C.A., Jr., 1976, The effect of lithium carbonate on the granulocyte phagocytic index, Experientia 32:238.

Sheard, M.H., 1971, Effect of lithium on human aggression, Nature 230:113.

Sheard, M.H., 1975, Lithium in the treatment of aggression, J. Nerv. Ment. Dis. 160:108.

Sinclair, J.D., 1974, Lithium-induced suppression of alcohol drinking by rats, Med. Biol. 52:133.

Tempel, R., Berman, M., Robbins, J., and Wolff, J., 1972, The use of lithium in the treatment of thyrotoxicosis, J. Clin. Invest. 51:2746.

Thomsen, J., Bech, P., Geisler, A., Jorgensen, M.B., Rafaelsen, O.J., Terkildsen, K., Udsen, J., and Zilstorff, K., 1974, Meniere's disease: Preliminary report of lithium treatment, Acta Otolaryngol. 78:59.

Tisman, G., Herbert, V. and Rosenblatt, S., 1973, Evidence that lithium induces human granulocyte proliferation: Elevated serum vitamin B12 binding capacity in vivo and granulocyte colony proliferation in vitro, Br. J. Haematol. 24:767.

Tyber, M.A., 1974, Treatment of painful shoulder syndrome with amitriptyline and lithium carbonate, Can. Med. Assoc. J. 111:137.

White, M.G. and Fetner, C.D., 1975, Treatment of the syndrome of inappropriate secretion of antidiuretic hormone with lithium carbonate, N. Engl. J. Med. 292:390.

DSM III Draft, 1978, Diagnostic and Statistical Manual of Mental Disorders, Third Edition.

Task Force on Lithium Therapy, 1975, The current status of lithium therapy, Report of the APA Task Force, Am. J. Psychiatry 132:997.

BIOLOGY OF THE LITHIUM ION

Ghanshyam N. Pandey and John M. Davis

Research Department
Illinois State Psychiatric Institute
1601 West Taylor Street
Chicago, Illinois 60612
and
Department of Psychiatry
Pritzker School of Medicine
University of Chicago
Chicago, Illinois

Lithium is used effectively in the treatment of acute mania. During maintenance therapy, it reduces the frequency of manic-depressive episodes. Lithium has also recently been used in the treatment of several other pathologic conditions such as schizophrenia, alcoholism, aggression, tardive dyskinesia, and Huntington's chorea; however, its therapeutic efficacy in such conditions may be controversial. Although lithium is one of the most effective drugs used in the treatment of manic-depressive illness, its mode of action remains unclear.

The physico-chemical properties of lithium are similar to those of sodium and potassium in some, but not all, respects. In certain ways, it is much more like alkaline earth metals such as magnesium. Lithium does not occur normally in biological material except in trace quantities; yet, it is tolerated in living systems in considerable amounts compared to other nonbiological metals. This reflects the similarity of lithium, sodium, potassium, magnesium and calcium. It is thus to be expected that lithium, when present in a living system, can either alter the functions performed by other cations or substitute in their place to perform the functions of such cations.

One important aspect of cation biology is the uneven distribution of the cations between intracellular (IC) and extracellular (EC) phases. This uneven distribution is the physico-chemical basis for membrane potentials and thereby for the functioning of nerves and muscles. It is not surprising, therefore, that studies on the mode of distribution of Li between intra- and extracellular phases have attracted the attention of several investigators. Initial studies indicated a lack of an active transport system for Li which could maintain a Li gradient between IC and EC phases, and it was believed that Li is distributed evenly by a passive diffusion process (Friedman, 1973; Anderson and Prockop, 1975).

Several investigations, however, indicated the existence of a Li gradient between red cells and plasma under steady-state conditions, suggesting active extrusion of Li from red cells. The mechanism by which such a Li gradient is maintained and the significance of such a distribution have been topics of interest in recent years. This aspect of Li biology is the main subject of this discussion. It is hoped that the current knowledge of Li transport in human red cells will be helpful not only in our understanding of the mechanism of action of Li, but that it can be used as a tool for studies of the biological factors associated with the etiology of affective illness.

Another important aspect of the biology of cations concerns their influence on a large number of enzymes. Many of the enzymes are known to be activated or inhibited by Na, K, Ca, and Mg. It has been shown that Li alters the activities of several enzymes associted with the biosynthesis and metabolism of biogenic amines. The effect of Li on the adenylate cyclase-cyclic AMP system appears to be of greatest interest, primarily because cyclic AMP has been shown to mediate the cellular effects of several hormones and neurotransmitters. Adenylate cyclase, which catalyzes the conversion of ATP to cyclic AMP, is closely coupled to the biogenic amine receptors. Therefore, the effect of Li on the cyclic AMP system will also be discussed.

LITHIUM TRANSPORT IN HUMAN RED BLOOD CELLS

The steady state distribution of Li between red cells and plasma (commonly referred to as Li ratio or Li_{IC}/Li_{EC}) has been related to clinical response to Li therapy (Mendels and Frazer, 1973; Ramsey *et al.*, 1976; Casper *et al.*, 1976), clinical diagnosis (Lyttkens *et al.*, 1973; Rybakowski *et al.*, 1978; Pandey *et al.*, in press), and side effects of lithium therapy (Elizur *et al.*, 1977; Hewick and Murray, 1976). Maggs (1963) was the first to report that patients with low intracellular Li levels tended to run a fluctuating clinical course during maintenance treatment. Mendels and associates (1973) observed that depressed patients who respond to long-term Li maintenance therapy have a higher IC/EC Li ratio than non-responders. Casper *et al.* (1976) reported that patients showing short-term responses to Li therapy had significantly higher mean Li ratios than patients who failed to respond. Several other investigators, however, have not confirmed these reports (Cazullo *et al.*, 1975; Rybakowski and Strzyzowski, 1976). Further interest in the Li ratio was generated by reports suggesting that the intracellular Li level was somewhat more reliable than the plasma level in predicting brain Li concentrations in the rat (Frazer *et al.*, 1973).

Although its clinical significance may be controversial, all investigators observe a large interindividual variation in the Li ratio in patients and normal controls. It has also been observed that the steady-state levels of Li in red cells are considerably lower than the plasma levels. If Li were distributed passively across the erythrocyte membrane, the Li distribution ratio between red cells and plasma would be equal to the Donnan ratio for chloride distribution, i.e. 1.2 (Tosteson and Hoffman, 1960). All investigators agree that the Li distribution ratio observed in patients is generally less than 1.0. It is clear, therefore, that some mechanism of Li transport across the erythrocyte membrane operates to keep the ratio below 1.0.

Several groups of investigators have studied Li transport in human red cells in order to examine the factors which are responsible for interindividual variations in the Li ratio. Schless et al. (1975) reported that the Li ratios obtained in vivo and in vitro in low-potassium sheep were higher than those obtained in high-potassium sheep. These observations suggested that Li transport in sheep red cells is coupled to the transport of Na; however, the nature of this coupling remained unclear. A major breakthrough in the understanding of Li transport in human red cells was provided by the work of Haas, Schooler, and Tosteson (1975), who demonstrated the presence of a Li-Na counterflow system in human red cells. This sytem, which is insensitive to ouabain, can drive Li against its own electrochemical gradient and is driven by an oppositely directed Na gradient. Subsequent work done by us and other investigators (Duhm and Becker, 1977a; Duhm and Becker, 1977b; Duhm and Becker, 1977c; Duhm et al., 1976; Duhham and Senyk, 1977; Frazer et al., 1977; Funder et al., 1978; Greil et al., 1977; Becker and Duhm, 1978; Haas et al., 1975; Meltzer et al., 1976; Pandey et al., 1977; Pandy et al., 1978; Sarkadi et al., 1978) resulted in the elucidation and characterization of at least four separate pathways of Li transport. These pathways, which are shown in Figure 1, and are described in detail in the following pages, are:

(1) Li-Na countertransport mediated by a phloretin-sensitive Li-Na exchange mechanism;

(2) ouabain-sensitive Li transport mediated by Na-K ATPase;

(3) passive diffusion which is insensitive to drugs;

(4) passive diffusion by ion pair formation in a bicarbonate-containing medium.

Li-Na Countertransport (Li-Na Exchange Pathway)

Haas et al. (1975) described the presence of a ouabain-insensitive Li-Na countertransport system in normal human red cells. Since ouabain inhibits Na-K ATPase, this system appears to be different from Na-K ATPase (Na-K pump). This system can move Li against its electrochemical potential gradient and is driven by an oppositely directed Na gradient. The presence of such a system was confirmed independently by Duhm et al. (1976). Further characteristics of this pathway of Li transport have been described by Pandey et al. (1977), Pandey et al. (1978), Sarkadi et al. (1978), and Duhm et al. (1976).

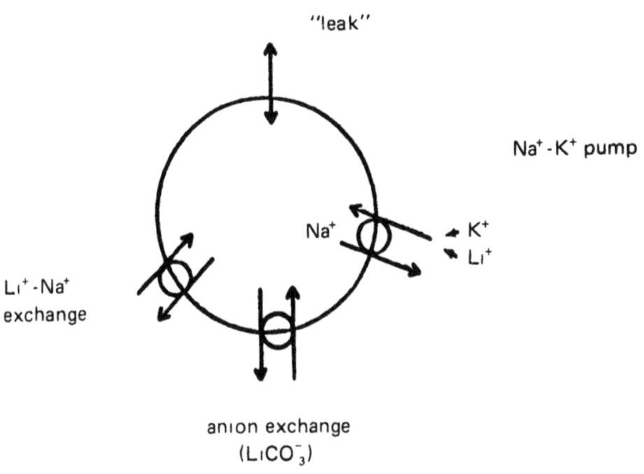

Figure 1. Pathways of Li transport in human red cell.

Uphill Li Efflux

The results of a simple experiment similar to that described by Haas et al. (1975), which demonstrates the presence of such a system, is shown in Figure 2. Human red cells are first loaded with Li to a level of 1 meq/liter of cells and are then incubated in two different media (one containing 10 mM NaCl and 1.5 mM LiCl, and the other containing 140 mM NaCl and 1.5 mM LiCl) for up to two hours. Assuming a 66% water content in human red cells, the concentration of Li inside a cell at 0 hour of incubation is almost equal to, or lower than, the concentration of Li in the medium. During two hours of incubation, the Li concentration in the red cells incubated in a high-sodium medium (medium A) gradually decreases, so that, at two hours, the red cell Li concentration is considerably lower than the Li concentration in the medium. However, a slight increase is observed in the Li concentration in the cells incubated in a low-sodium medium (medium B). These experiments demonstrate an uphill extrusion of Li from red cells that is driven by an oppositely directed Na gradient.

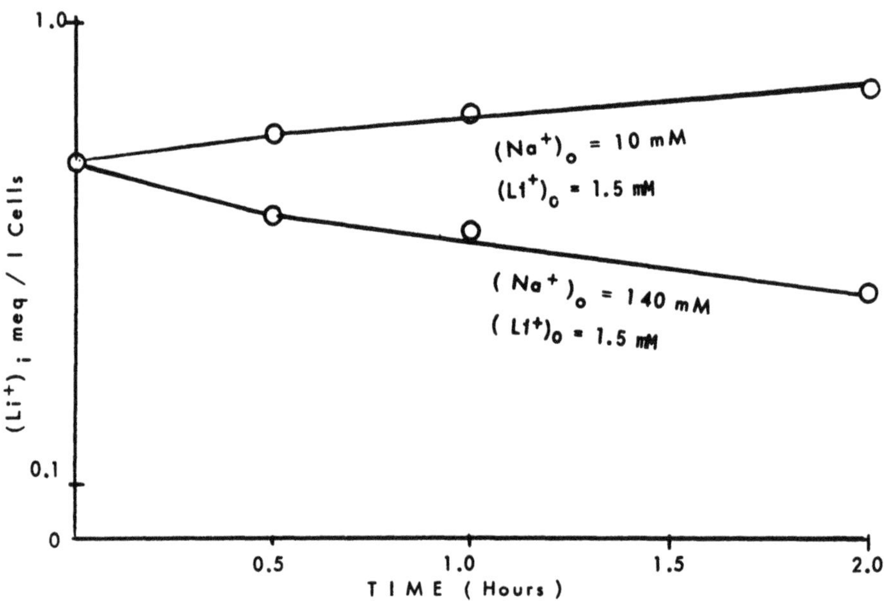

Figure 2. Li-Na counterflow system: Effect of external Na concentration.

Based on the results of experiments in which red cells are loaded with high Na (100 mmole/liter cells) and low Li (1.0 mmole/liter cells) concentrations and incubated in high- and low-sodium media, Haas et al. (1975) demonstrated that net uphill Li transport occurs in either direction across human red cell membranes, depending upon the direction of the Na electrochemical potential gradient.

Pandey et al. (1977) and Pandey et al. (1978) reported that the net uphill movement of Li can be inhibited by phloretin. Certain other compounds, e.g., furosemide, quinine, and quinidine, also inhibited Li countertransport, but were not as potent as phloretin. To demonstrate that this countertransport system does not require metabolic energy, we studied Na-dependent Li uphill movement in fresh cells and in ATP-depleted cells, and we observed that ATP depletion did not affect the net upward movement of Li across the erythrocyte membrane (Pandey et al., 1978). In experiments similar to that described above, we examined whether any other cation can substitute for Na in Li countertransport by substituting K^+, Mg^{++}, Ca^{++}, or choline for external Na^+. We observed no significant upward movement of Li^+ under these conditions. Our observations thus indicated the presence of a Na-dependent ouabain-insensitive Li-Na countertransport system in human red cells.

We studied the mechanism of Li transport in human red cells by investigating Li influx and efflux from human red cells under different conditions (Pandey et al., 1978).

Downhill Li Efflux

Lithium-loaded cells were incubated in Li-free media containing Na^+, K^+, Mg^{++}, or choline in the presence or absence of ouabain or phloretin or both. The highest rate of Li efflux, as shown in Figure 3, was observed in a medium containing a high Na^+ concentration, whereas Li efflux was approximately the same in several other media. Moreover, phloretin inhibited Li efflux when Li-loaded cells were incubated in the Na medium, but had no effect when the cells were incubated in media containing other cations. Ouabain had no significant effect on Li efflux under any of these conditions. The results indicated the presence of a component of Li efflux which is stimulated by Na, is insensitive to ouabain, and is inhibited by phloretin. By determining Li efflux from red cells which contained either Na or K along with Li (cells were loaded by the Nystatin technique) in a Na or K medium, we showed (Table I) that neither Na nor K in the red cells (cis side) has any significant effect on Na-dependent phloretin-sensitive Li efflux across the cell membrane. The absolute requirement of trans Na indicates that this component of Li efflux is mediated by a Li-Na exchange mechanism.

Since Li is not present in the human body under physiologic conditions, the presence of a specific Li-Na exchange pathway appeared unlikely. However,the presence of a Na-Na exchange diffusion pathway

TABLE I

LITHIUM EFFLUX IN HUMAN RED CELLS

EFFECT OF INTERNAL AND EXTERNAL CATIONS

Cation		Li efflux (m mol/l. cells/h)				Ouab. and Phlor. Sens. Li efflux		
External	Internal	Total	+Ouabain	+Phloretin	+Ouab. +Phlor.	Ouab. Sensitive	Phlor. Sens.	Insens.
K	Na	0.13	0.13	0.13	0.13	0.00	0.00	0.13
K	K	0.13	0.14	0.13	0.12	-0.01	0.02	0.12
Na	Na	0.40	0.38	0.20	0.20	0.02	0.18	0.20
Na	K	0.50	0.49	0.20	0.17	0.01	0.32	0.17

Red cells were loaded with Na or K by the nystatin method. In K cells, Na concentration was <0.1 m mol/liter of cells; in Na cells, K concentration was <1 mmol/liter of cells. For efflux experiments, the cells also contained 10 m mol Li/liter of cells. The nystatin loaded cells were incubated in 130 mM NaCl or 130 mM KCl media supplemented with 10 mM LiCl in the influx experiments, and in 140 mM/NaCl or 140 mM KCl media without external Li in the efflux experiments. The media also contained 20 mM glycylglycine buffered to pH 7.4. Hematocrit was 5%. Ouabain and Phloretin concentrations were 10^{-4}M.

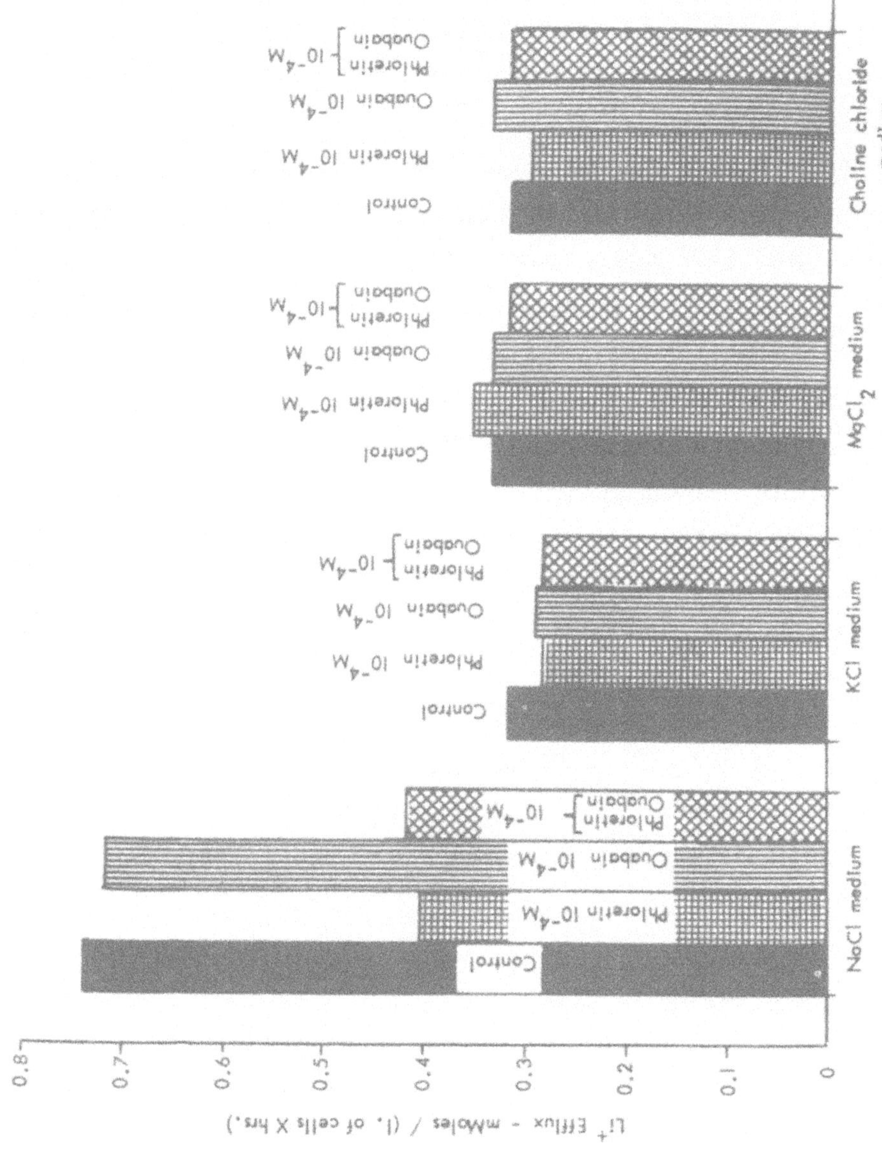

Figure 3. Lithium efflux: effect of counterion phloretin and ouabain.
At t = 0, intracellular Li concentration = 2.97 mmole/l cells.

had been characterized previously in red cells (Tosteson and Hoffman, 1960). Although the functional significance of this pathway has never been clear, it appears to be separate from the active Na-K transport system since it is insensitive to ouabain. It therefore appeared likely that the suggested Li-Na exchange pathway is probably the same one that operates Na-Na exchange diffusion; Li is annexed by the system and acts as a substitute for Na.

Evidence that Li-Na exchange is achieved by a Na-Na exchange diffusion pathway was provided by experiments in which the tracer ^{22}Na was used. Red cells loaded with ^{22}Na were incubated in a medium containing Na, K, or Li in the presence of ouabain and in the presence or absence of phloretin (Pandey et al., 1977). As shown in Table II, it was observed that the rate of ^{22}Na efflux was highest in Na media and lowest in K media. External Li stimulated ^{22}Na efflux. Phloretin inhibited ^{22}Na efflux in both the Na and Li media, but not in K medium. These results were thus compatible with the suggestion that Li can substitute for Na in the Na-Na exchange diffusion pathway, which is present in human red cells and operates under physiologic conditions.

The net uphill movement of Li can be directed inward or outward across the erythrocyte membrane, depending upon the direction of the Na gradient (Haas et al., 1975). If the red-cell Na concentration is higher than the EC concentration, uphill Li movement will be directed inward; if extracellular Na is higher than intracellular Na, uphill Li movement will be directed outward.

Downhill Lithium Influx

When fresh human red cells free of Li are incubated in a medium containing Li^+ and Mg^{++}, but not Na^+ or K^+ and bicarbonate, at least three components of Li, one which is inhibited by phloretin, one which is inhibited by ouabain, and one which is insensitive to both, can be identified. The effect of ouabain and phloretin on Li influx as a function of extracellular Li concentration is shown in Figure 4. The total Li influx increases with increasing external Li concentration. Ouabain partially

TABLE II

PHLORETIN SENSITIVE SODIUM EFFLUX FROM HUMAN RED CELLS: EFFECT OF EXTERNAL Na, K, AND Li

External Cation (140 mM)	Na^+ efflux (m mol/liter cells per hr)		
	Control	+Phloretin	Phloretin sens. Na efflux
Na	1.14	0.82	0.32
Li	0.45	0.35	0.10
K	0.26	0.22	0.04

Washed red cells were loaded with ^{22}Na by incubating them for 5 hours in an isotonic buffered media ($MgCl_2$ 95 mM, pH 7.4, 37°, 30% v/v). Cells were then washed free of the incubation media and aliquots were incubated in a medium containing NaCl (140 mM), KCl (140 mM) or LiCl (140 mM) at 10% (v/v). ^{22}Na efflux was measured at 0, 1, 2 and 3 hours of incubation at 37°. (For details, see Pandey et al., Proc. Natl. Acad. Sci. U.S.A. 74: 3607-3611, 1977).

inhibits Li influx; when phloretin is added, it causes further inhibition. These results thus indicate that a component of Li influx is insensitive to inhibition by ouabain but is inhibited by phloretin. Phloretin-sensitive downhill Li influx is not inhibited by external K^+ or Mg^{++}, although external Na^+ may have slight effects. However, when Li influx is determined in red cells which are loaded with either Na or K (Nystatin technique), it is observed, as shown in Table III, that Li influx in K^+-loaded cells is greatly reduced and is insensitive to inhibition by phloretin. The cation composition of the external medium has only marginal effects on ouabain-insensitive and phloretin-sensitive Li influx.

TABLE III

LITHIUM INFLUX IN HUMAN RED CELLS

EFFECT OF INTERNAL AND EXTERNAL CATIONS

Cation		Li influx (m mol/l. cells/h)				Ouab. and Phlor. Sens. Li influx		
External	Internal	Total	$^{+}$Ouabain	$^{+}$Phloretin	$^{+}$Ouab. $^{+}$Phlor.	Ouab. Sensitive	Phlor. Sens.	Insens.
K	Na	0.78	0.80	0.34	0.32	-0.02	0.48	0.32
K	K	0.13	0.13	0.13	0.13	0.00	0.00	0.13
Na	Na	0.77	0.50	0.50	0.27	0.27	0.23	0.27
Na	K	0.23	0.12	0.23	0.12	0.11	0.00	0.12

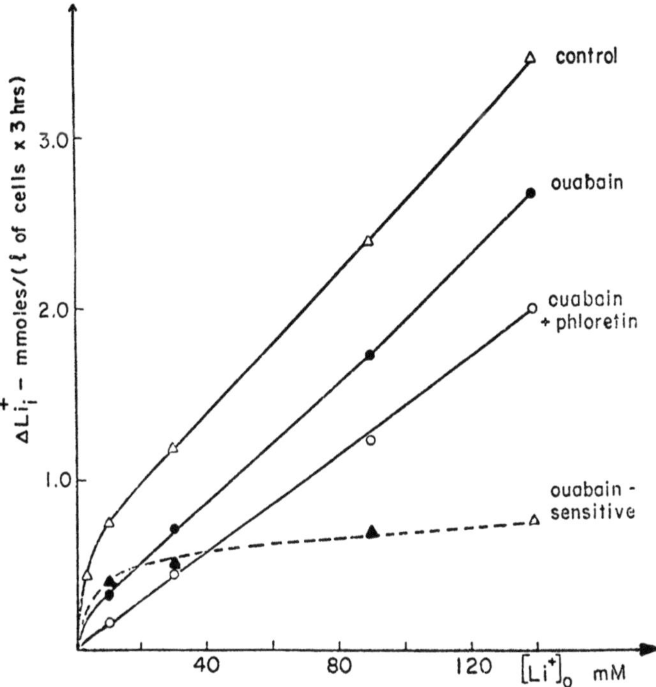

Figure 4. Lithium influx; effect of increasing extracellular Li on ouabain and phloretin sensitive Li influx.

The kinetics and stoichiometry of the Li-Na exchange system have been reported by Sarkadi et al. (1978). Based on the findings of Pandey et al. (1978), Duhm et al. (1976), and their own findings, they proposed a carrier model (Figure 5) for a tightly coupled, one-to-one Li-Na exchange system. The carrier reacts with the metal ions (Na^+, Li^+) on one side of the cell membrane and transfers the ions to the other side. However, the carrier cannot move across the membrane unless it is bound to a metal ion. The rate of ion transport depends on the concentrations of the transported species on both sides of the membrane, the rates of their reactions with the carrier, and the rate of translocation of the ion-carrier complex. The apparent affinities of the exchange system for Li are about 15-to-18-fold higher than for Na on either side of the membrane. Although this ratio is the same for both surfaces, the absolute affinities for Li and Na are three times greater for the internal sites. Measurements of the stoichiometry of the Li-Na exchange transport system indicated a 1:1 exchange of Na and Li moving in opposite directions across the red cell membrane.

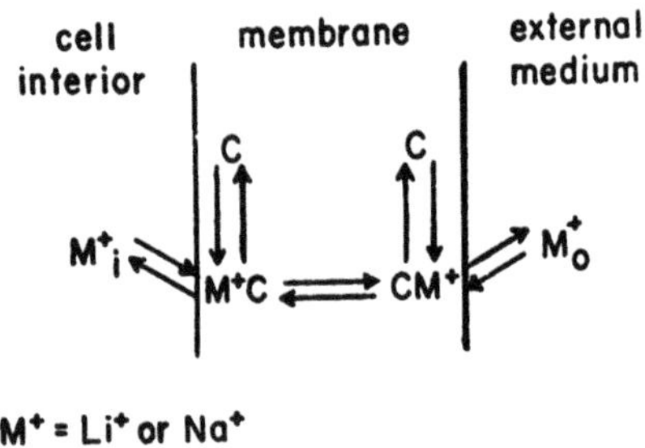

Figure 5. Carrier model for Li-Na exchange.

This exchange system can thus promote Li-Na heteroexchange in both inward and outward directions. In the presence of an oppositely directed Na gradient, it can also promote uphill movement of Li (Li-Na counter-flow). In the absence of Li, this sytem probably performs Na-Na exchange without a net gain of Na on either side of the membrane.

Ouabain Sensitive Lithium Transport by the Na-K Pump

Under certain conditions, another component of Li transport can be identified which is inhibited by ouabain and competitively inhibited by K and Na on cis side of the erythrocyte membrane, but is insensitive to inhibition by phloretin. This component of Li transport appears to be mediated by the Na-K pump which normally operates to transport Na and K, since ouabain also inhibits Na-K ATPase.

When normal red cells are incubated in a medium containing Na, K, or Mg, no significant effect of ouabain on Li efflux is observed (Figure 3). However, a component of Li efflux sensitive to ouabain can be identified in the red cells which contain neither Na nor K. It has been reported by Dunham and Senyk (1977) that in cells which are loaded with Li and choline and are free of internal K and Na and incubated in a Li free medium, Li efflux is partially inhibited by ouabain. Pandey et al. (1978) have reported similar results. They observed that ouabain partially inhibits Li efflux from red cells which have been loaded with Li, but contain no Na or K (Table IV). Ouabain-sensitive Li efflux was found to be higher in cells which were incubated in a KCl medium than in those incubated in a NaCl medium. It thus appeared that both internal Na and K competitively inhibited ouabain-sensitive Li efflux, whereas external K and external Na stimulated ouabain-sensitive Li efflux.

TABLE IV

EFFECT OF OUABAIN ON Li EFFLUX FROM Li-LOADED (Na- AND K-FREE) CELLS

Medium	Li efflux		
	Control	Oubain	Oubain-sensitive
		m mol (liter of cells x h)	
NaCl (140 mM)	3.05	2.47	0.58
KCl (140 mM)	3.46	2.36	1.10

Red cells were loaded with Li by the nystatin method. Intracellular Na concentration was < 0.1 m mol/liter of cells; K concentration < 1 m mol/liter of cells. Cells were incubated in either a 140 mM NaCl or in a 140 mM KCl medium supplemented with 20 mM glycylglycine, pH 7.4. Hematocrit was 5%, incubation temperature 37°C. The concentration of ouabain was 10^{-4}M.

Ouabain-sensitive Li influx also can be identified under certain conditions (Pandey, 1978). As shown in Figure 4, Li influx is partially inhibited by ouabain when normal cells are incubated in K- and Na-free media. This component of Li influx in insensitive to phloretin and can pump Li against its gradient. When Li-loaded cells (1.0 meq/liter cells) are

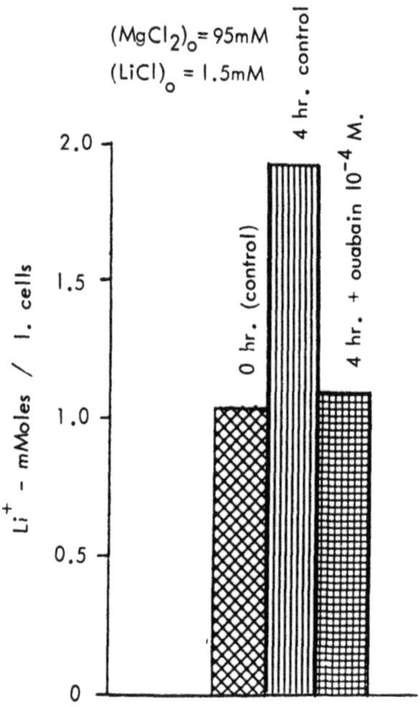

Figure 6. Ouabain sensitive uphill Li influx: effect of ouabain.

incubated in a $MgCl_2$ medium containing 1.5 mmole LiCl for four hours, the red cell Li level increases and is higher than the external Li concentration (Figure 6). This increase in red cell Li concentration is inhibited by ouabain. These results indicate that Li transport mediated by the Na-K pump can actively move Li against its gradient. In the absence of both Na and K in the external medium, Li influx into normal red cells through this mechanism has a maximum rate of approximately 0.5 nmole/liter of cells per hour and is half-maximally stimulated by approximately 15 mmoles of external Li. External K competitively inhibits ouabain-sensitive Li uptake, and half-maximal inhibition of ouabain-sensitive Li influx is caused by less than 2 mmoles K when the external Li concentration is 3.2 mmole. External Na also inhibits ouabain-sensitive Li uptake, but less so than K.

The above results are based on the reports of Pandey *et al.* (1978).

Lithium Transport by Passive Diffusion

In the absence of bicarbonate in the medium, another component of Li transport which is insensitive to ouabain and phloretin can be identified. Transport of Li through this pathway is a linear function of the Li concentration gradient (Figure 1) and appears to be mediated by passive leak diffusion.

Bicarbonate-Stimulated Li Transport by Passive Diffusion

The presence of bicarbonate in the medium results in another pathway by which Li is transported across the cell membrane as a result of ion pairing with HCO_3^- (Funder *et al.*, 1978; Sarkadi *et al.*, 1978; Becker and Duhm, 1978). This pathway, which cannot move Li against it electrical gradient, also appears to be mediated by passive leak diffusion.

Lithium Ratio and Lithium Transport Pathways In Vivo

The steady-state Li distribution between red cells and plasma, referred to as Li ratio, reflects the dynamic balance of all forms of Li transport across the red cell membrane. Alterations in Li transport mediated by any of the pathways can result in large variations in the Li ratio.

Under physiologic conditions, the Li influx through the ouabain-sensitive pathway is very small because of the high concentrations of Na and K in the plasma. The distribution of Li between red cells and plasma is thus determined by a balance between Li influx through leak pathways and an uphill Li efflux through Li-Na counterflow. There appear to be no large variations of the bicarbonate concentration in the plasma, and, hence, in the Li influx through this pathway. This suggests that interindividual variation in the Li ratio is caused by differences in Li transport through leakage, or through the Li-Na couterflow pathway.

To examine what aspects of Li transport cause interindividual variations in the Li ratio *in vivo*, we measured Li transport through different pathways in the red cells of normal controls and in the red cells of a manic patient who had an abnormally high Li ratio (0.97) in vivo (Pandey et al., 1977). The transport of Li through the ouabain-sensitive pathway and through leak diffusion in the red cells of this patient was similar to that observed in controls. However, transport by Li-Na exchange (Li-Na counterflow) was abnormally high. The patient's phloretin-sensitive Li-Na counterflow remained well below normal limits three months after Li treatment had stopped and at a time when his behavior was normal. Transport of Na through the Li-Na exchange mechanism was also significantly lower in the patient than in the control subjects.

These observations suggested that variations of the Li ratio in vivo among individuals are caused by variations in Li transport through the Li-Na exchange pathway. To confirm this assumption, we measured Li transport by Li-Na exchange and by passive leak diffusion in patients with affective disorders who had been admitted to our research wards and were subsequently treated with Li. As a measure of Li transport through Li-Na exchange, we determined net uphill Li efflux (Li-Na counterflow), total downhill efflux in NaCl media. Transport of Li by passive leak diffusion was measured by determination of Li efflux in KCl media. The difference in Li efflux in NaCl and KCl media provided a measure of Na dependent Li efflux.

Net Uphill Lithium Efflux

The net uphill Li efflux from red cells of the patients obtained before the start of Li therapy was measured by preloading of the cells with Li up to a level of 1 meq/liter of cells, followed by incubation for four hours in a buffered isotonic medium (pH 7.4) containing 135 mmole NaCl, 5 mmole KCl, and 1.5 mmole LiCl. The net extrusion of Li against its electrochemical gradient was determined and will be referred to as net uphill Li efflux (Li-Na counterflow). The net uphill Li efflux determined in red cells from 48 patients showed a significant inverse Pearson product-moment correlation (-0.91) with the mean Li ratio in vivo observed in these patients during the course of Li therapy (Figure 7). Those patients who had abnormally high Li ratios in vivo had a reduced uphill Li efflux, and those with normal or low Li ratios had a higher net uphill Li efflux.

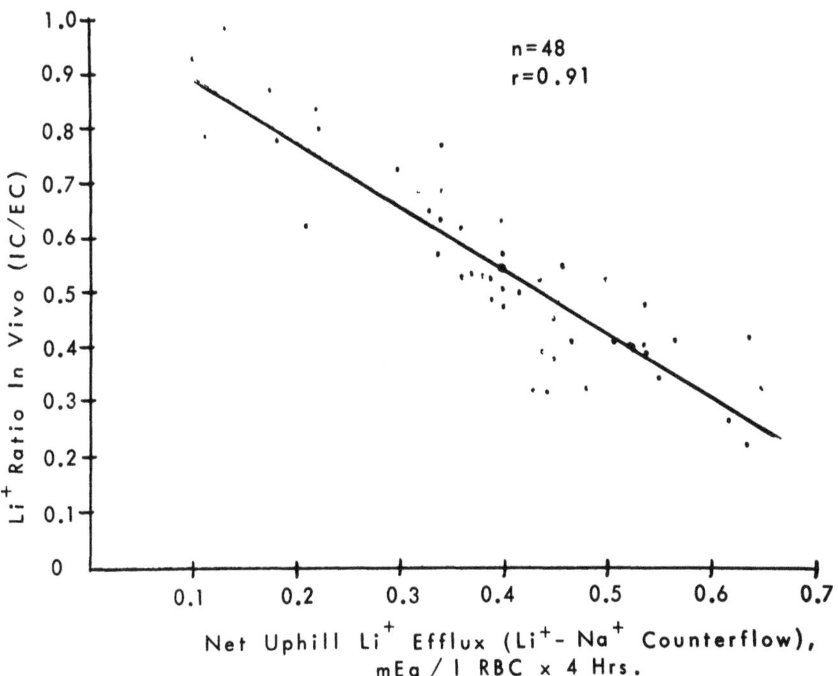

Figure 7. Correlation between counterflow (uphill Li efflux) and lithium ratio in vivo.

Downhill Li Efflux

The net uphill Li efflux determined by the above procedure is a measure of the difference between uphill Li efflux and downhill Li influx through passive leak diffusion. Thus, interindividual variation in net uphill Li efflux could be due to variation in either uphill efflux or downhill influx. To determine whether the variation in net uphill Li efflux was due to Li-Na exchange pathways, we measured the Li efflux from the red cells of patients in a NaCl or KCl medium. We preloaded the cells with Li to a level of about 1 meq/liter of cells, incubated them for up to four hours in a buffered (pH 7.4) isotonic medium containing 140 mmole NaCl or 140 mmole KCl, and then calculated the loss of Li from the cells.

The total downhill efflux from red cells incubated in NaCl medium was determined in 48 patients who were subsequently treated with Li. A highly significant correlation (0.91) was observed between total downhill Li efflux (NaCl medium), which is a measure of Li efflux via the Li-Na exchange mechanism and passive leak diffusion, and the mean Li ratio *in vivo* (Figure 8). This was not surprising, for under these conditions, passive leak diffusion contributed only up to 25% of the total Li efflux; thus, because of the predominant contribution by the Li-Na exchange pathway, a significant correlation was still observed.

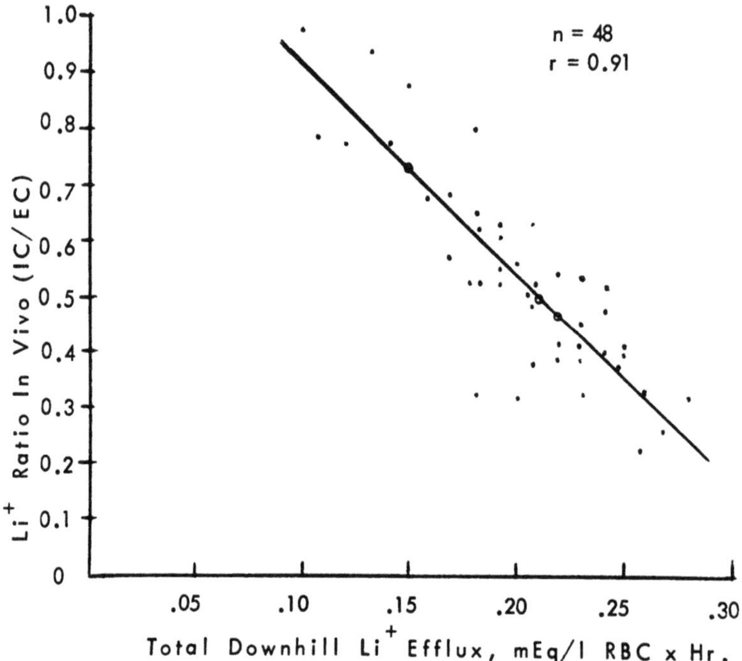

Figure 8. Correlation between downhill Li efflux. Total and *in vivo* ratio.

Sodium-dependent downhill Li efflux which is mediated by Li-Na exchange was determined as follows. Whereas downhill Li efflux in a high-Na medium is mediated by both pathways, downhill Li efflux in a Na-fee

KCl medium is mediated only by passive leak diffusion. Thus, the difference in Li efflux between NaCl and KCl media is a measure of Na-dependent Li efflux mediated by Li-Na exchange. The Na-dependent Li efflux showed a significant inverse correlation ($r = -0.81$, $p < 0.01$, $N=39$) with the Li ratio in vivo (Figure 9). No significant correlation ($r = 0.2$, $p < 0.10$, $N = 39$) was observed between Li efflux in KCl medium (passive leak diffusion) and the Li ratio in vivo.

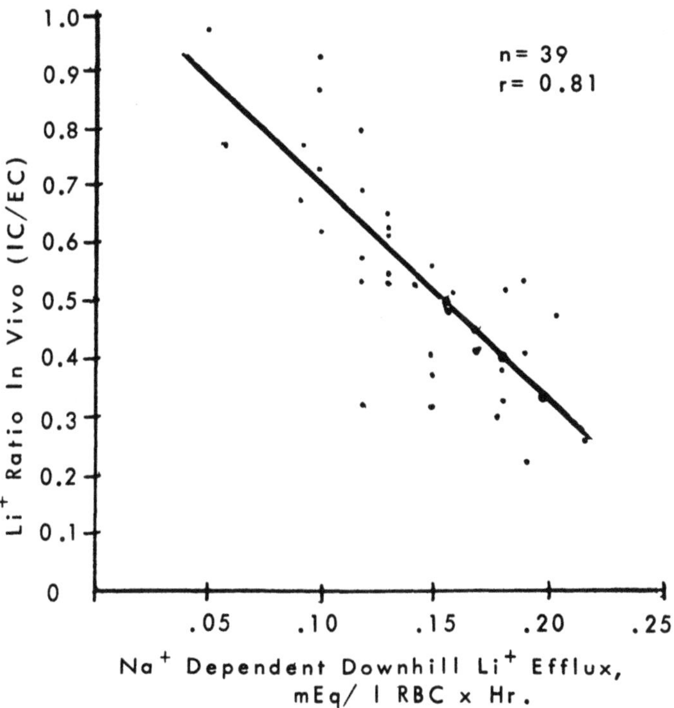

Figure 9. Correlation between Na-dependent Li efflux and Li ratio in vivo.

These results indicated that interindividual variation in the Li ratio is caused primarily by variation in Li transport from red cells which is mediated by the Li-Na exchange mechanism. Preliminary data have been reported before (Ostrow et al., 1978; Pandey et al., in press). Although alterations in Li transport mediated by Li-Na exchange may be the major cause of interindividual variations in the Li ratio, the possibility that these variations are caused by an alteration of Li transport which is mediated by other pathways cannot be ruled out. Small changes in plasma, potassium, or bicarbonate concentrations alter the Li influx mediated by ouabain-sensitive and leak diffusion pathways and, hence, could result in changes in red cell Li concentration. These possibilities need to be investigated further.

Li Ratio In Vitro

The Li ratio can be measured *in vitro* by incubation of red cells in a plasma-like medium containing LiCl. The steady-state distribution of Li *in vitro* between the medium and red cells is similar to that obtained *in vivo* and provides a simple method for predicting the Li ratio *in vivo*.

We have reported a procedure for the determination of the steady-state Li ratio *in vitro* in normal individuals. This ratio was significantly correlated with the Li ratio *in vivo* (Dorus *et al.*, 1975). In this procedure, we incubated red cells at 37°C in the presence of 1.5 mmole of LiCl for 24 hours. Based on our current understanding of the transport of Li in red cells, we recently modified this procedure (Pandey *et al.*, 1978). The cells are preloaded with Li up to a level of 1 meq/liter of red cells and then incubated for 24 hours in a physiologic buffered medium containing 1.5 mmole LiCl. At the end of this period, the ratio between red cell and extracellular Li is determined.

The Li ratio *in vitro* measured in 46 patients ranged from 0.15 to 0.59. A highly significant correlation (0.90, $p < 0.001$) was observed between the Li ratios *in vitro* and *in vivo*, as shown in Figure 10 (Pandey *et al.*, 1978). The mean Li ratio *in vitro*, determined during the course of Li treatment (0.40 ± 0.14, mean ± S.D.), was significantly higher than the mean ratio *in vitro* determined prior to the start of Li therapy, but also showed a significant correlation with the Li ratio *in vivo* (0.91, $p < 0.001$) (Pandey *et al.*, 1978). Since the Li ratio is negatively correlated with uphill and total downhill Li efflux, and since the Li ratio is significantly positively correlated with the ratio in vivo, the Li ratio provides an indirect measure of Li-Na exchange.

These results, and similar results obtained by other investigators (Greil et al., 1977), indicate that interindividual variation in the Li ratio is caused by variation in Li transport through the Li-Na exchange mechanism. Patients who have high Li ratios are likely to be deficient in the transport of Li via Li-Na exchange. Transport of Li by this pathway appears to be mediated by a carrier which probably is a small polypeptide. Sarkadi et al. (1978) have shown that differences in the affinity of such carrier sites among individuals are small. One can conclude, therefore, that patients who have high Li ratios have a smaller number of these carrier sites than do patients with low ratios.

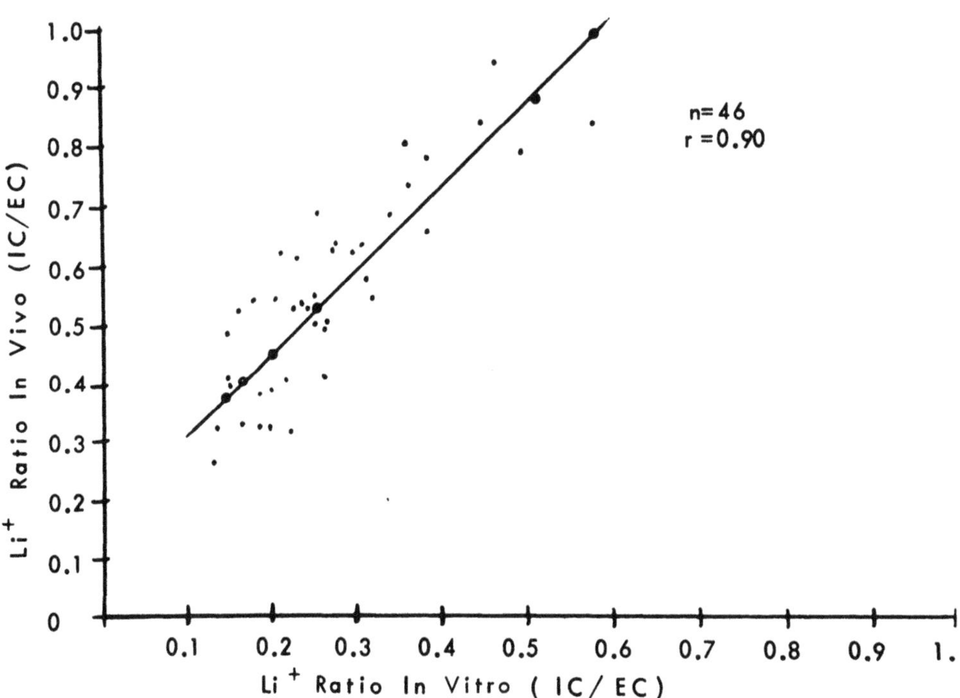

Figure 10. Correlation between Li ratio in vitro and in vivo.

Genetic Factors and Lithium Transport

The reports that a large interindividual variation in the Li^+ ratio is observed in patients during Li tretment (Mendels and Frazier, 1973; Casper, 1976) suggested that genetic factors may be responsible at least in part for such observed differences. Preliminary evidence for genetic control of the Li ratio was provided by the twin-study method carried out by Dorus *et al.* (1974) and Dorus *et al.* (1975). The Li ratio was first determined by *in vitro* by incubation, in a plasma-like medium containing 1.5 mM LiCl, of red cells obtained from normal monozygotic (MZ) and dizygotic (DZ) twin pairs. The Li^+ distribution ratio between erythrocytes and the medium was determined after 24 hours of incubation. In their first study, Dorus *et al.* (1974) determined the Li ratio *in vitro* in 10 MZ and 7 DZ twin pairs. The intra-pair differences in the Li ratio were significantly smaller in the MZ twin pairs than in the DZ twin pairs. In a subsequent study (Dorus *et al.*, 1975), Li was administered to MZ and DZ twin pairs for seven days, and the Li ratio was determined *in vivo* and *in vitro*. The variance in the Li ratio, *in vitro* and *in vivo*, in DZ twin pairs was significantly greater than that in MZ twin pairs. These results gave preliminary evidence of genetic control of the Li ratio.

To evaluate the degree of this genetic control, Dorus *et al.* (1979) studied the Li ratio in members of normal familes. In 291 members of 120 familes, they observed that parent-offspring and sibling-sibling correlations were significantly different from 0, but not significantly different from 0.5. If a quantitative trait is under complete polygenic control, the theoretically expected correlation for relatives who have, on the average, one half of their genes identical by descent (e.g., in parent-offspring and sibling-sibling pairs) is 0.50. There were no significant differences in the magnitude of the correlations between brother-brother, brother-sister, and sister-sister pairs. Similarly, there were no significant differences in the correlations between mother-son, mother-daughter, father-son, and father-daughter pairs, suggesting that sex-chromosome effects do not play a major role in determining the distribution of lithium. These results thus indicate that autosomal genetic factors contribute substantially to the interindividual variation observed in the Li ratio. It is not yet known, however, whether a single gene locus with a major effect or a number of gene loci with additive effects are involved.

The evidence that an abnormality of Li transport in human red cells, resulting in a high Li^+ ratio, is inherited was provided in a study of the family of a patient who had a high Li ratio *in vivo* (Pandey *et al*., 1977). This patient also had high Li ratio *in vitro* and the Li transport mediated by the Li^+-Na^+ exchange pathway (Li-Na counterflow) in his red cells was almost absent. The Na-Na exchange system was also found to be deficient in the red cells of this patient. Several members of his family, including his father, had Li^+ transport characteristics similar to his own, thus suggesting that a deficient Li transport in red cells mediated by the Li^+-Na^+ exchange pathway can be inherited. Similar results in several additional familes have been reported (Pandey *et al*., 1979).

Lithium Transport in Patients with Bipolar Illness

There is preliminary evidence that a cell membrane defect reflected in Li transport may be involved in the pathogenesis of at least a subgroup of patients with bipolar illness. Lyttkens *et al*. (1973) reported that bipolar patients have significantly higher Li ratios than do normal controls. Ostrow *et al*. (1978) found, in a previous study, that, on the average, bipolar patients did not differ from normal controls in uphill Li^+ transport from red cells (Li^+-Na^+ counterflow); a subgroup of patients with bipolar illness, however, had deficient counterflow.

We recently reported a comparison of Li^+ transport characteristics in red cells obtained from patients with bipolar illness and from normal controls (Pandey *et al*., 1979). The parameters studied were the Li^+ ratio *in vivo* and *in vitro*, and uphill and downhill Li^+ efflux. The results are shown in Table V.

Li Ratio In Vivo and In Vitro

The Li^+ ratio *in vivo* was measured in patients being treated with Li_2CO_3. The Li^+ ratio *in vitro* was determined in patients during a drug-

TABLE V

CHARACTERISTICS OF Li^+ TRANSPORT ACROSS THE HUMAN RED-CELL MEMBRANE

Pathway	Probably Mechanism	Characteristics
A. Ouabain-sensitive	Na^+-K^+ ATPase (Na^+-K^+ pump)	1. In the absence of K in the external medium, permits both downhill and uphill uptake (influx in the cells), but not extrusion (efflux). 2. Influx is inhibited by ouabain and ATP depletion and competitively inhibited by external K and Na. 3. Ouabain-sensitive Li transport is saturable at high external Li concentrations. 4. Can permit Li efflux in the absence of both K and Na in the cells.
B. Phloretin-sensitive	Carrier-mediated Li-Na exchange (Counterflow-countertransport)	1. Permits both uptake and extrusion; is inhibited by phloretin, quinine, quinidine, and by absence of contralateral Na.. 2. Absolute requirement of Na on trans side of membrane.

		3. Can move Li up its electrochemical potential which is driven by oppositely directed electrochemical potential for Na. 4. The uphill movement is not altered by ATP depletion; thus this sytem meets the criteria of Li-Na counter-flow (countertransport).
C. Insensitive to phloretin and ouabain	Passive diffusion	1. Permits only downhill influx and efflux. 2. Insensitive to ouabain and phloretin. 3. Not inhibited by Na or K. 4. Influx linearly related to external Li concentration and efflux to internal lithium concentration.
D. Ouabain insensitive anion exchange	Passive diffusion (anion pair formation)	1. Permits only downhill influx and efflux. 2. Requires HCO_3^- 3. Inhibited by phloretin and dipyridamole.

free baseline period and in normal controls according to the method described in Table V. The mean Li^+ ratio *in vivo* in the patients was 0.56 ± 0.19 (mean ± SD) and ranged from 0.32 to 0.97, with approximately 25% of the patients having ratios higher than 0.60. Since Li was not given to normals, their *in vivo* ratio was not determined. The mean Li^+ ratio *in vitro* of bipolar patients was significantly greater than the mean Li^+ ratio of normal controls ($t = 2.75$, $p < 0.01$). The variance within the bipolar patients was significantly greater than the variance within the normal controls (Bartlett's test for homogeneity of variance, $X^2 = 15.80$, $p < 0.001$).

Uphill and Downhill Li Efflux

For measurement of uphill Li^+ efflux, cells preloaded with Li^+ up to a level of 1.0 meq/liter were incubated in a high-Na^+ medium containing 1.5 meq LiCl. The mean uphill Li^+ efflux or Li^+-Na^+ counterflow of bipolar patients (Table V) was significantly lower than the mean of normal controls ($t = 1.99$, $p = 0.05$). The variance within bipolar patients also was significantly greater than the variance within normal controls ($X^2 = 7.43$, $p = 0.01$).

With respect to measures of downhill Li^+ efflux, the mean total and the mean Na-dependent Li^+ efflux for bipolar patients was significantly lower than the mean for normal controls ($t = 2.57$, $p = 0.02$ and $t = 1.99$, $p = 0.06$, respectively), although the variances did not differ. There were no significant differences between the means or variances of the bipolar patients and those of normal controls for the passive leak diffusion.

The above determinations of Li^+ transport, with the exception of passive leak diffusion, are either direct or indirect measures of Li^+-Na^+ exchange. Bipolar patients were significantly different from normal controls on all measures of Li^+-Na^+ exchange (Li^+ ratio *in vitro*, uphill Li^+ efflux and total downhill Li^+ efflux) except one (Na^+-stimulated Li^+ efflux), suggesting that bipolar patients have a deficiency in Li^+ transport by Li^+-Na^+ exchange. As anticipated, the groups did not differ in passive leak diffusion. Significant heterogeneity existed within the patient group for the Li^+ ratio *in vitro*, and Li^+-Na^+ counterflow. Most bipolar patients, rather than normal controls, had unusually high Li ratios and deficient Li^+-

Na^+ counterflow; other bipolar patients, however, had values in the normal range. In a recent study, we found that some patients who fall into other diagnostic groups, e.g., schizophrenia, also have high Li^+ ratios and deficient counterflow.

Our results indicate that there is no one-to-one relationship between bipolar illness and abnormalities of Li^+ transport; not all bipolar patients have high Li^+ ratios and deficient counterflow. On the other hand, the average for bipolar patients may differ from that for normal controls. More importantly, there is substantial heterogeneity within the bipolar groups with respect to Li^+ transport. This finding is consistent with data of Rybakowsky (1977), which indicate that bipolar patients with first-degree relatives who have a history of affective illnesses have a higher mean Li^+ ratio than those with no such family history. Frazer et al. (1978) have also reported heterogeneity of bipolar patients, those with lower schizoid indices having significantly higher Li^+ ratios, on the average, than patients with higher schizoid indices.

Rybakowski et al. (1978), in a recent report, compared Li^+ ratios in bipolar patients, depressed patients, and normal controls. They observed a significantly higher Li^+ ratio in bipolar patients than in normal controls. They also observed a significantly higher Li^+ ratio in male bipolar patients than in male unipolar depressed patients. The results are very similar to those reported by Pandey et al. (1979).

These observations suggest that it would be useful to characterize patients with high Li^+ ratios and deficient Li^+ ratios and deficient Li^+ efflux, regardless of their diagnosis, by means of a range of biochemical, clinical, and pharmacologic parameters.

LITHIUM TRANSPORT IN OTHER TISSUES

The mechanism of Li transport in human red cells and the factors that regulate the distribution of Li across the erythrocyte membrane are fairly well established, but the mechanism of Li^+ transport in other human tissues remains obscure. This is so primarily because of the nonavailability of such tissues and their unsuitability for Li^+ flux studies. Attempts have been made, however, to study Li^+ transport in tissues obtained from experimental animals.

Wraae et al. (1976) have reported Li^+ uptake (influx) characteristics in slices of cortex obtained from rat brains. Using lower external Li^+ concentrations (0.5-2 mM), they observed, at steady-state levels, that the concentration of Li^+ in the slices was linearly related to the concentration of Li^+ in the external medium. A steady-state distribution was achieved within one hour of incubation. Saturation of Li^+ uptake was not observed with the range of external Li^+ concentrations used. They therefore assumed that, if the system was saturable, the K_m must be well above the concentration used clinically. In the absence of K^+ in the medium, Li uptake in the cortex slices was 50% higher than in the presence of 4.9 mM K^+. Lithium uptake in the slices increased with gradual lowering of K^+ in the external medium. Increasing the Mg^{++} concentration in the medium resulted in an increase of Li^+ uptake.

These results were not conclusive in elucidating the pathways involved in Li^+ transport in the rat cortex. However, the interaction of K^+ with Li^+ and of Mg^{++} with Li^+ observed in Li^+ influx was similar to that observed in red cells and suggests that the trasnsport of Li^+ mediated by the Na-K pump may be similar in the two systems.

Lithium entry (influx) into an electrically active adrenergic clone of mouse neuroblastoma cells was studied by Richelson (1977). He observed that the alkaloid vertridine stimulated Li^+ influx in the neuroblastoma cells, and that this increase was inhibited by tetradotoxin. Since veratridine selectively increases the permeability of electrically excited membranes to sodium and tetrodotoxin blocks the fast sodium channels, Richelson concluded that one of the major pathways of Li^+ entry to these cells is through the sodium channel.

Kinsey and McLean (1974) have reported a ouabain-sensitive component of Li^+ transport in the lens of the rabbit eye. They found that ouabain inhibits Li influx and efflux from the rabbit lens. Potassium was a potent competitive inhibitor of the carrier-mediated transport of Li^+ in the cells.

Lithium transport studies in other tissues thus do not provide adequate information on the various pathways which may be involved in the transport of Li^+. However, striking similarities in Li^+ transport in red cells, brain slices, and the rabbit lens were observed with respect to Li's competitive inhibition by K^+ and its transport inhibition by ouabain.

LITHIUM AND THE CYCLIC AMP SYSTEM

Lithium has been shown to alter the activity of several enzymes; of particular interest are its effect on the responsiveness of the enzyme adenylate cyclase to neurotransmitters and hormones. Adenylate cyclase is a membrane bound enzyme which catalyzes the conversion of adenosine-5'-triphosphate (ATP) to cyclic AMP. Cyclic AMP mediates the cellular effects of several hormones and neurotransmitters and plays an important role in synaptic transmission (Greengard et al., 1972). Adenylate cyclase has been closely linked with adrenergic receptors (Lefkowitz, 1975) and may even be an integral part of the adrenergic receptor system. It is, therefore, quite possible that lithium's effect on the adenylate cyclase - cyclic AMP system may be related to its therapeutic mode of action.

The effect of Li on adenylate cyclase has been studied in various tissues obtained from both animals and humans and has been elegantly reviewed by Friedman (1973) and Forn (1975). The effect of Li on adenylate cyclase and cyclic AMP in humans will be briefly discussed. It is generally established that Li inhibits adenylate cyclase activity as well as the hormone stimulated synthesis of cyclic AMP in preparations obtained from a variety of tissues (Friedman, 1973; Forn, 1975).

Lithium and Platelet Adenylate Cyclase

Human platelets have been shown to have an adenylate cyclase system which is sensitive to stimulation by prostaglandin E_1 (PGE_1) and by prostacyclins. Norepinephrine (NE) has, however, only marginal effects on basal platelet adenylate cyclase activity but significantly inhibits the increase of cyclic AMP synthesis stimulated by PGE_1 (Murphy et al., 1973; Wang et al., 1974). The inhibition produced by NE on PGE_1 stimulation of platelet adenylate cyclase is blocked by the α-adrenergic antagonist phentolamine (Robison, et al., 1969; Wang et al., 1974). The NE induced inhibition of PGE_1 stimulated platelet adenylate cyclase, which is blocked by phentolamine, suggests that the responses produced by NE in human platelets are primarily α-adrenergic responses.

The effects of Li and other cations on platelet adenylate cyclase have been studied by Wang et al. (1974) and Murphy et al. (1973). Wang et al. (1974) studied the in vitro effects of Li on adenylate cyclase in both intact and fragmented platelet preparations. They observed that Li^+ had no significant effect on basal adenylate cyclase activity but it produced a significant inhibition of PGE_1 stimulated platelet adenylate cyclase activity in a dose dependent fashion. Concentrations of Li^+ as low as 1 mM inhibited about 14 percent of the PGE_1 stimulated activity. This inhibitory effect of Li^+ was not affected by phentolamine as shown in Figure 11, suggesting that Li^+ and NE act at separate sites. It was also observed that increasing the concentration of Mg^{++} in the incubation media resulted in a reduction in the magnitude of inhibition produced by Li^+. In the absence of Mg^{++}, 6 mM Li produced a 22 percent inhibition of PGE_1 stimulated ^3H-cyclic AMP synthesis; however, in the presence of 6 mM Mg^{++}, only 8 percent inhibition was observed.

Murphy et al. (1973) studied the effect of Li^+ treatment on platelet adenylate cyclase in patients. They observed that the mean PGE_1 stimulated synthesis of ^3H-cyclic AMP determined in platelets obtained from 16 Li treated patients was about 50 percent lower than those determined in the platelets obtained from 19 normal controls. These results indicate that Li^+ therapy decreases platelet adenylate cyclase responsiveness to PGE_1.

Effect of Lithium Treatment on Cyclic AMP

The effect of Li treatment on urinary, plasma, and CSF cyclic AMP

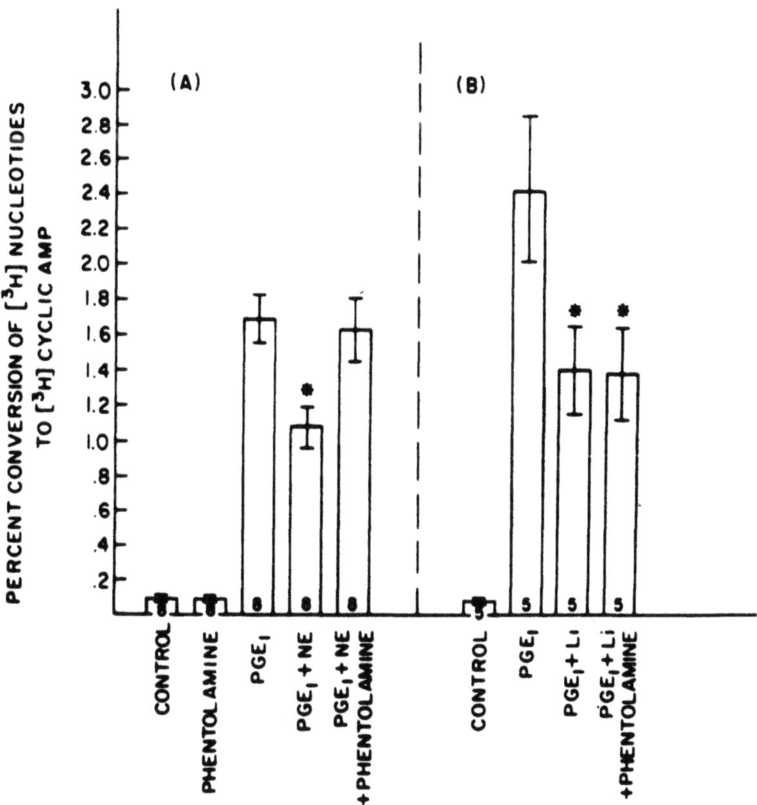

Figure 11. Effect of lithium on PGE_1-sensitive cyclase in human platelets.

levels has been studied by some investigators. Paul et al. (1971) studied the effect of Li treatment on urinary cyclic AMP levels in six patients before and during treatment with Li. In three of the patients, cyclic AMP excretion during Li treatment was increased, whereas it was decreased in the other three patients. They, however, observed that the direction of urinary cyclic AMP changes was related to changes in the clinical status. It increased as depression improved and decreased as mania improved. Sen et al. (1976) did not find any relationship between clinical changes and cyclic AMP excretion during Li treatment

Smith et al. (1976) studied the effect of Li treatment on CSF cyclic AMP levels but did not find any significant differences in patients treated with Li as compared to patients receiving other psychotropic drugs or in patients taking no drugs. One of the more fruitful strategies for studying neuroendocrine systems has been the use of provocating pharmacological agents which alter the levels of such hormones. For example, no significant differences in the basal levels of hormones are obtained between populations of patients; however, drug stimulated release or inhibition of these hormones may be different in the psychiatric subgroups. Pandey et al. (1977) using this strategy have shown that apomorphine induced human growth hormone release is significantly higher in acute schizophrenic patients as compared to normal subjects.

A similar strategy has been used by Ebstein et al. (1976) for studying the effect of Li treatment on plasma cyclic AMP levels. They observed that subcutaneous administration of 0.5 mg of adrenaline results in an increase of plasma cyclic AMP levels, the peak levels being observed at about 40 minutes after the administration of adrenaline. They observed that the adrenaline induced increase in plasma cyclic AMP levels was significantly lower in patients during Li^+ therapy as compared to the drug-free control subjects. Nine Li treated patients showed no increase in plasma cyclic AMP levels after adrenaline administratioin. Although the specific mechanism by which Li^+ treatment produces such decrease is not known, it has been suggested by these investigators that Li^+ inhibits adrenaline stimulated cyclic AMP increase due to its effect on α-adrenergic receptors.

Geisler et al. (1976) and Ebstein et al. (1977) found no significant effects of Li treatment on glucagon stimulated cyclic AMP secretion in man. Similarly, Speigel et al. (1976) did not observe any significant effect of Li treatment on parathyroid hormone (PTH) stimulated increase in urinary cyclic AMP excretion, studied in 4 patients before and during Li treatment.

These results thus suggest that Li may inhibit adrenaline stimulated cyclic AMP release in vivo but has no effect on glucagon or parathyroid hormone stimulated cyclic AMP release. As suggested by Ebstein et al. (1977), it is quite possible that Li may interact with adrenergic receptors in vivo and can produce alterations in cyclic AMP synthesis, but may not have any pronounced effect on other hormone receptors coupled to adenylate cyclase. This aspect of Li effect obviously needs to be investigated further.

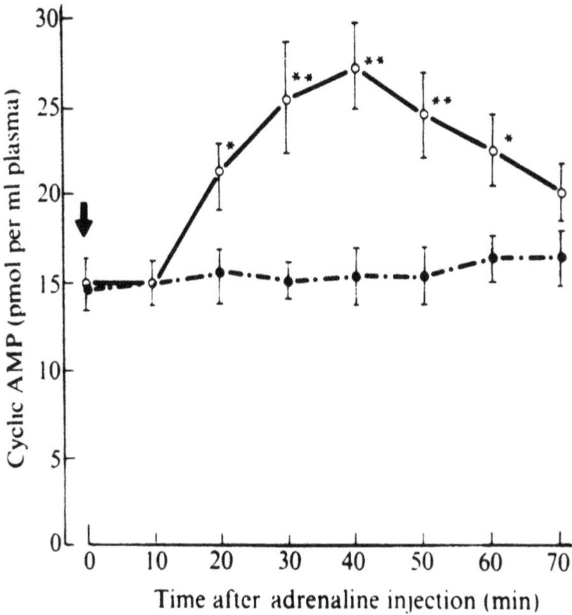

Figure 12. Effect of lithium on adrenaline-stimulated cyclic AMP release.

LITHIUM DOSAGE, PLASMA LEVELS, AND PHARMACOKINETICS

The therapeutic response to a particular drug, in most cases, is dependent on the body levels of the drug. As a measure of the body levels, plasma concentrations of the drug are generally monitored, although tissue levels, such as red cell levels in certain cases, may be more appropriate. The plasma levels of drugs are dependent on many processes: absorption of the drug; metabolism; reabsorption in the tissues; and elimination or excretion. In some cases, too little drug in the plasma may be a reason for an inadequate response to the drug, whereas too much drug in the plasma may result in the development of toxic side effects. It is therefore desired that the plasma levels of the drug are maintained within the therapeutic range. (For details of dosage, serum lithium levels, and patient management, also see Schou, 1973; Kerry, 1975; and Grof, 1979).

Dosage

Several salts of Li are used for treatment purposes; the most common preparation, however, is Li carbonate. Since large inter-individual variations exist in the absorption, redistribution in the tissues, and elimination of lithium, the dosage of Li required to achieve a desired plasma Li level differs from individual to individual. It has been suggested that plasma lithium levels determined 10-14 hours after the last intake of lithium should be between 0.8 to 1.5 meq/l plasma (Prien et al., 1971; Schou, 1973). Initial treatment with Li is started with a daily dose of 30-60 mMole (900-2400 mg Li carbonate), depending on the patient's age and body weight. Steady state between intake and elimination is reached within 5-6 days. The dosage of Li is subsequently adjusted according to the observed plasma levels of Li. Lithium is administered in multiple daily dosages. Recently, some investigators have described methods for predicting optimal Li dosage based on single dose pharmacokinetic studies. During maintenance therapy, the intake of Li should be equal to the elimination of Li. Since Li is primarily eliminated by the kidneys, it is the renal Li clearance which determines the maintenance dose. During maintenance therapy the Li dose should be adjusted according to the observed plasma levels.

It has been reported that the doses of Li required to treat manic patients were higher than normal subjects would tolerate (Trautner et al., 1955). Several investigators have suggested the need to reduce the dose of Li after recovery from an acute manic attack. Consequently, plasma Li levels and Li dosage must be carefully regulated in those cases other than psychiatric illness, e.g., its use in cancer chemotherapy. It may be advisable in such cases to stay in the lower side of the therapeutic range.

Plasma-Serum Lithium Levels and Pharmacokinetics

When given in a readily absorbed form, except for the slow releasing capsules, Li is rapidly absorbed and the serum Li level starts rising quickly and peaks within 1-2 hours after the intake (Figure 13). The maximum concentration is high compared to the dosage and body weight. After the peak serum Li concentration has been established, there is a quick decrease due to simultaneous renal excretion and the distribution of Li into other tissues. During this elimination phase, serum Li has a half life of approximately 10-20 hours. Li is generally administered in divided dosage. Steady state between elimination and intake is achieved after 5-6 days of treatment. The interval between Li intake and blood withdrawal for serum Li determinations should be uniform and standardized. Since there is an initial rapid increase after Li intake, the Li levels determined during the first 4 hours after intake give Li levels which are higher than the steady-state levels and show large variations. It has been recommended that blood samples should be drawn after 10-16 hours of Li intake for steady-state plasma Li determinations.

The initial dosage of Li should be adjusted to give a serum Li level in the range of 0.9 to 1.4 meq/l plasma. This range may differ slightly during maintenance therapy. The optimal Li dosage required to achieve a desired Li level can be predicted by an acute pharmacokinetic study (Cooper et al., 1973; Cooper and Simpson, 1976; Chang et al., 1979). Serum Li levels should be monitored at least weekly in the initial phases of treatment and monthly during the maintenance therapy.

CONCLUSIONS

Two aspects of the biology of Li ion have been described. The first one is the mechanism of Li transport in human red cells. Recent studies resulting in the characterization of the various pathways involved in the transfer of Li across erythrocyte membrane, and the factors which regulate Li distribution between red cells and plasma have been discussed. The other aspect discussed briefly is the effect of Li on the adenylate cyclase-cyclic AMP system in humans.

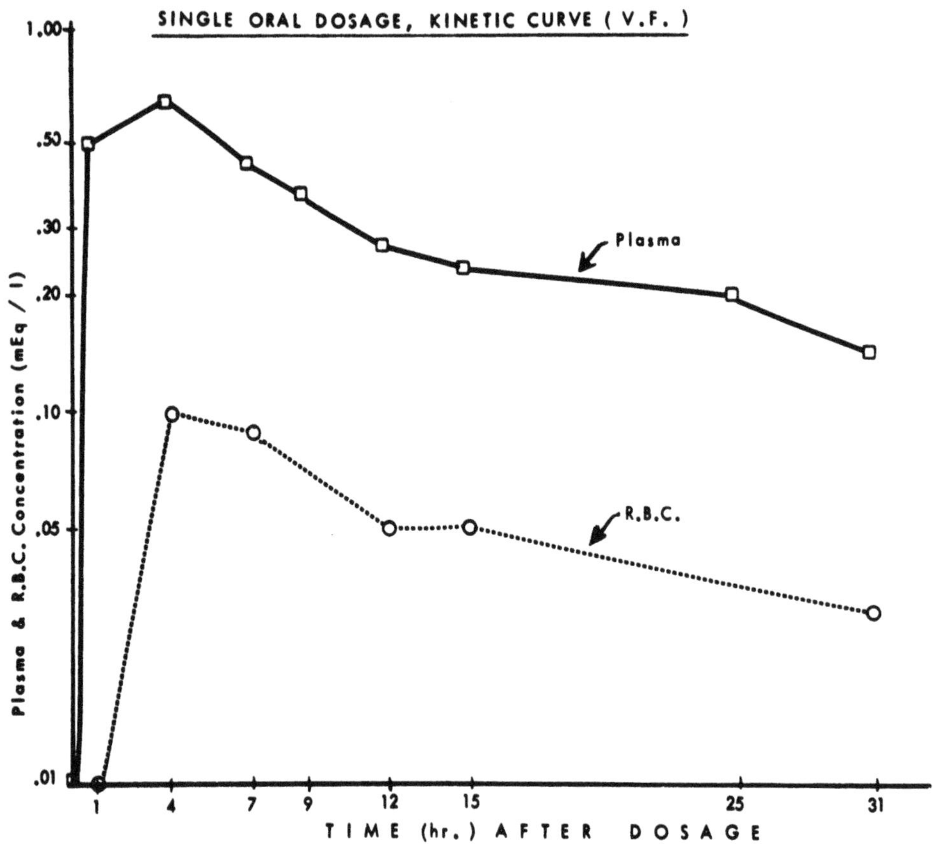

Figure 13. Plasma and red blood cell lithium curves after administration of lithium carbonate.

Studies of Li transport in human red cells have resulted in the elucidation of at least four distinct pathways of Li transport and have provided an understanding of the factors which regulate distribution of Li across the erythrocyte membrane. The most significant finding resulting from these studies is the discovery of a Li-Na countertransport system which is mediated by a Li-Na exchange mechanism. Li transport mediated by this pathway is reduced significantly in bipolar patients, and this deficiency may be inherited, or genetic factors may substantially contribute toward the variability of this system. These observations may provide useful leads not only to a better understanding of the mechanism of action of Li, but also to our understanding of the pathophysiology of bipolar illness.

One question of interest concerns the mechanism of pharmacological action of Li. Li transport studies have provided the evidence for the existence of a Na-Na exchange system in human red cells. This exchange system normally does not promote net transport of Na across the red cell membrane, and hence the physiological significance remains unclear. It is, possible, however, that this exchange system is involved in the transport of other physiologically active cations like Ca^{++} or positively charged neurotransmitters. Since this system can also accept Li, Li itself might compete with and thus alter the effect of some physiologically active ion at its effector site. Alternatively, Li might alter the transport and thus the concentration of physiologically active cations in the region of their receptors.

Another question concerns the relationship between abnormalities of the Na-Na exchange system and brain function. If a deficiency in this transport system alters the distribution of physiologically active cations, it could alter the effects of such substances.

Li has been shown generally to inhibit adenylate cyclase in various tissues, but only a few human studies have been reported. Of these human studies, two studies indicate that Li inhibites PGE_1 sensitive adenylate cyclase in human platelets under in vitro conditions and one study indicates such inhibition under in vivo conditions. Whereas Li treatment decreases adrenalin stimulated plasma cyclic AMP levels, it has no significant effects on glucagon stimulated and parathyroid hormone stimulated urinary cyclic AMP excretion. Whereas some of the side effects of Li therapy may be related to its effect on the adenylate cyclase system, it is not clear if the clinical effects of Li therapy are mediated by such mechanisms.

Future studies of Li distribution will probably be directed toward elucidating the functional significance of a Li-Na or a Na-Na exchange system present in red cells. Is this sytem present in other tissues, especially the neuronal tissues? Is this sytem also involved in the transport of neurotransmitters or other physiologically active cations? Does Li treatment restore the imbalance in the transport of these physiologically active compounds present in a subgroup of psychiatric patients? It is hoped that future studies will provide answers to some of these questions.

In order to avoid side effects and achieve maximum therapeutic response, plasma Li levels should be monitored regularly by a standardized procedure. Steady-state plasma levels are achieved 5-6 days after the start of therapy and should be determined in blood samples drawn 10-16 hours after lithium intake.

REFERENCES

Anderson, D.K. and Prockop, Q.D., 1975, Lithium absorption and distribution in body tissues, in "Lithium Research and Therapy," (F.N. Johnson, ed.), pp. 267-278, London, Academic Press.

Becker, B.F. and Duhm J., 1978, Evidence for anionic cation transport of lithium, sodium, and potassium across the human erythrocyte membrane induced by divalant anions, J. Physiol. 282:149.

Casper, R.C., Pandey, G., Gosenfeld, L., and Davis, J.M., 1976, Intracellular lithium and clinical response, Lancet 2:418.

Cazzullo, C.L., Smeraldi, E., and Sacchetti, E., 1975, Intracellular lithium concentration and clinical response, Br. J. Psychiatry 126:298.

Chang, S.S., Pandey, G.N., Casper, R.C., Kinard, C.O., and Davis, J.M., Pharmacokinetics of lithium: Predicting optimal dosage, in "Lithium: Controversies and Unresolved Issues" (Cooper, T.B., Gershon, S., Kline, N.S., et al., eds.), Excerpta Medica, in press.

Cooper, T.B. and Simpson, G.M., 1976, The 24-hour lithium level as a prognosticator of dosage requirements. A 2-year follow-up study, Amer. J. Psychiat. 133:440.

Dorus, E., Pandey, G.N., Frazer, A., and Mendels, J., 1974, Genetic determinant of lithium ion distribution. I. An in vitro monozygotic-dizygotic twin study, Arch. Gen. Psychiatry 31:463.

Dorus, E., Pandey, G.N., and Davis, J.M., 1975, Genetic determinant of lithium ion distribution. An in vivo monozygotic-dizygotic twin study, Arch. Gen. Psychiatry 32:1097.

Dorus, E., Pandey, G.N., Shaughnessy, R., and Davis, J.M., 1979, Lithium transport across the reo cell membrane: A study of genetic factors, Arch. Gen. Psych., in press.

Duhm, J. and Becker, B.F., 1977a, Studies on the lithium transport across the red cell membrane II. Characterization of ouabain-sensitive and ouabain insensitive Li transport. Effects of biocarbonate and dipyridamole, Pfluegers Arch. Eur. J. Physiol. 367:211.

Duhm, J. and Becker, B.F., 1977b, Studies on the lithium transport across the red cell membrane III. Factors contributing to the inter-individual variability of the in vitro Li distribution across the human red cell membrane, Pfluegers Arch. Eur. J. Physiol. 368:203.

Duhm, J. and Becker, F.B., 1977c, Studies on the lithium transport across the red cell membrane IV. Inter-individual variations in the Na-dependent Li countertransport system of human erythrocytes, Pfluegers Arch. Eur. J. Physiol. 370:211.

Duhm, J., Eisenried, F., Becker, B.F., and Greil, W., 1976, Studies on the lithium transport across the red cell membrane. I. Li uphill transport by the Na-dependent Li countertransport system of human erythrocytes, Pfluegers Arch. Eur. J. Physiol. 364:147.

Dunham, P.B. and Senyk, O., 1977, Lithium efflux through Na-K pump in human erythrocytes, Proc. Natl. Acad. Sci. U.S.A. 74:3099.

Ebstein, R.P., Kara, T., and Belmaker, R.H., 1977, The effect of Li on the glucagon-sensitive adenylate cyclase in vivo in man, Acta Pharmacol. Toxicol. 41:80.

Ebstein, R.P., Belmaker, R.H., Grunhaus, L., and Rimon, R., 1976, Lithium inhibition of adrenaline-stimulated adenylate cyclase in humans, Nature 259:411.

Elizur, A., Gaff, E., and Steiner, M., 1977, Intra/extra red blood cell lithium and electrolyte distributions as correlates of neurotoxic reactions during therapy, in "The Impact of Biology on Modern Psychiatry" (Gershon, E.S., Belmaker, R.H., and Kety, S.S., eds.), pp. 555-64, Plenum Press, New York.

Form, J., 1975, Lithium and cyclic AMP, in "Lithium Research and Therapy" (F.N. Johnson, ed.), pp. 485-497, Academic Press, London.

Frazer, A., London, J., Mendels, J., and Ramsey, A., 1978, Cell membranes, lithium and affective disorders. Paper presented at 131st annual meeting of the American Psychiatric Association, Atlanta, May 8-12.

Frazer, A., Mendels, J., and Brunswick, D., 1977, Transfer of lithium ions across the erythrocyte membrane, Comms. Psychopharm. 1:255.

Frazer, A., Mendels, J., Secunda, S.K., Cochrane, C.M., and Bianchi, C.P., 1973, The prediction of brain lithium concentrations from plasma or erythrocyte measures, J. Psychiat. Res. 10:1.

Friedman, E., 1973, Lithium's effects on cyclic AMP, membrane transport, and cholinergic mechanisms, in "Lithium: Its Role in Psychiatric Research and Treatment" (S. Gershon and B. Shopsin, eds.), pp 75-82, Plenum Press, New York.

Funder, J., Tosteson, D.C., and Wieth, J.O., 1978, Effects of bicarbonate on lithium transport in human red cells, J. Gen. Physiol. 11:721.

Geisler, A., Vendsborg, P.B., Johannesen, M., Klysner, R., and Thomsen, J., 1976, The effect of lithium on unstimulated and glucagon-stimulated urinary cyclic AMP excretion in rat and man, Acta Pharmacol. Toxicol. 38:433.

Greil, W., Eisenreid, F., Becker, B.F., and Duhm, J., 1977, Interindividual differences in the Na^+ dependent Li^+ countertransport system and in the Li^+ distribution ratio across the red cell membrane among Li^+-treated patients, Psychopharmacology 53:19.

Greengard, P., McAfee, D.W., and Kebabian, J.W., 1972, On the mechanism of action of cyclic AMP and its role in synaptic transmission, in "Advances in Cyclic Nucleotide Research, Vol. 1," (P. Greengard and B.A. Robison, eds.), pp. 337-355, Raven Press, New York.

Grof, P., 1979, Some practical aspects of lithium treatment, Arch. Gen. Psychiat. 36:891.

Haas, M., Schooler, J., and Tosteson, D.C., 1975, Coupling of lithium to sodium transport in human red cells, Nature 258:424.

Hewick, D.S. and Murray, N., 1976, Red blood cell levels and lithium toxicity, Lancet 2:473.

Kerry, R.J., 1975, The management of patients receiving lithium treatment, in "Lithium: Research and Therapy" (Johnson, F.N., ed.), pp. 143-163, Academic Press, New York.

Kinsey, V.E. and McLean, I.W., 1974, Studies on the crystalline lens. XXI. Bidirectional carrier-mediated transport of lithium, Invest. Ophthalmol. 13:784.

Lefkowitz, R.J., 1975, Heterogeneity of adenylate cyclase-coupled β-adrenergic receptors, Biochem. Pharmacol. 24:583.

Lyttkens, L., Soderberg, U., and Wetterberg, L., 1973, Increased lithium erythrocyte/plasma ratio in manic-depressive psychosis, Lancet 1:40.

Maggs, R., 1963, Treatment of manic illness with lithium carbonate, Brit. J. Psychiatry 109:56.

Meltzer, H.L., Rosoff, C.J., Kassir, S., and Fieve, R.R., 1976, Active efflux of lithium from erythrocytes of manic-depressive subjects, Life Sci. 19:371.

Mendels, J. and Frazer, A., 1973, Intracellular lithium concentration and clinical response: Towards a membrane theory of depression, J. Psychiatr. Res. 10:9.

Murphy, D.L., Donnelly, C., and Moskowitz, J., 1973, Inhibition by lithium of prostaglandin E1 and norepinephrine effects on cyclic adenosine monophosphate production in human platelets, Clin. Pharmacol. Ther. 14:810.

Ostrow, D.G., Pandey, G.N., Davis, J.M., Hurt, S.W., and Tosteson, D.C., 1978, A heritable disorder of lithium transport in the red blood cells of a subpopulation of manic patients, Am. J. Psychiatry 135:1070.

Pandey, G.N., Garver, D.L., Tamminga, C., Erickson, S., Ali, S.I., and Davis, J.M., 1977, Postsynaptic supersensitivity in schizophrenia, Am. J. Psychiat. 134:518.

Pandey, G.N., Ostrow, D.G., Haas, M., Dorus, E., Casper, R.C., Davis, J.M., and Tosteson, D.C., 1977, Abnormal lithium and sodium transport in erythrocytes of a manic patient and some members of his family, Proc. Natl. Acad. Sci. U.S.A. 74:3607.

Pandey, G.N., Sarkadi, B., Haas, M., Gunn, R.B., Davis, J.M., and Tosteson, D.C., 1978, Lithium transport pathways in human red blood cells, J. Gen. Physiol. 72:233.

Pandey, G.N., Baker, J., Chang, S., and Davis, J.M., 1978, Prediction of red cell-plasma Li^+ ratio in vivo by in vitro methods, Clin. Pharmacol. Ther. 24:343.

Pandey, G.N., Dorus, E., Davis, J.M., and Tosteson, D.C., 1979, Lithium transport in human red cells: Genetic and clinical aspects, Arch. Gen. Psychiat., in press.

Paul, M.I., Games, H., and Goodwin, F.K., 1971, Urinary cyclic AMP excretion in depression and mania, Arch. Gen. Psychiat. 24:327.

Prien, R.F., Caffey, E.M., and Klett, C.J., 1972, The relationship between lithium level and clinical response in acute manics treated with lithium carbonate, Cooperative Studies in Psychiatry, Report No. 91, VA-NIMH Collaborative Study Group, Perry Point, Md.

Ramsey, T.A., Frazer, A., Dyson, W.L., and Mendels, J., 1976, Intracellular lithium and clinical response, Br. J. Psychiatry 128:103.

Richelson, E., 1977, Lithium ion entry through the sodium channel of cultured mouse neuroblastoma cells: A biochemical study, Science 196:1001.

Robison, G.A., Arnold, A., and Hartman, R.C., 1969, Divergent effects of epinephrine and prostaglandin E1 on the level of cyclic AMP in human blood platelets, Pharm. Res. Commun. 1:325.

Rybakowski, J. amd Strzyzewski, W., 1976, Red blood cell lithium index and long-term maintenance treatment, Lancet 1:1408.

Rybakowski, J., 1977, Pharmacogenetic aspect of red blood cell lithium index in manic-depressive psychosis, Biol. Psychiatry, 12:425.

Rybakowski, J., Frazer, A., Mendels, J., and Ramsey, T.A., 1978, Erythrocyte accumulation of the lithium ion in control subjects and patients with primary affective disorder, Comm. Psychopharmacol. 2:99.

Sarkadi, B., Alifimoff, J.K., Gunn, R.B., and Tosteson, D.C., 1978, Kinetics and stoichiometry of Na-dependent Li transport in human red blood cells, J. Gen. Physiol. 72:249.

Schless, A.P., Frazer, A., Mendels, J., Pandey, G.N., and Theodorides, V.J., 1975, Genetic determination of lithium ion metabolism, II. An in vitro study of lithium ion distribution across erythrocyte membranes, Arch. Gen. Psychait. 32:337.

Schou, M., 1973, Preparation, dosage and control, in "Lithium: Its Role in Psychiatric Research and Treatment" (S. Gershon and B. Shopsin, eds.), pp 189-199, Plenum Press, New York.

Sen, A.K., Awad, A.G., Stancer, H.C., and Godse, D.C., 1976, Urinary cyclic AMP in relation to lithium treatment in manic depressive illness, J. Nerv. Ment. Dis. 163:210.

Spiegel, A.M., Gerner, R.H., Murphy, D.L., and Aurbach, G.D., 1976, Lithium does not inhibit the parathyroid hormone-mediated rise in urinary cyclic AMP and phosphate in humans, J. Clin. Endocrinol. Metabol. 43:1390.

Smith, C.C., Tallman, J.F., Post, R.M., VanKammen, D.P., Jimmerson, D.C., and Brown, G.L., 1976, An examiniation of base-line and drug induced levels of cyclic nucleotides in the cerebrospinal fluid of control and psychiatric patients, Life Sci. 19:131.

Spitzer, R., Endicott, J., and Robbins, L., 1975, "Research Diagnostic Criteria (RDC) for a Selected Group of Functional Disorders," 2nd ed., New York State Psychiatric Institute, Biometrics Research, New York.

Tosteson, D.C. and Hoffman, J.F., 1960, Regulation of cell volume by active cation transport in high and low potassium sheep red cells, J. Gen. Physiol. 44:169.

Trautner, E.M., Morris, R., Noack, C.H., and Gershon, S., 1955, Med. J. Aust. 2:280.

Wang, Y.C., Pandey, G.N., Mendels, J., and Frazer, A., 1974, Effect of lithium on prostaglandin E1-stimulated adenylate cyclase activity of human platelets, Biochem. Pharmacol. 23:845.

Wraae, O., Hillman, H., and Round, E., 1976, The uptake of low concentrations of lithium ions into rat cerebral cortex slices and its dependence on cations, J. Neurochemistry 26:835.

Zakowska-Dabrowska, T. and Rybakowski, J., 1973, Lithium-induced EEG changes: Relation to lithium level in serum and red blood cells, Acta Psychiatr. Scand. 49:457.

RELEASE OF VITAMIN BINDING PROTEINS FROM GRANULOCYTES BY LITHIUM: VITAMIN B_{12} AND FOLATE BINDING PROTEINS

Victor Herbert and Neville Colman

Hematology and Nutrition Laboratory
Bronx Veterans Administration Medical Center
Bronx, New York, and
Department of Medicine
SUNY - Downstate Medical Center
Brooklyn, New York

In 1968, Dr. Seymour Rosenblatt, a psychiatrist using lithium in the treatment of manic-depressive psychosis at the Mount Sinai Hospital in New York City called our attention to the fact that some of his patients receiving lithium appeared to have mild leukocytosis. Joint investigation of this phenomenon with him confirmed that such was the case, and we learned that this phenomenon had been observed as far back as 1955 (Bille and Plum).

Since various agents are known to induce peripheral blood granulocytosis by bringing about demargination of leukocytes from blood vessel walls into the bloodstream, without stimulation of granulopoiesis or retardation of granulocyte egress from the bloodstream (Boggs and Winkelstein, 1975), we first addressed ourselves to the question of whether the effect of lithium was simply to induce demargination. Since lithium was known to produce a rise in serum cortisol (Platman and Fieve, 1968), and cortisol was known to induce demargination, this seemed a likely explanation, and indeed was suggested by Shopsin _et al_. (1971).

If the sole effect of lithium was to induce demargination, lithium should not stimulate an increase in granulocyte pool size. We chose measurement of B_{12} binding capacity to measure granulocyte pool size, since our laboratory had at that time just demonstrated that transcobalamins I and III, which constituted a significant portion of vitamin B_{12} binding protein in human serum, were largely products of granulocytes (Corcino et al., 1970) and, when used as an index of granulocyte pool size, gave results essentially identical to those of the more elaborate DFP^{32} labelling procedure (Chikkappa et al., 1969; Chikkappa et al., 1971). Vitamin B_{12} binding capacity proved to be elevated in patients receiving lithium therapy, supporting the concept that lithium in fact did enlarge the granulocyte pool and therefore must in some direct or indirect way stimulate granulopoiesis.

At this point in January, 1970, we moved our laboratory from Mount Sinai Hospital to the Bronx VA Medical Center, where after six months we were joined by Dr. Glenn Tisman, a highly enthusiastic, energetic and bright young research fellow. He quickly set up leukocyte cultures by the technique of Kurnick and Robinson (1971) and demonstrated that adding lithium to such cultures significantly increased new colony formation. These data, along with those on the elevated serum vitamin B_{12} binding protein levels produced by lithium therapy (and the granulocytosis so produced) were finally published in 1973 in the British Journal of Haematology (Tisman et al., 1973) after being rejected in 1972 by two American journals, as was our application to a major granting agency to fund further studies. Were it not for the British Journal of Haematology, there might have been no Workshop on "Effects of Lithium on Granulopoiesis and Immune Function" here at Eagle River.

In that article, as in our preliminary report in 1972 (Tisman et al., 1972), we first proposed the use of lithium to treat cyclic and other neutropenias, including those induced by chemotherapy and, Dr. Tisman having by then gone off to California, he and we continued to investigate the use of lithium in treating various neutropenias, including those associated with chemotherapy and malignancies (Jacob and Herbert, 1974; Tisman, 1974). In our preliminary clinical studies, oral doses of lithium carbonate sufficient to sustain a serum lithium level of 0.5 to 1.5 meq/l appeared to improve effective granulopoieisis in subjects with neutropenia alone, neutropenia and splenomegaly due to cirrhosis and portal hypertension, and neutropenia anticipated during a course of cyclophosphamide therapy (Jacob and Herbert, 1974).

Our eight years of experience in treating various neutropenias with lithium has not yet been prepared for publication, beyond our first preliminary report (Jacob and Herbert, 1974), but it may be of value to mention a patient of Dr. E. Amorosi of New York University Medical Center. This young man had cyclic neutropenia with recurrent infections, and, when treated in 1975 through one cycle with lithium, still had his neutropenia but did not get his usual infections and showed some rise in plasma vitamin B_{12} binding protein before, during, and after his neutropenic phase. Now we are discussing with Dr. Amorosi re-treating him through a number of cycles, in view of the report by Hammond and Dale (1979) that the cyclic neutropenia of grey collie dogs is favorably influenced by lithium in terms of measurable neutrophil count only after several cycles, but clinical infections during neutropenic periods did not occur, the report by Perez et al. (1979) that lithium can correct defective chemotaxis in human neutrophils and the report by Buckley et al. (1978) that elevated cyclic AMP in granulocytes reduces their adherence and their migration into infected tissues. Lithium lowers adenylate cyclase (Perez et al. 1979), and may modulate cyclic AMP-dependent effects in leukocytes (Gelfand et al., 1979).

LITHIUM AND HEMATOLOGIC MALIGNANCIES

We early feared (Tisman et al., 1972; Tisman et al., 1973) that lithium might induce leukemia, and so carried out with Frenkel in Texas a study of the frequency of granulocytic leukemia in populations drinking high- vs low-lithium content water (Frenkel and Herbert, 1974). Communities with high and low lithium content of their drinking water were initially identified from the U.S. Geologic Survey of the 100 largest cities in the United States (Durfor and Becker, 1964). This survey identified two cities in Texas with a consistent lithium content of their water supply considerably higher than any of the rest: El Paso and Amarillo. Of the other 100 cities surveyed, only Los Angeles, California, had a consistently elevated value in the range identified for these Texas cities. A more extensive and current analysis of the lithium content of drinking waters carried out by the more sensitive atomic absorption spectrophotometry demonstrated that the high levels of lithium in El Paso and Amarillo were unchanged over the past decade. The water supply has multiple origins in El Paso, Texas but the year-round average drinking water lithium content for the average El Pasoan is 66 µg/L (Trieff et al., 1973). These more recent, careful and serial studies further identified Amarillo, Texas as another geographic area with a consistently high lithium content (44 µg/L) in the drinking water (Trieff et al., 1973). Data from this same study revealed that the average lithium content of water supplying the Dallas - Fort Worth area was 1.8 µg/L and current weekly assays since that survey have been below the level of detection (Frenkel, personal communication).

The cases of leukemia from the Dallas - Fort Worth Metropolitan Area were compiled from the data from the Third National Cancer Survey (1975) which utilized this area as one data base (Frenkel, 1975). The El Paso data were compiled from the El Paso County Tumor Registry and Survey and corroborated by Epidemiologic Survey for El Paso conducted through M.D. Anderson Hospital, Houston, Texas (data provided by Dr. E.J. MacDonald of M.D. Anderson Hospital). Leukemia incidence data and the population base covered for Amarillo, Texas were obtained from the Texas Department of Health Resources Cancer Surveillance Program and corroborated by Cancer Registry evaluation. In each geographic area, only resident cases were recorded.

The levels of lithium ingested by residents of El Paso did not approach the usual therapeutic dose. At 66 &g/L, and an intake of three liters a day, this is only 200 µg of lithium per day, or 0.2 mg. Lithium carbonate is supplied in 300 mg tablets, and the usual daily dose is 900 mg, or 170 mg of lithium, over 800 times the dose from El Paso water.

The frequency of chronic (CGL) and acute (AGL) granulocytic leukemia was determined in the population of Dallas - Fort Worth (no lithium in water) vs El Paso (mean 66 μg/L Li in water). As shown in Table I, the frequency of AGL was substantially lower in the population drinking water containing lithium. The frequency of CGL was similar in both populations. Whether these findings were irrelevant coincidence or represent a lower incidence of AGL in populations with drinking water containing lithium awaits study of a larger number of paired populations in whom mean granulocyte and lymphocyte levels would also be of interest (Tisman et al., 1973). Other cities with high lithium-content drinking water include Phoenix, Los Angeles, and Lubbock. Cities with low lithium-content water include San Francisco, New York, Memphis, and Milwaukee. According to Durfor and Becker (1964), content does not change much from year to year, but most cities have more than one major source of drinking water. For example, the Croton supply to New York City has only 0.16 μg Li/L but the Catskill and Delaware supply has 0.27 μg Li/L and the Jamaica Wells supply has 1.5 μg Li/L (personal communication from L.J. McCabe, Water Supply Research Laboratory, US EPA, National Environmental Research Center, Cincinnati, Ohio 45268). McCabe indicated the highest content in the U.S. water was 170 μg Li/L at the Rio Grande treatment plant at El Paso, Texas. Should such Li intake prove to be associated with lower incidence of AGL, this could support the possibility that such doses of Li may stimulate blast cell differentiation and maturation, and thereby protect against AGL.

It is possible that therapeutic doses of lithium may have effects in terms of frequency of neoplasia different from the benign effects of much smaller quantities in municipal water supplies (which have been alleged to be protective against mental illness (Dawson et al., 1970; Voors, 1972) as well as against AGL). However, El Paso is located at some 4,000 feet in dry western Texas and Dallas at some 700 feet in relatively moist northern Texas. Second, Dallas has more than six times the total population and El Paso has many more Mexican-Americans than Dallas. These and other differences might account for the different numbers in Table I.

Although the frequency of leukemia is much lower in El Paso than in Dallas, if one adjusts for 6.4-fold difference in the populations, there is no consistent difference in the frequency of chronic granulocytic leukemia, and a smaller but consistently lower rate of acute leukemia:

	CGL		
2.32 m	24	30	22
0.36 m	6.4 x 3 = 19	6.4 x 7 = 45	6.4 x 4 = 26

	AGL		
2.32 m	63	64	49
0.36 m	6.4 x 1 = 6	6.4 x 4 = 26	6.4 x 2 = 13

TABLE I

FREQUENCY OF CHRONIC GRANULOCYTIC LEUKEMIA (CGL) AND ACUTE GRANULOCYTIC LEUKEMIA (AGL) IN POPULATIONS DRINKING HIGH (EL PASO) VS LOW (DALLAS/FT. WORTH) LITHIUM CONTENT WATER (FRENKEL AND HERBERT, 1974)

	Population Base	1969	1970	1971
		CGL[a]		
Dallas/Ft. Worth	2,318,036[b]	24	30	22
El Paso	359,291[b]	8	7	4
		AGL		
Dallas/Ft. Worth	2,318,036	63	64	49
El Paso	359,291	1	4	2

[a] All cases of CGL were in patients > 15 years old.

[b] Counting only residents of the 2 respective geographic areas. Based on 1970 Census figures.

Obviously, the data must be considered in the light of the actual and considerable demographic differences; perhaps the geographical differences are relevant, too.

The frequency of CGL and other hematologic neoplasms in patients taking lithium in therapeutic doses of 300 mg lithium carbonate thrice daily (or more) for periods of a year or more may be greater than chance, and further study is required of this possibility by statistical evaluation of adequate numbers of psychiatric patients receiving long-term lithium vs those not receiving such therapy. We had observed myeloblastic proliferation in a patient receiving long-term lithium therapy in 1972, and, in 1975, Dr. M. Goldstein of Montefiore Hospital in the Bronx, New York City, brought to our attention the second such case of which we are aware, in a 46 year-old milkman who, after being treated with 300 mg lithium carbonate four times daily for three years, developed CGL. Jim (1979) reported the appearance of CGL in a patient who had received 900 mg of lithium daily for 11 months, and mentioned the patient of Tosato et al. (1978) in whom CGL appeared after two years of lithium. Additionally, with Dr. Seymour Rosenblatt of Mount Sinai Hospital in New York, we noted in 1972 a 52 year-old female patient who developed asymptomatic kappa chain myeloma after four years of 300 mg Li_2CO_3 four times daily for manic-depressive psychosis (Tisman et al., 1972).

However, patients with infection-threatening neutropenia in association with multiple myeloma or macroglobulinemia may have increased neutrophil production to levels adequately protective against infection when treated with lithium, as occurred in a macroglobulinemia patient of Dr. Edward Amorosi of New York University Medical Center in 1975 in consultation with us.

No measurable lithium was found by Dr. Leslie Baer and Dr. Mort Levitt of Psychiatric Institute, Columbia Presbyterian Medical Center, in samples of plasma or fingernail clippings from ten patients with acute and ten with chronic granulocytic leukemia. The samples were provided to us by Dr. Hamid Al-Mondhiry and Dr. Bayard Clarkson of Memorial Hospital for Cancer and Allied Diseases.

RELATIONS OF NUTRIENT BINDING PROTEINS, LITHIUM, AND CELL PROLIFERATION

Recent studies have suggested a manner whereby the above-mentioned effects of lithium on granulocytes, in part mediated by colony-stimulating factor, might be related to the ability of lithium to initiate or enhance the release of crucial nutrient-binding proteins from granulocytes. This recent information has been provided in part by identification of lactoferrin as the granulocyte-derived inhibitor of colony-stimulating activity production (Broxmeyer et al., 1978). Since lactoferrin is contained in the secondary or specific granules of the rabbit heterophil (Baggiolini et al., 1970) and the human neutrophil (Spitznagel et al., 1974), and since the granulocyte binders for vitamin B_{12} and folate are also contained within these granules (Kane and Peters, 1975; Colman and Herbert, 1979b), it seems likely that there is a relationship between the effects of lithium which cause granulocytes to proliferate and that which causes these cells to release binders for nutrients crucial to DNA synthesis, such as vitamin B_{12} and folate. Indeed, a correlation does appear to exist between levels of vitamin B_{12} binding protein and colony-stimulating factor in human urine (Gibson et al., 1974).

Our studies of the release of vitamin binders from granulocytes under the influence of lithium arose with our discovery that the unsaturated vitamin B_{12} binding capacity (UBBC) of human serum increased with increasing in vitro exposure of granulocytes to certain anticoagulants, especially those containing lithium (Bloomfield et al., 1973) and that these in vitro effects could be totally abolished by the addition of an agent which blocked leukocyte degranulation, namely, sodium fluoride (Herbert et al., 1973). In whole blood, the lithium concentration which effected optimal release of vitamin B_{12} binder was 75 - 90 meq/L, and 50 meq/L was chosen as a suitable working concentration (Scott et al., 1974). When whole blood was incubated at room temperature, the vitamin B_{12} binder was released from granulocytes both in the presence and absence of lithium, but study of the time course of this release (Figure 1) indicated that the action of lithium was to accelerate the process greatly without significantly increasing the total amount of binder eventually released from cells. The type of binder released under these conditions by granulocytes was transcobalamin III (TC III), which elutes early with β-globulins from ion exchange columns together with the polypeptide binder (Scott et al., 1974). Although 47 mM sodium fluoride completely inhibited B_{12} binder release, even in the presence of lithium, 1 mM sodium fluoride had less effect, permitting a substantial amount of binder release on lithium stimulation. Sodium arsenate at a comparable concentration was equally effective, but other inhibitors such as KCN, sodium azide, 2,4-dinitrophenol, 2-deoxyglucose, and methotrexate were ineffective at 1 mM concentration in preventing lithium-stimulated B_{12} binder release from granulocytes in whole blood. Since our prior studies demonstrated a correlation between the total blood granulocyte pool and the serum UBBC (see Figure 2), suggesting that the B_{12} binders are released by granulocytes into extracellular compartments in vivo (Chikkappa et al., 1971), an anticipated effect of lithium would be to accelerate such release in vivo.

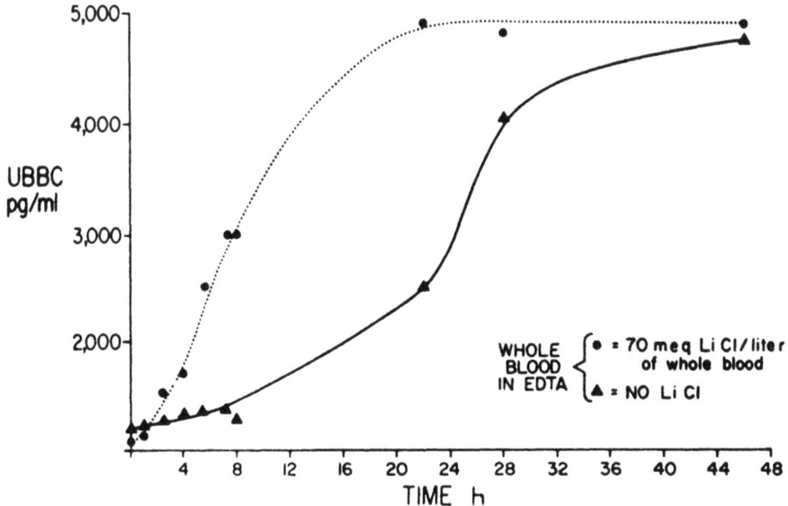

Figure 1. Effect of time on release of vitamin B_{12} binder from granulocytes at 22°C. The data show a comparison between tubes containing no additive compared with the tubes containing 70 meq lithium/L. (From Scott et al., 1974).

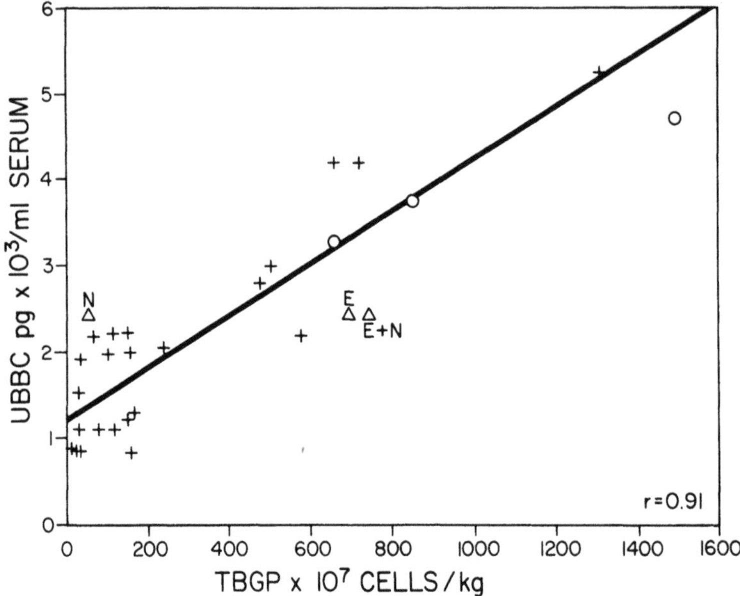

Figure 2. The correlation between total body granulocyte pool (TBGP) and serum UBBC. The points shown as N, E and E + N represent the neutrophil pool, eosinophil pool, and sum in a patient with eosinophilic leukemia. (From Chikkappa et al., 1971).

Although lithium-induced release of B_{12} binding protein can be detected in all subjects, release of folate binder is only detectable at present in 15 - 30% of subjects, usually being present in those who have relatively high serum folate binders; in these subjects, lithium produced striking enhancement of folate binder release with characteristics very similar to those described above for vitamin B_{12} binder (Colman and Herbert, 1974a). In some subjects receiving lithium therapy for neutropenia an elevation in circulating plasma folate binding protein was observed (Colman and Herbert, 1974a). The study of folate binding protein released from granulocytes in the presence of lithium was important in identifying differences between granulocyte binder and total plasma binder in pH optimum for binding and relative affinity for different folate analogues (Colman and Herbert, 1974b). These differences were subsequently borne out by our demonstration that serum folate binders elute as two peaks from ion exchange columns, whereas granulocyte folate binder elutes as a single peak (Colman and Herbert, 1979a).

In recent studies, we have used the calcium ionophore A23187 as a new tool to study the phemenoma previously investigated using lithium. Simon et al. (1978) had found that this ionophore was relatively specific in causing the release of vitamin B_{12} binder, a specific granule marker, from isolated granulocytes incubated at 37° for 30 minutes, whereas less than 10% of the cell content of an azurophilic marker, β-glucuronidase, was released under the same conditions. Using the same system as Simon et al. (1978), we have observed that folate binder release under the influence of the calcium ionophore A23187 correlated very closely with that of the vitamin B_{12} binder used as a marker for specific granules. The parallelism included similar optimal concentrations of A23187 and calcium chloride for release, similar temperature dependence, similar virtual complete inhibition of release by deoxyglucose, and similar time of peak release. In these studies, we found that the optimal effect of lithium could occur within 30 minutes when isolated cells were incubated at 37°C (Colman and Herbert, 1979b). Thus, the granulocyte binders for folate and vitamin B_{12} released under the influence of lithium are extremely similar in homogeneity, elution pattern from ion exchange columns, in the manner in which lithium effects their release, and in being ineffective in delivery of bound vitamin to bone marrow and other dividing cells (see Figure 3 and Table II). It is of interest that A23187 which has little effect without Ca^{++}, increased the lithium-stimulated release by ten percent in the absence of Ca^{++}, suggesting that it may directly enhance the lithium effect.

There is considerable indirect information that the effects of lithium upon granulocyte binders might be mediated via cyclic AMP metabolism. Gelfand et al. (1979) have again drawn attention to the fact that lithium may impair cyclic AMP production by interfering with the activation of adenylate cyclase, and the reverse effects of fluoride could similarly be associated with its stimulation of this enzyme (Robison et al., 1971). For these reason, we studied the effect of cyclic AMP and a number of substances known to elevate cellular cyclic AMP levels, such as dibutyryl cyclic AMP, and were unable to inhibit the enhancement of B_{12} binder released by these cells (Stebbins and Herbert, 1974). In recent preliminary studies geared to parallel those reported for vitamin B_{12} binder, folate binder release from granulocytes was similarly unaffected by 0.1 mM concentrations of cyclic AMP, dibutyryl cyclic AMP and isoproteronol (Table III). We have thus been unable to demonstrate that cyclic AMP mediates the lithium stimulated release of vitamin binding proteins from granulocytes in the manner which Gelfand et al. (1979) found it to mediate certain lithium effects in lymphocytes.

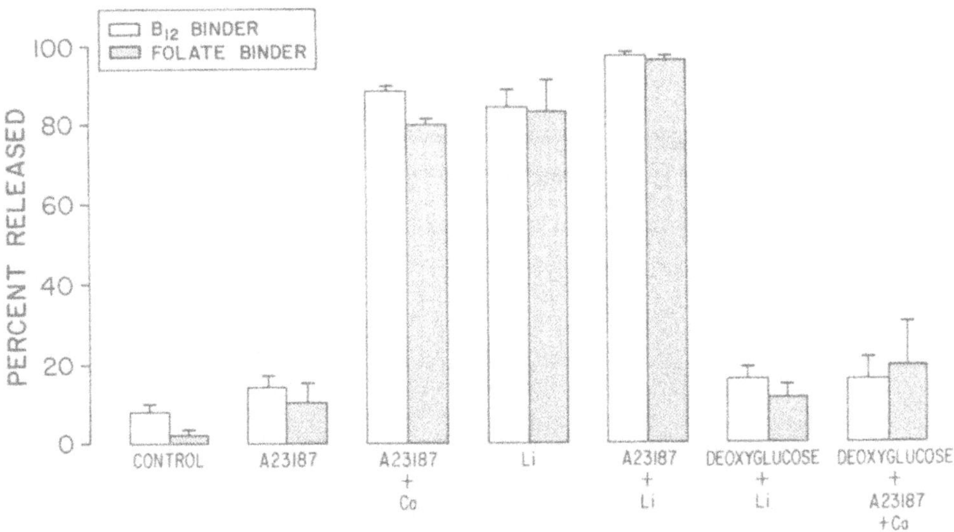

Figure 3. Percentage of total granulocyte folate and B_{12}-binder release in the presence of lithium and A23187, alone and in combination, and in the presence of 2'-deoxyglucose. (From Colman and Herbert, 1979b).

TABLE II

EFFECT OF FLUORIDE AND LITHIUM ON GRANULOCYTE RELEASE OF TRANSCOBALAMINS (TC) AND FOLATE BINDER (F.B.).

	time (hrs)	TC I	TC II	TC III	F.B.
EDTA, $0^{o}C$*		61	1308	93	148
EDTA	0	62	1274	248	210
	24	52	1233	424	249
EDTA + NaF	0	53	1124	64	126
	24	53	1237	73	121
EDTA + LiCl	0	59	1262	85	132
	24	94	1309	2888	749
EDTA + NaF + LiCl	0	38	915	39	103
	24	44	1155	348	111

*All samples incubated at room temperature unless otherwise stated.

Concentrations were 1.5 mg/ml EDTA, 2 mg/ml NaF and 2.14 mg/ml LiCl.

TABLE III

VITAMIN BINDER RELEASE FROM GRANULOCYTE SUSPENSION DURING THE 24 HOURS AFTER ADDITION OF AGENTS AFFECTING CYCLIC AMP LEVELS

	UBBC		UFBC	
	No Li	50 mg/l Li	No Li	50 mg/l Li
Control	1008	4408	84	392
Cyclic AMP (10^{-4}M)	947	3904	86	305
Dibutyryl cyclic AMP (10^{-4}M)	981	4654	93	227
Isoproteronol (10^{-4}M)	978	4269	76	249
NaF (47 mM)	793	756	70	86

UBBC: Unsaturated B_{12} Binding Capacity

UFBC: Unsaturated Folate Binding Capacity

It is unclear why the specific granules of granulocytes contain proteins which bind the two vitamins most intimately involved in DNA synthesis and render these metabolically unavailable for hematopoiesis and, presumably, for other forms of cell division. One apparent possibility is that they may interfere with the proliferation of organisms, i.e., they may be bacteriostatic when they are released by activated granulocytes (Gilbert, 1974; Ford et al., 1974). Since lithium stimulates colony formation, it is appropriate to mention that the specific granule constituents released by lithium include not only an inhibitor of the production and release of colony-stimulating activity, namely lactoferrin (Broxmeyer et al., 1978), but also the vitamin B_{12} binder which seemed to correlate with urinary colony-stimulating factor (Gibson et al., 1974), which Toohey (1976) showed to be separable in the mouse from colony-stimulating factor. In the same year, Dr. Richard Shadduck of Montefiore Hospital in Pittsburgh and we found almost no vitamin B_{12} binding protein in 20 ml of serum-free mouse L-cell conditioned media CMRL 1066, which bound only 5.9 pg radioactive B_{12} per ml, but had CSF activity of approximately 100 colonies/0.1 ml. Human CSF and inhibitors therefore need to be studied for crucial nutrient-binding proteins. Since all three of the binders of hematinics (lactoferrin, TC III, and folate binder) appear to derive from the same specific (secondary) granule, it is probable that their release is generally triggered together and that they all serve to modulate similar physiologic events in the regulation of cellular proliferation.

ACKNOWLEDGEMENT

This work was supported by the Veterans Administration and by USPHS Grant AM20526 from the National Institutes of Health.

REFERENCES

Baggiolini, M., deDuve, C., Masson, P.L., and Heremans, J.F., 1970, Association of lactoferrin with specific granules in rabbit heterophil leukocytes, J. Exp. Med. 131:559.

Bille, M. and Plum, C.M., 1955, Komplikationer ved lithium-behandling, Ugeskrift for Laeger 117:293.

Bloomfield, J., Scott, J., Herbert, V., and Stebbins, R., 1973, Human serum unsaturated B12-binding capacity (UBBC) increases with increasing length of in vitro presence of granulocytes and certain anticoagulants especially those containing lithium, Fed. Proc. 32:892A.

Boggs, D.R. and Winkelstein, A., 1975, "White Cell Manual", 3rd Edition, F.A. Davis Company, Philadelphia.

Broxmeyer, H.E., Smithyman, A., Eger, R.R., Myers, P.A., and de Sousa, M., 1978, Identification of lactoferrin as the granulocyte-derived inhibitor of colony-stimulating activity production, J. Exp. Med. 148:1052.

Buckley, R.M., Ventura, E.S., and MacGregor, R.R., 1978, Propranolol antagonizes the anti-inflammatory effect of alcohol and improves survival of infected intoxicated rabbits, J. Clin. Invest. 62(3):554.

Chikkappa, G., Corcino, J., Greenberg, M., and Herbert, V., 1969, Correlation of total blood leukocyte pools with B12 binding proteins, Blood 34:828.

Chikkappa, G., Corcino, J., Greenberg, M., and Herbert, V., 1971, Correlation between various blood white cell pools and the serum B12-binding capacities, Blood 37:142.

Colman, N. and Herbert, V., 1974a, Release of folate-binding protein (FBP) from granulocytes: Enhancement by lithium and elimination by fluoride; studies with normal, pregnant, chirrhotic, and uremic persons, Proc. 17th Ann. Mtg., Am. Soc. Hemat., Atlanta, Georgia, December 7-10.

Colman, N. and Herbert, V., 1974b, Evidence for "granulocyte-related" and "liver-related" folate binders in human serum and renal glomerular filtration of folate binder, Clin. Res. 22:700A.

Colman, N. and Herbert, V., 1979a, Kinetic and chromatographic evidence for heterogeneity of high affinity folate binding proteins in serum, in: "Chemistry and Biology of Pteridines," (R. Kisliuk and G. Brown, eds.) p. 525, Elsevier/North Holland, New York.

Colman, N. and Herbert, V., 1979b, Studies using the calcium ionophore A23187 suggest localization of the human granulocyte folate binder in specific (secondary) granules, Clin. Res. 27:291A.

Corcino, J., Krauss, S., Waxman, S., and Herbert, V., 1970, Release of vitamin B12-binding protein by human leukocytes in vitro, J. Clin. Invest. 49:2250.

Cutler, S.J. and Young, J.L., Jr., eds., 1975, Third National Cancer Survey: Incidence Data, DHEW Publication No. (NIH) 75-787, National Cancer Institute Monograph 41.

Dawson, E.B., Moore, T.D., and McGanity, W.J., 1970, The mathematical relationship of drinking water lithium and rainfall to mental hospital admission, Dis. Nerv. Syst. 21:811.

Durfor, C.N. and Becker, E., 1964, Public water supplies of the hundred largest cities in the United States, 1962, in: "Geological Survey Water Supply Paper 1812," U.S. Government Printing Office.

Ford, J.E., 1974, Some observations on the possible nutritional significance of vitamin B12- and folate-binding proteins in milk, Brit. J. Nutr. 31:243.

Frenkel, E.P., 1975, Cancer in the Dallas - Fort Worth Metropolitan Area, in: "The Third National Cancer Survey Advanced Three Year Report (1969 - 1971 Incidence)," DHEW Publcation No. (NIH) 75-641.

Frenkel, E.P. and Herbert, V., 1974, Frequency of granulocytic leukemia in populations drinking high vs low lithium water, Clin. Res. 22:390A.

Gelfand, E.W., Dosch, H.-M., Hastings, D., and Shore, A., 1979, Lithium: A modulator of cyclic AMP-dependent events in lymphocytes, Science 203:365.

Gibson, E.L., Herbert, V., and Robinson, W.A., 1974, Granulocyte colony stimulating activity and vitamin B12 binding proteins in human urine, Brit. J. Haemat. 28:193.

Gilbert, H.S., 1974, Proposal of a possible function for granulocyte vitamin B12 binding proteins in host defense against bacteria, Blood 44:926.

Hammond, W.P. and Dale, D.C., 1979, Canine cyclic hematopoiesis (CH): Treatment with lithium, Clin. Res. 27:461A.

Herbert, V., Bloomfield, J., Stebbins, R., and Scott, J., 1973, Use of fluoride to prevent erroneously high measurements of human serum unsaturated B12-binding capacity (UBBC); evidence that granulocyte-derived binders (Transcobalamin I and III) (TC I and III) are a smaller component of normal circulating UBBC than previously believed, J. Clin. Invest. 52:39a.

Jacob, E. and Herbert, V., 1974, Lithium therapy for neutropenias, J. Clin. Invest. 53:359.

Jim, R.T.S., 1979, Letter to the Editor, Blood 53:1031.

Kane, S.P. and Peters, T.J., 1975, Analytical subcellular fractionation of human granulocytes with reference to the localization of vitamin B12 binding protein, Clin. Sci. Molec. Med. 49:171.

Kurnick, J.E. and Robinson, W.A., 1971, Colony growth of human peripheral white blood cells in vitro, Blood 37:136.

Perez, H.D., Kaplan, H., Shenkman, L., Borkowsky, W., and Goldstein, I., 1979, Reversal of an abnormality of polymophonuclear leukocyte chemotaxis with lithium, Clin. Res. 27:353A.

Platman, S.R. and Fieve, R.R., 1968, Lithium carbonate and plasma cortisol response in the affective disorders, Arch. Gen. Psychiat. 18:591.

Robison, G.A., Butcher, R.W., and Sutherland, E.W., 1971, "Cyclic AMP," Academic Press, New York.

Scott, J.M., Bloomfield, F.J., Stebbins, R., and Herbert, V., 1974, Studies of derivation of transcobalamin III from granulocytes. Enhancement by lithium and elimination by fluoride of in vitro increments in vitamin B12-binding capacity, J. Clin. Invest. 53:228.

Shopsin, V., Friedmann, R., and Gershon, S., 1971, Lithium and leukocytosis, Clin. Pharmacol. Therap. 12:293.

Simon, J.D., Houck, W.D., and Albala, M.M., 1978, The effect of the calcium ionophore A23187 on the release of azurophilic and specific granule constituents of human granulocytes, Fed. Proc. 37:233.

Spitznagel, J.K., Dalldorf, F.G., Leffell, M.S., Folds, J.D., Welsh, I.R., Cooney, M.H., and Martin, I.E., 1974, Character of azurophil and specific granules purified from human polymophonuclear leukocytes, Lab. Invest. 30:774.

Stebbins, R. and Herbert, V., 1974, Studies of cyclic AMP effect on release of unsaturated vitamin B12 binding capacity from human blood cells, Proc. Soc. Exp. Biol. Med. 145:734.

Tisman, G., 1974, Lithium carbonate protection against drug-induced leukopenia in lymphosarcoma patients, IRCS 2:1509.

Tisman, G., Herbert, V., and Rosenblatt, S., 1972, Stimulation of granulocyte proliferation by lithium, Proc. 15th Ann. Mtg., Am. Soc. Hemat., Hollywood, Florida, December 3 - 6, 1972.

Tisman, G., Herbert, V., and Rosenblatt, S., 1973, Evidence that lithium induces human granulocyte proliferation: Elevated serum B12 binding capacity in vivo and granulocyte colony proliferation in vitro, Brit. J. Haemat. 24:767.

Toohey, J.L., 1976, Letter to the Editor, Blood 47:166.

Tosato, G., Whang-Peng, J., Levine, A.S., and Poplack, D.G., 1978, Acute lymphoblastic leukemia followed by chronic myelogenous leukemia, Blood 52:1033.

Trieff, N.M., Frey, S.M., Rao, M.S., Bunce, H., III, and Herman, B., 1973, Analysis for lithium in Texas drinking waters, Texas Rpts. Biol. Med. 31:55.

U.S. Bureau of Census, 1970, "Census of Population: 1970, General Population Characteristics, Final Report PC(1)-B1:U.S. Summary," U.S. Government Printing Office.

Voors, A.W., 1972, Drinking water lithium and mental hospital admission in North Carolina, N. Car. Med. J. 33:597.

THE EFFECT OF LITHIUM ON RELEASE OF GRANULOCYTE COLONY STIMULATING ACTIVITY *IN VITRO*

Robert A. Joyce and Paul A. Chervenick

University of Pittsburgh School of Medicine
Pittsburgh, Pennsylvania 15261

Blood neutrophil concentration increases when lithium carbonate (Li) is given to hematologically normal subjects (O'Connell, 1970; Shopsin and Friedman, 1971). Recent reports (Hammond and Dale, 1979) have suggested that Li may increase blood neutrophils in gray collie dogs with cyclic hematopoiesis and may attenuate the neutropenia induced by cytotoxic chemotherapy (Stein *et al.*, 1977; Fehir and Rossof, 1977; Lyman *et al.*, 1978; Joyce and Chervenick, 1979). Following reports (Tisman *et al.*, 1973) that lithium enhances granulocyte production *in vitro* and increases release of colony stimulating activity (CSA) (Joyce and Chervenick, 1975a), Rothstein *et al.*, (1978) demonstrated increased granulocyte production and expanded blood granulocyte pools in psychiatric patients receiving Li. Malloy *et al.*, (1978) studied normal subjects given Li and found increased marrow neutrophils and neutrophil progenitor cells and increased levels of urinary CSA. Increased levels of urine CSA have been reported in patients with Felty's syndrome given Li (Gupta *et al.*, 1976) and addition of Li to media conditioned by murine lung tissue has been demonstrated to enhance release of CSA (Harker *et al.*, 1977). Blood monocytes and mitogen stimulated lymphocytes are major sources of CSA in man (Chervenick and LoBuglio, 1972; Cline and Golde, 1974). The increased release of CSA from leukocytes in the presence of Li forms the basis of this report.

METHODS

Blood was collected from normal donors and separated into leukocyte fractions. Mixed leukocytes were collected after sedimentation of whole blood for one hour at room temperature. Mononuclear cells were separated by Ficoll-Hypaque density centrifugation. Monocytes were isolated by attachment of mononuclear cells, 4×10^6/ml, for 2 hours in 35 by 10mm plastic tissue culture dishes followed by removal of nonadherent lymphocytes. Nonadherent lymphocytes were separated by incubating mononuclear cells in plastic tissue culture dishes for 30 minutes. Nonadherent cells were removed, incubated an additional 90 minutes in fresh culture dishes and collected. Mitogen stimulation of lymphocytes was achieved by adding PHA (Wellcome Laboratories), 1 μg/ml, to samples of nonadherent lymphocytes.

Conditioned media (CM) were prepared from the isolated leukocytes as described previously (Joyce and Chervenick, 1975). Except for monocytes, cells were suspended in McCoy's tissue culture medium containing 15% fetal calf serum with and without Li in combination with 10^6 cells/ml and were incubated at 37°C in 7.5% CO_2. CM from monocytes were prepared by overlaying the attached cells with one ml culture medium with and without Li. After 7 days incubation, media were collected, filtered and stored frozen until tested for CSA.

Feeder layers were prepared by the method described by Pike and Robinson (1970). Feeder layers of monocytes were prepared by overlaying the attached monocyte monolayer with one ml of 0.5% agar in McCoy's culture medium with and without Li. The remaining fractions of separated cells were suspended in agar with and without Li and were plated in tissue culture dishes. Lithium carbonate (Sigma Chemical Company, St. Louis, MO) was dissolved in distilled water and buffered to pH 7.4 for use in these studies.

CM were tested for CSA by their ability to stimulate colony formation from mouse marrow cells. To 0.9 ml marrow cells suspended in methylcellulose, fetal calf serum and culture media, 0.1 ml of the CM was added and the marrow cell mixture was incubated at 37°C in 7.5% CO_2 for

7 days. Feeder layers were tested for CSA by overlaying one ml of mouse or human nonadherent marrow cell mixture and incubating for 7 or 14 days respectively. The number of colonies containing more than 50 cells was then recorded and used as a measure of CSA.

RESULTS

The increase in CSA with addition of Li to media conditioned by blood mononuclear cells collected from 2 normal donors is seen in Table I. A significant incrase in colony formation from mouse marrow cells was observed with media conditioned by mononuclear cells with Li, 1 meq/L, compared with colony formation using CM from mononuclear cells without Li ($p < 0.05$). There was no further increase in levels of CSA with higher concentrations of Li and increase in CSA was detected with concentrations of Li less than 1 meq/L. Colony formation was not observed when Li was added to marrow cell cultures without CM. The media were also dialyzed prior to use to remove Li and no change in levels of CSA was noted.

Levels of CSA in media conditioned by isolated blood leukocytes are seen in Figure 1. There was a significant increment in CSA in media conditioned by monocytes with Li, 35 ± 2 colonies/10^5 marrow cells compared with 24 ± 3 colonies without Li ($p < 0.05$). There was no increase in CSA with addition of Li to media containing granulocytes or nonadherent unstimulated lymphocytes. PHA stimulated lymphocytes without Li released low levels of CSA (9 ± 1 colonies/10^5 marrow cells). However, CSA was significantly increased when Li was added to lymphocytes (22 ± 4 colonies, $p < 0.01$). Studies with lymphocytes were done at concentrations of 10^6 cells/ml to minimize the contribution of CSA by small numbers of contaminating monocytes. Similar changes in colony formation were detected with addition of Li to feeder layers prepared from isolated fractions of blood leukocytes.

To determine the effect of Li on the ability of blood leukocytes to stimulate human marrow colony formation, feeder layers of leukocytes collected from normal donors were prepared with and without Li. The

TABLE I

LITHIUM EFFECT ON CSA RELEASE

Sources of Conditioned Media[a]	Lithium meq/L	Colonies/10^5 mouse marrow cells[b]
Mononuclear cells	----	47 ± 4
Mononuclear cells	0.5	42 ± 5
Mononuclear cells	1.0	69 ± 4
Mononuclear cells	5.0	76 ± 4
L-cell	----	85 ± 5
L-cell	0.1[c]	90 ± 3
----	----	0
----	0.1[c]	0

[a] Concentration of human mononuclear cells to condition media was 10^6/ml.

[b] Number stimulated by 0.1 ml conditioned media in 2 separate studies plated in triplicate and expressed as mean ± standard error.

[c] Concentration of lithium carbonate added to marrow cell culture.

effect on colony formation from nonadherent human marrow cells is seen in Table II. No colony formation was observed from unstimulated marrow. There was significantly greater colony formation using feeder layers containing 0.5 x 10^5 leukocytes and Li 2 meq/L compared with feeder layers without Li ($p < 0.05$). The number of colonies observed with lithium was similar to values using twice the concentration of feeder leukocytes. Enhanced colony formation was not observed with lower concentrations of Li and there was no significant increase with higher concentrations.

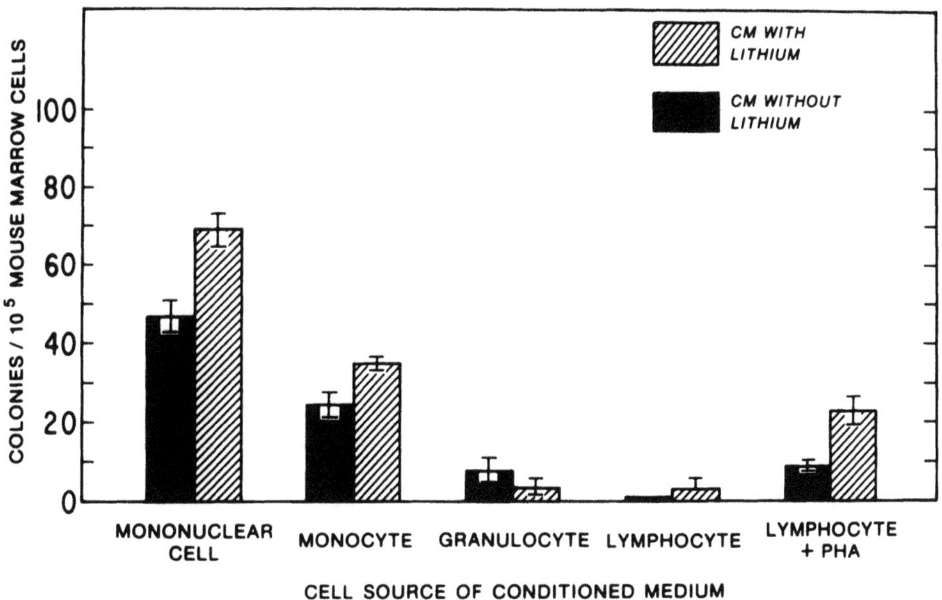

Figure 1. Levels of colony stimulating activity in conditioned media prepared from separated human blood leukocytes and expressed as mean ± standard error of the number of colonies/10^5 mouse marrow cells with addition of 10% conditioned media.

A similar increase in colony formation from human marrow was noted when Li was added to isolated mononuclear cells, monocytes or PHA sitmulated lymphocytes. There was no colony formation from human marrow cells with feeder layers containing unstimulated lymphocytes with or without Li.

TABLE II

LITHIUM EFFECT ON HUMAN MARROW COLONY FORMATION

Leukocytes per feeder layer[a]	Li (meq/L)	Colonies/10^5 human marrow cells[c]
0.5×10^6	----	43 ± 6
0.5×10^6	0.5[b]	39 ± 3
0.5×10^6	1.0	39 ± 4
0.5×10^6	2.0	60 ± 3
0.5×10^6	5.0	47 ± 3
1.0×10^6	----	67 ± 6
-----	----	0

[a] Leukocytes for feeder layers collected from 2 normal donors.

[b] Concentrations of lithium carbonate added to feeder layers.

[c] Data represent mean ± SE of values from nonadherent marrow cells from 3 normal controls.

DISCUSSION

The results of these studies indicate that Li increases release of CSA from human blood leukocytes. This response is limited to isolated cell fractions containing monocytes or PHA stimulated lymphocytes. Li added to human leukocytes enhances CSA stimulation of both murine and human marrow cell colony formation with a higher concentration of Li required for human marrow response.

REFERENCES

Chervenick, P.A. and LoBuglio, A.F., 1972, Human blood monocytes: stimulators of granulocyte and mononuclear colony formation in vitro, Sicence 178:164.

Cline, M.J. and Golde, D.W., 1974, Production of colony stimulating activity by human lymphocytes, Nature 248:703.

Fehir, K.M. and Rossof, A.H., 1977, Lithium carbonate protects canine granulopoiesis from damage by cyclophosphamide, Clin. Res. 26:434A.

Gupta, R.C., Robinson, W.A., and Kurnick, J.E., 1976, Felty's syndrome: Effect of lithium on granulopoiesis, Am. J. Med. 61:29.

Hammond, W.P. and Dale, D.C., 1979, Canine cyclic hematopoiesis: treatment with lithium, Clin. Res. 27:461A.

Harker, W.G., Rothstein, G., Clarkson, D., Athens, J.W., and MacFarlane, J.L., 1977, Enhancement of colony stimulating activity production by lithium, Blood 49:263.

Joyce, R.A. and Chervenick, P.A., 1975a, Effect of lithium on the release of colony stimulating activity from blood leukocytes, Proc. Am. Soc. Hematol. 18:126.

Joyce, R.A. and Chervenick, P.A., 1975b, Stimulation of granulopoiesis by liver macrophages, J. Lab. Clin. Med. 86:112.

Joyce, R.A. and Chervenick, P.A., 1979, Lithium effect on granulopoiesis following vinblastine, Clin. Res. 27:388A.

Lyman, G.H., Williams, C.C., and Preston, D., 1978, A prospective randomized study of the effect of lithium carbonate on the granulocytopenia and incidence of infection associated with intensive chemotherapy and radiation therapy for undifferentiated small cell bronchogenic carcinoma, Blood 52:228 (Supplement 1).

Malloy, E.L., Zauber, N.P., and Chervenick, P.A., 1978, The effect of lithium on blood and marrow neutrophils, Blood 52:228 (Supplement 1).

O'Connell, R.A., 1970, Leukocytosis during lithium carbonate treatment, Int. J. Pharmacopsychiatry 4:30.

Pike, B. and Robinson, W.A., 1970, Bone marrow colony growth in agar gel, J. Cell. Physiol. 76:77.

Rothstein, G., Clarkson, D.R., Larsen, W., Grosser, B.I., and Athens, J.W., 1978, Effect of lithium on neutrophil mass and production, N. Engl. J. Med. 298:178.

Shopsin, B. and Friedman, R., 1971, Lithium and leukocytosis, Clin. Pharmacol. Ther. 12:923.

Stein, R.S., Beaman, D., Ali, M.Y., Hansen, R., Jenkins, D.D., and Jume'an, H.G., 1977, Lithium carbonate attenuation of chemotherapy-induced neutropenia, N. Engl. J. Med. 297:430.

Tisman, G., Herbert, V., and Rosenblatt, S., 1973, Evidence that lithium induces human granulocyte proliferation: Elevated serum vitamin B12 binding capacity in vivo and granulocyte colony proliferation in vitro, Brit. J. Haemat. 24:767.

THE EFFECT OF LITHIUM UPON GRANULOCYTE PRODUCTION *IN VITRO* AND *IN VIVO* IN THE MOUSE

G. Rothstein, A.K. Oshita, W.G. Harker,
G. Lonngi, and R.D. Christensen

Howard Hughes Medical Institute Laboratories
Department of Medicine
University of Utah
Salt Lake City, Utah 84132

Following the institution of lithium therapy in the management of manic states, observers noted that leukocytosis and neutrophilia frequently occurred (Risetto and Gassano, 1952; Mayfield and Brown, 1966; O'Connell, 1970; Murphy and Goodwin, 1971; Shopsin and Friedman, 1971). In 1973, Tisman *et al.* postulated that the neutrophilia was due to an increase in the total blood granulocyte pool and also demonstrated augmentation of granulocyte proliferation *in vitro* (Tisman *et al.*, 1973). In 1975, it was demonstrated that lithium enhanced colony stimulating activity (CSA) production in mice (Harker *et al.*, 1975), and humans (Joyce and Chervenick, 1975), suggesting that this CSA alteration had a mechanistic role *in vivo*. In the present study, we have examined the action of lithium upon murine granulocytopoiesis *in vivo* and *in vitro* in order to: 1) further define the action of lithium upon CSA production by lung, adherent peritoneal cells, and marrow; 2) to examine the direct effect of lithium upon the proliferation of colony forming cells (CFC) or their progeny; and 3) to test the hypothesis that lithium stimulation of CSA production is due to modulation of cellular cyclic AMP (cAMP) levels.

MATERIALS AND METHODS

Adult male CBA or DBA/2 mice were used in all experiments. Bone marrow was obtained by flushing the hind-limb bones with McCoy's 5A medium (M5A) with 15% fetal calf serum (FCS). Clumps of cells were eliminated by aspirating repeatedly through a 25-gauge needle. The cell concentrations of the marrow suspensions were measured electronically using a Coulter Counter (Coulter Electronics, Hialeah, Fla.) and the means of triplicate counts were determined. The cell concentrations were adjusted with M5A and 50,000 marrow cells were then cultured in individual 35-mm plastic dishes in a manner similar to that previously described (Pluznik and Sachs, 1965; Bradley and Metcalf, 1966; Iscove, 1972). After incubation at 37°C, 7% CO_2 in a high humidity incubator, the colonies (greater than 50 cells) were scored with the aid of a stereomicroscope. LiCl was dissolved in distilled water in appropriate concentrations for use in cultures. With the lithium concentrations employed, the pH of M5A was not altered. Serum rich in CSA was generated by injecting mice with 25 µg of Salmonella endotoxin and collecting the serum 3 hours later. The post endotoxin serum (PES) was pooled and stored at -80°C until used. When PES was added to cultures, the appropriate volume of PES to yield a final desired concentration throughout the culture was added to the lower layer before the upper layer was poured. For example, the addition of 0.1 ml PES to the lower layer of culture whose final volume was 2 ml resulted in a culture containing 5% PES.

CSA produced by mouse lungs was obtained by the metod of Sheridan and Metcalf (1974). For each 40 mg of lung, 1 ml of serum-free M5A was used. Lung conditioned medium (LCM) was collected after 48 hours of incubation and was heated to 56°C for 30 minutes before it was centrifuged at 12,000 g for 15 minutes at 4°C. Then the LCM was dialyzed against distilled water containing 200,000 units/liter penicillin and 200 mg/liter streptomycin. The dialyzed LCM was centrifuged at 4°C for 15 minutes at 12,000 g. Finally, LCM was assayed for CSA by adding 0.1 ml aliquots to the underlayers of marrow cultures which did not contain lithium. Peritoneal cells were collected by lavage with M5A, allowed to adhere to plastic dishes for two hours and the non-adherent cells washed away. Then, the cells were incubated in M5A with 15% FCS for 5 days. Conditioned medium was then prepared for use as described above. Concentrated solutions of cyclic nucleotides or other culture additives were prepared in distilled water prior to their use.

The vena caval blood neutrophils were quantified by triplicate electronic counting and differential counting of Wright's stained smears. Femoral marrow was flushed from the femurs, counted electronically and 1000 cell differential counts performed to determine the absolute cell numbers/femur. The morphologic criteria of Chervenick and Boggs (1973) were employed.

RESULTS

The Effect of Lithium Upon Proliferative Granulocytes In Vitro

The action of Li upon the granulocyte colony forming cell (CFC) or its mitosis-capable progeny was examined by adding LiCl to cultures containing approximately 50,000 mouse marrow cells. In the absence of added CSA or CSA producing tissue, 0.5-3.0 mM Li did not stimulate colony or cluster formation in any of 20 individual cultures. The effect of 1 or 3 mM Li in cultures containing submaximal concentrations of CSA (post endotoxin serum) was also investigated. In other experiments, 1 or 3 mM Li was included in methylcellulose cultures with added PES. Six-7 days later, the cultures were scored for colony formation, after which the contents of the plates were removed, employing a teflon policeman, and diluted for cell counting in a hemocytometer chamber. The results, shown in Figure 1, reveal that Li did not significantly alter colony formation, but it did inhibit the net production of cells. Similar results were noted with PES concentrations of 1,3,5, and 10%.

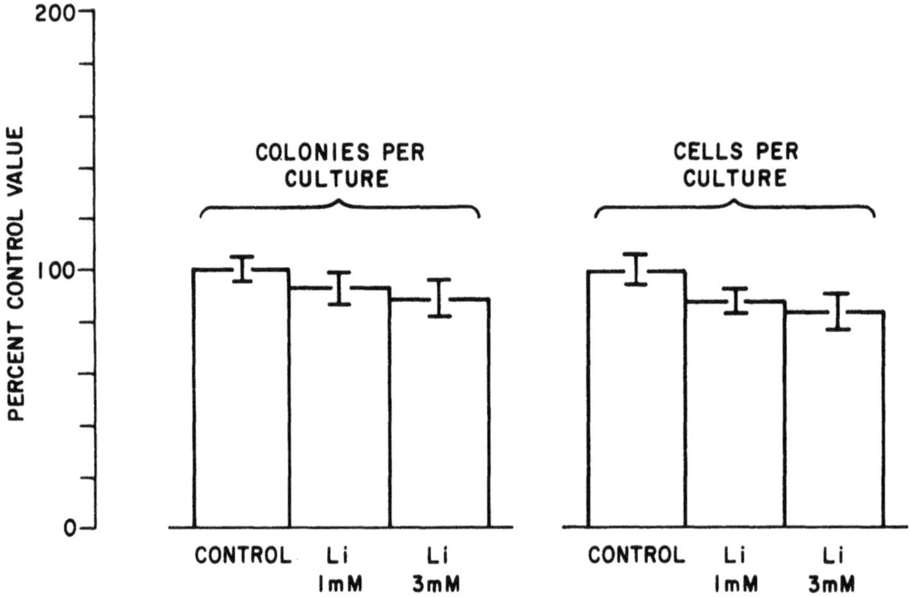

Figure 1. The effect of lithium upon semisolid cultures containing preformed CSA. Each bar represents the mean value for groups of 12 cultures. The brackets delineate the standard error. The values for cell number in cultures containing 1 and 3 mM Li were significantly lower than the controls ($p < 0.025$ and $p < 0.05$ respectively).

The Effect of Lithium Upon CSA Production

Marrow, adherent peritoneal cells, and mouse lung were studied. When 1-3 mM LiCl was added to cultures of $1\text{-}5 \times 10^6$ marrow cells, no CSA could be detected in the medium after a 5 day incubation period. Similarly, 1-3 mM Li, failed to induce colony formation in semisolid cultures of 50,000-300,000 marrow cells over a 7 - 10 day period. Thus, no evidence of CSA production by mouse marrow was noted. When cultures of marrow were supplied with mouse lung feeder layers, colony formation increased from a mean of 24 ± 2 (SD) colonies in controls to 51 ± 6 in cultures with 3 mM Li ($p < 0.005$). The addition of Li to incubation mixtures with 40 mg of lung/ml similarly increased CSA production, as was the case in incubates containing 1 x 10^6 adherent peritoneal cells/ml (Figure 1).

The Effect of Cyclic Nucleotide Altering Agents Upon CSA Production

Because Li can antagonize cyclic AMP (cAMP) mediated cell processes (Lee et al., 1971; Singer and Rotenberg, 1973), we explored the possibility that alteration in cellular cAMP might modulate CSA production. Two maneuvers were employed: 1) the addition of dibutyryl cAMP (db cAMP) to elevate cellular cAMP; and 2) the addition of cGMP or addition of its agonist carbamylcholine, to increase the cGMP concentration. Agents were included in the lung or peritoneal cell incubates, and following the incubation period, dialysis was employed to remove residual additives. The results of groups of 6-15 replicates are shown in Table I.

TABLE I

CSA (% CONTROL VALUE FOR VARIOUS ADDITIVES)

Tissue Source	No additive	db cAMP 10^{-6}M	Li 3 mM	Carbamylcholine 10^{-8}M
Lung	100 ± 8	63 ± 16*	164 ± 19**	174 ± 23**
Peritoneal cells	100 ± 5	75 ± 6^+	157 ± 14**	146 ± 11^+

Table I. The effect of cyclic nucleotide altering maneuvers upon CSA production. The means and standard errors for groups of 6-15 values are shown.

+ $p < 0.05$

* $p < 0.025$

** $p < 0.01$

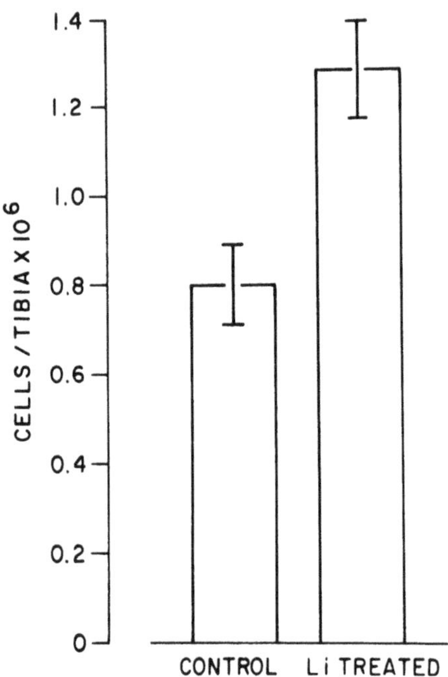

Figure 2. The effect of lithium treatment upon marrow proliferative granulocytes. The bars represent the mean values for groups of five mice. The brackets indicate the standard deviation. The lithium treated group had significantly more granulocytes that its corresponding control ($p < 0.01$).

The Effect of Lithium Upon In Vivo Granulocyte Production

In order to compare the *in vivo* and *in vitro* effects of lithium, groups of mice were given 50-100 mg/kg of LiCl via gastric instillation once or twice daily. Dose alterations were carried out to maintain blood Li levels at 4.0 meq/liter 1 hour after instillation and 1.0 - 1.5 meq/liter before the next dose. Blood levels were monitored in a separate group of treated mice who were sacrificed at the time caval blood was sampled. Animals given the same volume of water via gastric tube served as controls. Eighteen days after the institution of Li treatment, groups of five animals were sacrificed and blood and marrow cellularity were quantified. The blood neutrophil concentration of the lithium treated group controls

(1170/μl) (mean) did not differ from the control group (1100/μl). However, the number of mature femoral marrow neutrophils (Figure 2) and proliferative granulocytes (Figure 3) were greater in the Li group than in the controls.

Five days after Li treatment was stopped, the proliferative and mature marrow granulocyte pools had returned to control levels. These data demonstrate that Li treatment of mice results in increased in vivo marrow granulocyte numbers similar to the effect of Li in vitro. However, blood neutrophilia was not observed.

DISCUSSION

The recognition that lithium could induce neutrophilia in human subjects (Risetto and Gassano, 1952; Mayfield and Brown, 1966; O'Connell, 1970; Murphy and Goodwin, 1971; Shopsin and Friedman, 1971; Tisman et al. 1973) has stimulated considerable interest in lithium as a neutropoietic agent. The studies of Gupta et al. (1976) first illustrated that lithium could augment the blood neutrophil concentration in subjects with the neutropenia of Felty's syndrome and the increase in urinary CSA which these authors found was consistent with previous observations that lithium increased the production of CSA in vitro in mice (Harker et al., 1977) and in human tissue (Joyce and Chervenick, 1975). Indeed, subsequent reports suggest that lithium can attenuate the hematotoxic effect of cancer chemotherapy (Stein et al., 1977). In addition, the report of Hammond and Dale (1979) indicates that lithium suppresses cyclic neutropenia in collie dogs. These observations provide evidence in favor of the usefulness of lithium as a therapeutic agent in the stimulation of granulocyte production. In addition, the reports of Joyce and Chervenick (1979) and Fehir and Rossof (1977) indicate the development of animal models with which in vivo effects can be further studied.

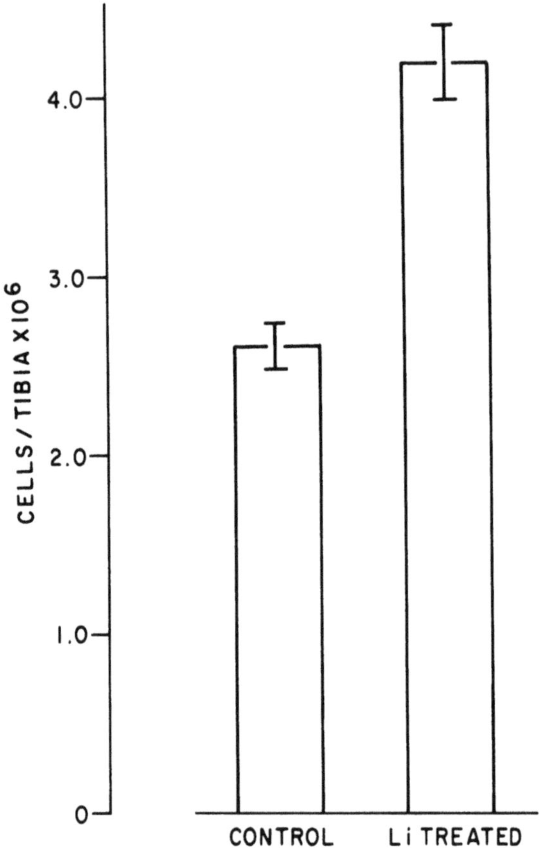

Figure 3. The effect of lithium treatment upon marrow mature granulocytes. The bars represent the mean values for groups of five mice. The brackets indicate the standard deviation. The lithium treated group had significantly more granulocytes than its corresponding control ($p < 0.05$).

Concomitant with in vivo observations, the effect of lithium in vitro has been under investigation. In the mouse, lithium did not directly stimulate CFC in agar cultues (Harker et al., 1977); thus, in mice, the granulocytopoietic effect appeared to be restricted to stimulation of CSA production. Further study revealed that the effect of lithium upon CSA production required the synthesis of new protein, as evidenced by the observation that the addition of puromycin to lung incubates ablated the production of CSA in cultures with added lithium (Harker et al., 1977).

In the present study, we extended our previous experiments in order to investigate the effect of lithium upon CSA production by lung, peritoneal cells, and marrow, as well as the possible interrelationship between lithium action and cellular cAMP. In addition, we studied the effect of lithium upon cell proliferation in methylcellulose cultures, a setting which allowed not only an assessment of colony formation, but by washout techniques, cell number as well. Finally, we explored the possibility that a granulocytopoietic effect of lithium in vivo might parallel the in vitro stimulation of granulocyte production. It was found that lithium did stimulate CSA production by lung and peritoneal cell preparations, but not by marrow, whether studied in conditioned medium experiments, or in semisolid cultures for autostimulatory effect. Even so, the administration of lithium to mice did result in increased marrow granulocyte numbers, a finding in keeping with previous studies demonstrating increased effective granulocyte production in humans (Rothstein et al., 1978). However, if CSA is the mediator of lithium effect in vivo in the mouse, the CSA responsible for the increased granulocyte numbers likely originates in sites other than the marrow.

Enhancement of CSA production by lithium is of particular interest because this phenomenon may provide information as to the mechanism by which CSA production is regulated. Lithium is known to modify a number of cAMP mediated cellular functions, presumably via its ability to inhibit the cAMP synthetic enzyme, adenylate cyclase (Lee et al., 1971). Thus we postulated that the action of lithium upon CSA producing cells might involve the same mechanism. When cells were incubated with lithium, CSA production was enhanced. Conversely, the addition of cAMP suppressed CSA production. In other studies, cGMP and the cGMP agonist carbamylcholine stimulated CSA production indicating another cyclic nucleotide alteration which enhances CSA production. Therefore, it appears that the production of CSA can be modulated by variations in cellular cyclic nucleotide levels, with cAMP antagonism, a property of lithium, being a stimulator. It is postulated that the anti-cAMP action of lithium may be responsible for its CSA production stimulation. The pattern of response to cyclic nucleotide altering maneuvers is itself of interest, because of its similarity to those involved in the secretory process of polymorphonuclear leukocytes (PMN). PMN have been shown to release lysosomal enzymes in response to cGMP, while enzyme release is inhibited by cAMP and its agonists (Zurier et al., 1974). Thus, the response of CSA production to cyclic nucleotide alteration resembles that of the PMN secretory process, suggesting that the mechanisms and controls of secretion in the CSA producing cell may be similar to those of the PMN. In the further study of the intracellular events which accompany CSA production, lithium may be a useful investigatory tool.

ACKNOWLEDGEMENTS

Dr. Rothstein is an Investigator, Howard Hughes Medical Institute and Dr. Christensen is a Research Associate, Howard Hughes Medical Institute.

REFERENCES

Bradley, T.R. and Metcalf, D. 1966, The growth of mouse bone marrow cells in vitro, Aust. J. Exp. Biol. Med. Sci. 44:287.

Chervenick, P.A., Boggs, D.R., Marsh, J.C., Cartwright, G.E. and Wintrobe, M.M., 1973, Quantitative studies of blood and bone marrow neutrophils in normal mice, Amer. Jour. Phys. 215:353.

Fehir, K.M. and Rossof, A.H., 1977, Lithium carbonate stimulation of marrow colony forming units and peripheral granulocytes in a canine model, Blood 50:145 (Supplement 1).

Gupta, R.C., Robinson, W.A. and Kurnick, J.E., 1976, Felty's syndrome: effect of lithium on granulopoiesis, Am. J. Med. 61:29.

Hammond, W.P. and Dale, D.C., 1979, Canine cyclic hematopoiesis: Treatment with lithium, Clin. Res. 27:461A.

Harker, G.W., Rothstein, G., Clarkson, D.W. and Athens, J.W., 1975, Stimulation of neutrophil production by lithium, Clin. Res. 23:103A.

Harker, W.G., Rothstein, G., Clarkson, J., Athens, J.W., and MacFarlane, J.L., 1977, Enhancement of colony-stimulating activity production by lithium, Blood 49:263.

Iscove, N.N., 1972, Technique for culture of human CFU-c, in "In vitro culture of hemopoietic cells," (Van Bekkum, D.W. and Dicke, K.A., eds.), Rijswijk Radiobiol. Inst. TNO.

Joyce, R.A. and Chervenick, P.A., 1975, Effect of lihtium on the release of colony-stimulating activity (CSA) from blood leukocytes, Proc. Amer. Soc. Hematol. 18:126.

Joyce, R.A. and Chervenick, P.A., 1979, Lithium effect on granulopoiesis following vinblastine, Clin. Res. 27:388A.

Lee, R.V., Jampol, L.M. and Brown, W.V., 1971, Nephrogenic diabetes insipidus and lithium intoxication - complications of lithium carbonate therapy, N. Engl. J. Med. 284:93.

Mayfield, D. and Brown, R.G., 1966, The clinical laboratory and electroencephalographic effects of lithium, J. Psychiatr. Res. 4:207.

Murphy, D.L. and Goodwin, F.K., 1971, Leukocytosis during lithium treatment, J. Psych. Res. 127:1559.

O'Connell, R.A., 1970, Leukocytosis during lithium carbonate treatment, Int. J. Pharmacopsychiatry 4:30.

Pluznik, D.H. and Sachs, L., 1965, The cloning of normal mast cells in tissue culture, J. Cell Comp. Physiol. 66:319.

Risetto, G. and Gassano, G., 1952, Variazioni del sanque perifico nella intossicazione sperimentale da sali di litio, Riv. Patol. Clin. Sper. 7:202.

Rothstein, G., Clarkson, D.R., Larsen, W., Grosser, B.I., and Athens, J.W., 1978, Effect of lithium on neutrophil mass and production, New Engl. J. Med. 298:178.

Sheridan, J.W. and Metcalf, D., 1974, CSF production and release following endotoxin, in "Hemopoiesis in Culture, 2nd International Workshop," (Robinson, W.A., ed.), Washington, D.C., NIH 74-205.

Shopsin, B. and Friedman, R., 1971, Lithium and leukocytosis, Clin. Pharmacol. Ther. 12:923.

Singer, I. and Rotenberg, D., 1973, Mechanisms of lithium action, New Eng. J. Med. 289:254.

Stein, R.S., Beaman, C., Ali, M.Y., Hansen, R., Jenkins, D.D. and Jum'ean, H.G., 1977, Lithium carbonate attenuation of chemotherapy-induced neutropenia, New Engl. J. Med. 297:430.

Tisman, G., Herbert, V., and Rosenblatt, S., 1973, Evidence that lithium induces human granulocyte proliferation: Elevated serum vitamin B12 binding capacity in vivo and granulocyte colony proliferation in vitro, Br. J. Haematol. 24:767.

Zurier, R.B., Weissmann, G., Hoffstein, S., Kammerman, S., and Tai, H.H., 1974, Mechanisms of lysosomal enzyme release from human leukocytes. II. Effects of cAMP and cGMP, autonomic agonists, and agents which affect microtubule function, J. Clin. Invest. 53:297.

EFFECT OF LITHIUM ON COLONY FORMATION AND PRODUCTION OF COLONY-STIMULATING FACTOR

Peter R. Galbraith

Department of Medicine
Queen's University
Kingston, Ontario K7L 2V6
Canada

Lithium is a unique and simple agent which has depressant effects on a wide variety of synthetic processes in different organs (Singer and Rotenberg, 1973), and yet has a stimulatory effect on granulopoiesis (Murphy et al., 1971; Tisman et al., 1973; Gupta et al., 1976). Its potential as a therapeutic agent in Felty's syndrome is now well known, and future uses remain to be clearly defined. Lithium has been reported to stimulate production of colony-stimulating factor (CSF), a putative regulator of granulopoiesis (Gupta et al., 1976; Harker et al., 1977). Lithium has also been reported to enhance the action of CSF (Morley and Galbraith, 1978).

In this study the action of lithium has been investigated in a human bone marrow culture system designed to minimize effects attributable to interacting cell populations (Haskill et al., 1972) and serum factors (Baker and Galbraith, 1978; Baker and Galbraith, 1979). Experience with this dynamic system has shown that the time at which cultures are evaluated influences the results because cell proliferation, maturation and death occur concommitantly, as in the mouse system (Metcalf, 1969). It was therefore necessary to re-assess the effect of lithium on growth of granulocytic colonies and the amount of CSF produced by mononuclear leukocytes (MNL), bearing these kinetic features in mind.

METHODS

Collection of Cells

Venous blood samples and bone marrow aspirates were collected from informed, healthy volunteers as described previously (Galbraith *et al.*, 1979). Citrate phosphate dextrose solution USP (Fenwal Laboratories, Division of Baxter Travenol Laboratories of Canada, Ltd., Malton, Ontario) was the anticoagulant, and 3% dextran was used to accelerate the sedimentation of erythrocytes. The nucleated cell-rich suspensions were washed three times in CMRL-1066 tissue culture medium (Grand Island Biological Company, Grand Island, New York), and then subjected to cell separations based on cell density in Ficoll^R (density 1.070 g/ml) (Pharmacia Fine Chemicals, Uppsala, Sweden) and adhesiveness to plastic (Galbraith *et al.*, 1979). The following fractions were collected:

(1) The non-adherent light density nucleated cell fraction of normal human bone marrow cells which served as the source of target colony-forming cells (CFC).

(2) The light density mononuclear leukocyte (MNL) fraction of normal blood leukocyte suspensions, which was used to make CSF.

Preparation of Cultures

The semi-solid agar culture system was used. Non-adherent light density bone marrow cells (10^5) were suspended in a 1 ml agar layer. This contained 0.3% agar in CMRL-1066 tissue culture medium, supplemented with 30% normal human serum previously inactivated by heating to 58^oC for 150 minutes (Galbraith *et al.*, 1979).

Preparation of CSF

Mononuclear leukocyte-conditioned medium was prepared by incubating 2×10^6 normal light density blood MNL/ml in CMRL-1066 tissue culture medium supplemented with 30% heat-inactivated human serum for 7 days at 37^oC (Galbraith *et al.*, 1979).

Experimental Design

Lithium chloride was added in concentrations of 0 - 4 mM/1 to semi-solid bone marrow cell cultures stimulated by CSF in order to determine the effects of lithium on CFC proliferation; and to liquid cultures of 2 x 10^6 blood MNL/ml in order to examine the effects of lithium on CSF production. CSF was assayed in separate cultures. Aggregates were counted at intervals (triplicate plates), and their size was determined by examining 100 consecutive aggregates under the high power objective (100X).

RESULTS

The culture is a dynamic system in which aggregates of granulocytic cells make their appearance as doublets on day 1. The number of aggregates increases to a maximum between the third and fourth day and thereafter declines. Throughout culture periods of up to 14 days the size of surviving aggregates increases. Disappearance of aggregates is not due to depletion of CSF or other nutritional factors since the system gives similar results when non-adherent light density marrow cells are seeded in culture over the range 0.25 to 4.0 x 10^5 cells per 1 ml culture. The following brief account of the kinetic features of the culture system is necessary in order to understand how lithium acts in it.

Effect of CSF Concentration on Number and Size of Aggregates

Figures 1 - 3 shows typical results obtained in a single experiment. In cultures evaluated 4 and 7 days from inception, all aggregates of 2 or more cells were counted. Their number was little influenced by CSF on the 4th day, but on the 7th day it was reduced in a dose-related fashion; their size was directly related to CSF and was greater on the 7th day. During the interval between the 4th and 7th day, the relative increase in the size of surviving aggregates was similar at all CSF concentrations (Figure 1).

As a result of these kinetic features, total cells per culture (calculated from the product of mean aggregate number and mean aggregate size) increased in proportion to CSF only in early cultures (Figure 2).

Comment: Traditional evaluation on the 7th day of the number of colonies, by whatever criterion used to define the clone, may not yield interpretable results because the number of colonies is, by then, declining (Figure 3). The decline is accelerated by increasing the level of stimulator, and conversely, may be retarded when inhibitor is added to the system (unpublished). Earlier evaluation of the cultures and/or an estimation of mean aggregate size may be more appropriate measurements because, even in declining cultures, the size of surviving aggregates is quantitatively related to the concentration of CSF. CSF dose response curves (Figure 1) may be employed to give semi-quantitative estimations of the effect of enhancing and inhibiting factors.

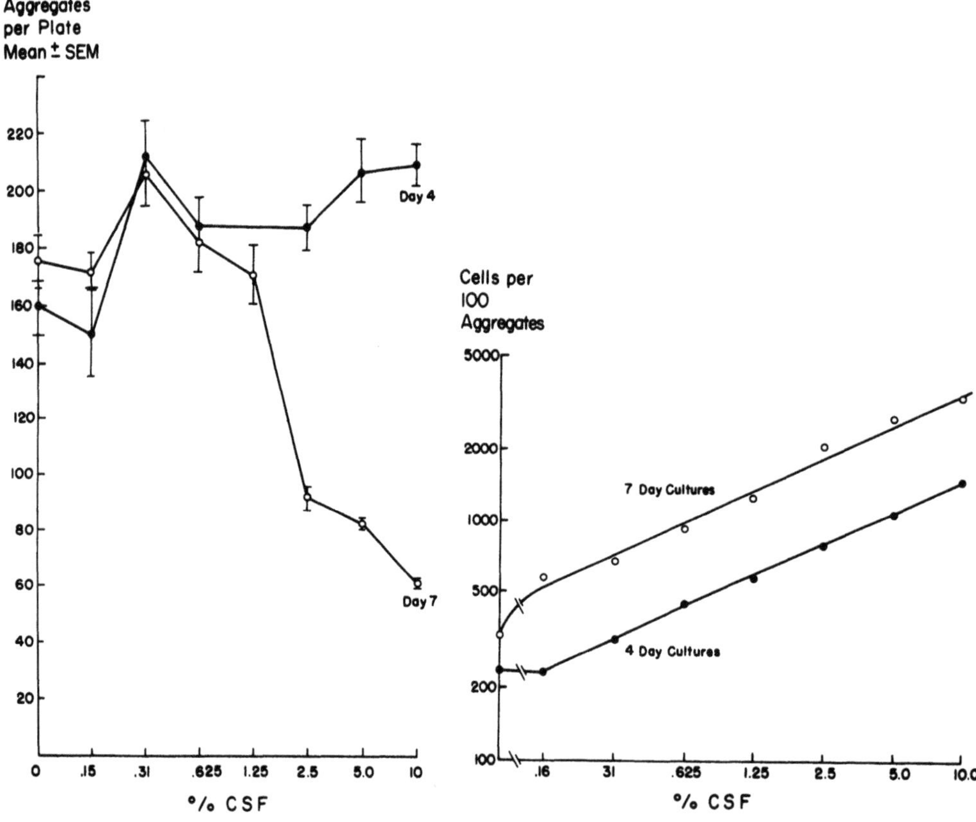

Figure 1. Effect of CSF concentration (MNL-conditioned medium) on the number of aggregates of 2 or more cells contained in 100 consecutive aggregates (right). Cultures were evaluated 4 and 7 days from inception.

Effects of Lithium

Preliminary experiments showed the effects of lithium were similar over a range of CSF concentrations (MNL-conditioned medium, 1.25 - 10%). Therefore a single concentration of CSF (5%) was used in the following experiment. Lithium (0 - 4 mM/l final concentration) was added to cultures evaluated over a 7 day period. The number and size of all aggregates of 4 or more cells were recorded. In cultures without lithium, aggregates appeared and peaked on the third day (Figure 4). In cultures with lithium, aggregates appeared one day earlier, and were initially larger than those in cultures without lithium (Figures 4 and 5). This was followed by earlier appearance (and disappearance) of aggregates composed of 20 or more cells (Figure 6). Although aggregates reached their maximum size at an earlier time, they did not exceed the size of those found in control cultures (Figure 5). Consequently, total cells per culture, relative to control, were greater in early cultures and less in later cultures (Figure 7). From the dose response curve relating aggregate size to CSF concentration, it was estimated that 1, 2 and 4 mM lithium had an effect comparable to increasing the concentration of CSF from 5% to 5.5, 7.8, and 7.4% respectively.

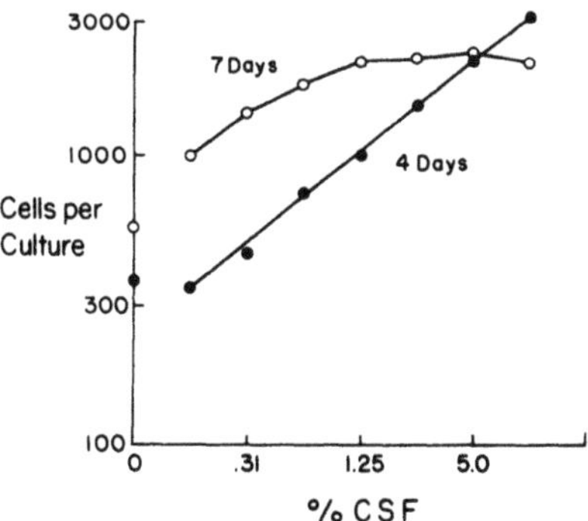

Figure 2. Effect of CSF concentration on total cells per culture (the product of mean aggregate number and mean aggregate size) in cultures assessed 4 and 7 days from inception.

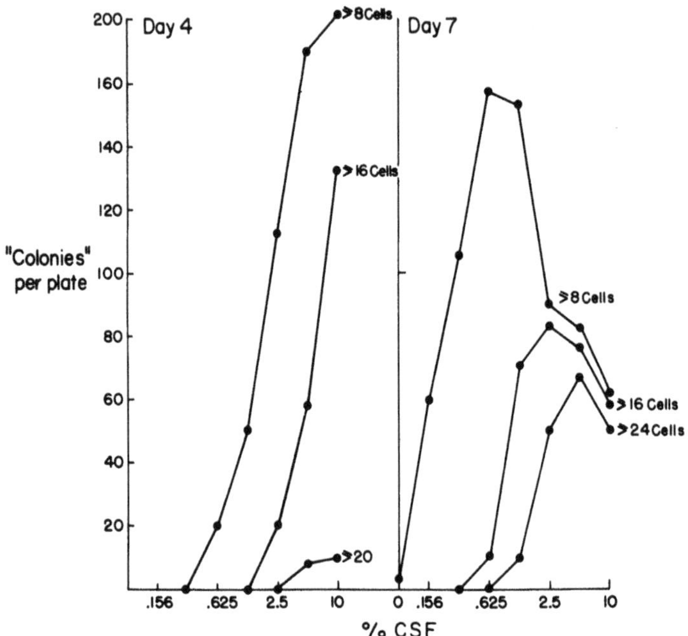

Figure 3. Effect of CSF on the number of colonies of different size in cultures assessed 4 and 7 days from inception.

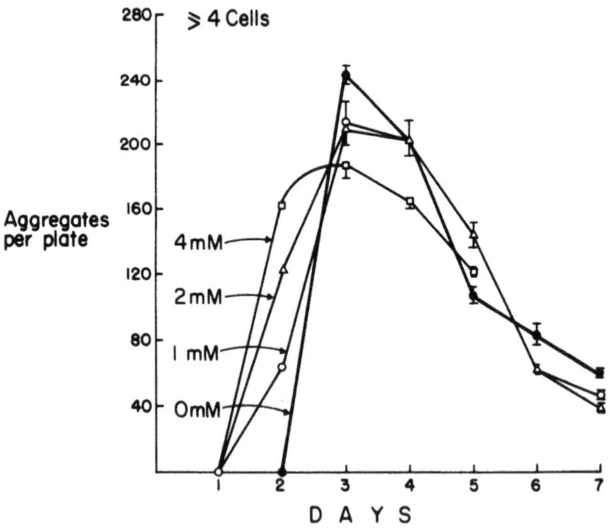

Figure 4. Effect of lithium (0 - 4 mM) in cultures stimulated with 5% CSF (MNL-conditioned medium). Only aggregates containing 4 or more cells were counted.

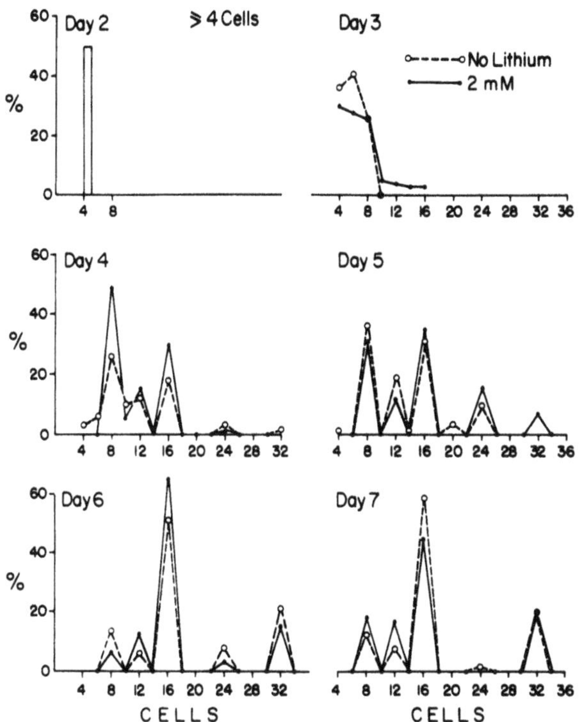

Figure 5. Histogram showing the incidence of different sized aggregates in cultures containing 5% CSF plus 0 and 2 mM lithium

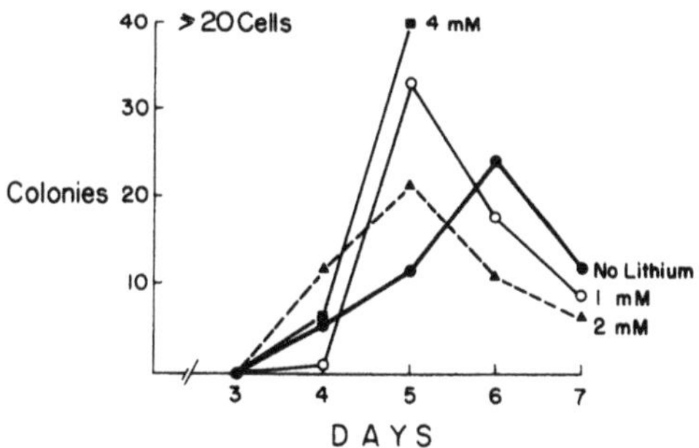

Figure 6. Effect of lithium (0 - 4 mM) on the formation and disappearance of colonies composed of 20 or more cells in cultures stimulated by 5% CSF.

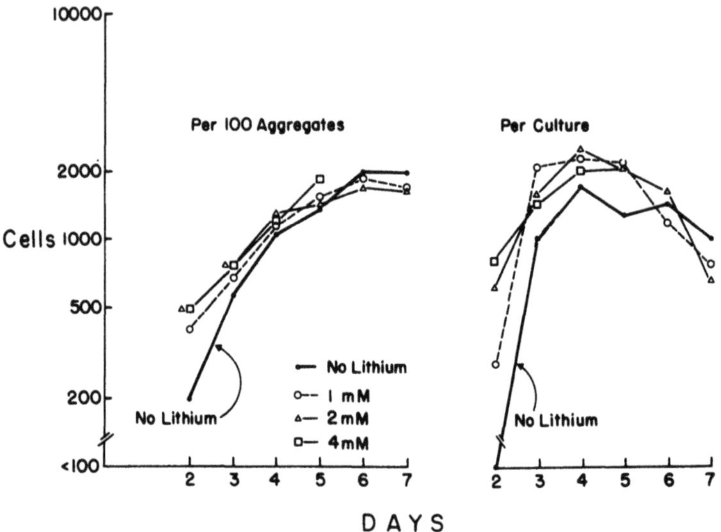

Figure 7. Effect of lithium (0 - 4 mM) on total cells per 100 aggregates (left) and per culture (right). Cultures were stimulated by 5% CSF.

Effect of Lithium in CSF Production

In four separate experiments, lithium (0 - 4 mM) was added to 24 hour liquid cultures containing mononuclear leukocytes suspended in culture medium supplemented with 30% heat-inactivated serum. Lithium was also added to control cultures at the completion of the 24 hour incubation period. Cells were removed by millipore filtration and CSF content of each filtrate was assayed (5%) in marrow cultures shown to respond appropriately to CSF. Representative results from a single experiment presented in tabular form showed that the effects of lithium were equivocal: 1 mM neither enhanced nor inhibited CSF production; 2 mM increased CSF production slightly (10%); and 4 mM reduced CSF production by approximately 25% (assessed from effects on mean aggregate size from the control CSF dose response curve). (See Table I).

DISCUSSION

I have emphasized some of the kinetic features of a culture system developed to investigate factors influencing granulopoiesis. This is a sensitive system because it has been depleted of neutrophil- and serum-derived inhibitors, and endogenous CSF production has been virtually eliminated. However, there are problems related to the dynamic nature of the system itself. These must be appreciated if it is to be applied appropriately. Results are time-dependent, and clearly it is preferable to make observations during the growing phase of the cultures rather than later, when clonal disappearance has become a major factor.

TABLE I

EFFECT OF LITHIUM ON CSF PRODUCTION BY MNL DURING 24 HOURS OF INCUBATION

	Concentration of Lithium (mM)	Control (Lithium added at harvest of CSF)	Effect of Lithium (Added at Inception of Cultures)
Aggregates mean ± SEM	0	290 ± 8	290 ± 8
	1	289 ± 12.4	257 ± 6
	2	290 ± 10	273 ± 11
	4	265 ± 6	289 ± 7
Cells per aggregate (mean) *	0	7.71	7.71
	1	7.31	7.33
	2	7.01	7.15
	4	7.53	6.44⁺

* Average of 100 consecutive aggregates.

⁺ Equivalent to a reduction of approximately 25% as determined by CSF dose response curve.

A discussion of clonal disappearance, while beyond the scope of this paper, deserves brief comment. It probably indicates heterogeneity of seeded CFC with respect to the number of times they have already divided, assuming that they have a pre-programmed limited capacity for self-renewal. Once this capacity has been exceeded, their progeny proceed down the maturation pathway, and disperse. The clone disappears in toto. The size of surviving clones is determined by the balance between proliferation of CFC and their progeny on the one hand, and terminal differentiation and migration of end stage cells on the other hand. Consequently, the lifespan and size of granulocytic colonies is susceptible to the influence of factors which influence cell proliferation and maturation. In cultures declining with respect to colony number, the size of surviving clones increases in proportion to CSF stimulation and thus, an estimation of mean colony size still provides a realistic method of evaluation.

This study suggests that lithium shortens the cycle time of cells proliferating in response to CSF. Aggregates of more than 2 cells appeared earlier and reached a maximum with respect to number and size earlier than in control cultures, and they disappeared sooner. Therefore, lithium, like CSF, accelerates amplification and terminal differentiation, but does not increase the number of cells produced per CFC. Neither agent is able to re-program committed granulocytic precursors to increase their yield of end stage cells. Therefore, other explanations should be sought for the clinical effects of lithium on granulopoiesis.

To sustain granulopoiesis at a higher than normal level for prolonged periods of time would require either increased recruitment of CFC from uncommitted precursors, or decreased peripheral loss. Theoretically, lithium could act either directly or indirectly via feedback mechanisms to achieve increased recruitment. Possibly CSF could also act in this way. Unfortunately, the observed effects of CSF and lithium on the amplification process do not provide details concerning in vivo mechanisms.

ACKNOWLEDGEMENT

This work was supported by Grant 309 from the Ontario Cancer Treatment and Research Foundation.

REFERENCES

Baker, F.L. and Galbraith, P.R., 1978, Nutritional and regulatory roles of human serum in cultures of human granulopoietic cells, Blood 52:241.

Baker, F.L. and Galbraith, P.R., 1979, Mechanism of action of serum factors that regulate granulopoiesis in vitro: Possible physiologic role of serum-inhibiting activity, Blood 53:304.

Galbraith, P.R., Cooke, L.J., and Baker, F.L., 1979, Action of inhibitor released from neutrophils and leukemic blast cells, Can. Med. Assn. J. 120:545.

Gupta, R.C., Robinson, W.A., and Kurnick, J.W., 1976, Felty's syndrome. Effect of lithium on granulopoiesis, Am. J. Med. 61:29.

Harker, W.G., Rothstein, G., and Clarkson, D., 1977, Enhancement of colony-stimulating activity production by lithium, Blood 49:263.

Haskill, J.S., McKnight, R.D., and Galbraith, P.R., 1972, Cell-cell interaction in vitro: Studied by density separation of colony-forming, stimulating, and inhibiting cells from human bone marrow, Blood 40:394.

Metcalf, D., 1969, Studies on colony formation in vitro by mouse bone marrow cells 1. Continuous cluster formation and relation of clusters to colonies, J. Cell Physiol. 74:323.

Morley, D.C., Jr. and Galbraith, P.R., 1978, Effect of lithium on granulopoiesis in culture, Can. Med. Assn. J. 118:288.

Murphy, D.L., Goodwin, F.K., and Bunney, W.E., Jr., 1971, Leukocytosis during lithium treatment, Am. J. Psychiatry 127:1559.

Singer, I. and Rottenberg, D., 1973, Mechanisms of lithium action, N. Eng. J. Med. 289:254.

Tisman, G., Herbert, V., and Rosenblatt, S., 1973, Evidence that lithium induces human granulocyte proliferation: elevated serum vitamin B12 binding capacity in vivo and granulocyte colony proliferation in vitro, Br. J. Haematol. 24:767.

MYELOPOIETIC MODULATION BY LITHIUM: *IN VITRO* EXPERIMENTS ON ITS MECHANISMS OF ACTION IN MAN

Dharmvir S. Verma, Gary Spitzer, Axel R. Zander,
Miloslav A. Beran, and Karel A. Dicke

Department of Developmental Therapeutics
The University of Texas System Cancer Center
M.D. Anderson Hospital and Tumor Institute
6723 Bertner Avenue
Houston, Texas 77030

Various reports have described consistent elevation of granulocytes accompanying lithium administratioin in psychiatric patients (Mayfield and Brown, 1966; O'Connell, 1970; Shopsin *et al.*, 1971). In 1975 Gupta *et al.* reported that lithium increased the leukocyte count in patients with Felty's syndrome. They also documented increase in colony stimulating activity (CSA) active against murine bone marrow cells in the urine of these patients (Gupta *et al.*, 1976). Recently, several authors have reported that lithium, when administered to patients with various malignancies, may ameliorate chemotherapy induced myelosuppression (Catane *et al.*, 1976; Greco *et al.*, 1976; Stein *et al.*, 1977; Tisman, 1974; Tisman and Wu, 1977) and reduce the duration of granulocytopenia induced by chemotherapy in acute myeloid leukemia (Charron *et al.*, 1977). Lithium has also been used to elevate leukocytes, platelets and hemoglobin levels in aplastic anemia with some success (Barrett *et al.*, 1977).

Recently, Rothstein et al. (1978) have shown that the increase in blood neutrophil count seen after lithium administration is not merely due to demargination, but is a result of enlargement of the total blood neutrophil mass and increased neutrophil production.

Studies in mice have revealed that lithium enhances CSA production by lung tissue (Harker et al., 1975; Harker et al., 1977). Using human peripheral leukocyte underlayers, lithium has been shown to increase colony formation in the in vitro agar culture system (Tisman et al., 1973). Thus far, however, the exact mechanism(s) involved have not been clearly elucidated. Herein, we report in vitro experiments performed to delineate these mechanisms in detail using human bone marrow cells.

MATERIALS AND METHODS

These investigations were performed after approval by the local Human Investigations Committee. All patients donating their marrow were informed about the nature of the investigation.

Acquisition of marrow specimens

Human marrow specimens were routinely obtained from patients with non-hematological malignancies without bone marrow involvement or prior chemotherapy at the time of diagnostic bone marrow aspirations. Marrow was aspirated from the posterior iliac spine. Approximately 1 ml of marrow was placed into a tissue culture tube containing preservative free heparin (300 units in 2 ml of phosphate buffered saline).

Marrow cell preparation used in various experiments

Buffy coat cells were used for the experiments designed to elicit the enhancement of spontaneous colony formation by lithium and the abrogation of this effect by removal of adherent cells. Buffy coat cells were also used in those experiments showing the effect of lithium on human placental conditioned medium (HPCM) stimulated marrow cells. HPCM was prepared as described previously (Burgess et al., 1977).

Ficoll-Hypaque interface cells were used in the experiments designed to show the release of colony stimulating activity by lithium.

Preparation of buffy coat cells

Marrow specimens were centrifuged at 1200 g for 10 minutes in plastic culture tubes. The buffy coat was aspirated gently with a pasteur pipette and subsequently used for various experiments.

Preparation of light density cells

Marrow specimens were diluted in equal volumes of α-MEM (modified Eagle's medium) with 15% fetal calf serum (FCS) and centrifuged at 400 g for 35 minutes after layering over a cushion of Ficoll-Hypaque (density 1.077 g/ml) contained in a conical plastic tube (Boyum, 1977). The interface cells were aspirated gently with a pasteur pipette, washed with phosphate buffered saline, resuspended in α-MEM and used for the experiments mentioned later.

Culture procedure

The culture procedure has been described before except for using HPCM as a source of CSA instead of peripheral blood leukocytes (Spitzer et al., 1976). Briefly, the marrow preparations were cultured in equal volumes of double-strength α-MEM with 30% FCS and 0.6% Bacto-agar (Difco), giving a final concentration of 0.3% agar with single strength α-MEM and 15% FCS. For all cultures 0.1 ml HPCM was used as a source of CSA in underlayers of 0.5% agar and α-MEM with 15% FCS. The same batch of HPCM was used throughout the study. All cultures were plated in triplicate for 7 days in a fully humidified atmosphere of 7% CO_2 in air at $37^{o}C$.

Culture scoring

Cultures were scored on day 7 using a dissecting microscope at 25-40x. They were analyzed for total number of colonies (per plate). The final colony incidence was the mean of the colony incidence from each plate for that particular observation in the study.

Removal of adherent cells

Removal of adherent cell population was achieved by incubating 2 x 10^6 buffy coat cells per ml of α-MEM and 15% FCS, total volume of 2 ml, in 35 mm plastic petri dishes for 3 hours. Non-adherent cells for culture were obtained as described below.

Preparation of conditioned media

In the experiments designed to examine the release of CSA, light density marrow cells were obtained by Ficoll-Hypaque gradient centrifugation (density 1.077 g/ml) as described above.

To prepare the conditioned media 2 x 10^6 interface cells from a Ficoll-Hypaque gradient were incubated per 1 ml of α-MEM and 15% FCS (total volume of 2 ml, total cells 4 x 10^6/dish). To obtain adherent cell conditioned media, 2 x 10^6/ml of interface cells were subjected to the adherence procedure as described above (4 x 10^6 cells/dish) and non-adherent cells were removed by two thorough washings of petri dishes with α-MEM. Subsequently, the petri dishes with adherent cells were incubated (each dish containing 2 ml of α-MEM with 15% FCS) for varying periods in a fully humidified atmosphere of 7% CO_2 at 37^oC. Conditioned media from non-adherent cells were prepared by centrifuging the aspirated non-adherent cells, removing the supernatant, resuspending the cells to a volume of 2 ml in α-MEM and 15% FCS and reseeding into new 35 mm plastic petri dishes.

Conditioned media (CM) were harvested at specific times and prepared by centrifuging at 1200 g for 10 minutes and passing through a millipore filter (0.22μ). CM were stored at -20^oC until assayed on 1.0 x 10^5 non-adherent light density (< 1.077 g/ml) human marrow cells from a single donor.

Agents used

Lithium carbonate (lot 763970, Fisher Scientific Co., N.Y.) was dissolved in α-MEM in a stock solution of 1000 meq/l of lithium. A lithium concentration of 1 meq/l was used in those experiments designed to examine spontaneous colony formation and the effect of spontaneous colony formation after removal of adherent cells. This concentration is equivalent to serum lithium concentrations achieved in man with oral lithium carbonate.

Lithium carbonate was used at concentrations of 1.0, 2.0, and 4.0 meq/l in experiments examining CSA release.

Statistics

Differences between the results of experiments with and without lithium were examined by using a Student's two sample test.

RESULTS

Lithium effects on human marrow cells: with and without HPCM

To explore the effect of lithium on *in vitro* culture growth of human myeloid progenitor cells, lithium was used at a concentration of 1 meq/l with varying cell numbers (1×10^5 to 7.5×10^5 per dish) obtained from buffy coat preparations of human bone marrow. Simultaneous experiments were performed using HPCM alone and HPCM with lithium. A total of 9 experiments of this design showed no definite pattern of stimulation with lithium in the presence of HPCM over that achieved with HPCM alone. Because of this unexpected finding we next examined the effect of lithium on spontaneous colony formation. Twelve experiments were performed at a cell number of 5×10^5 per plate, a dose which routinely induces spontaneous colony formation, ten experiments incorporating lithium in culture plates with and without HPCM, and two experiments examining spontaneous colony formation alone. In other experiments we also examined the effect of lithium at other cell concentrations on both stimulated and unstimulated colony formation. A total of two experiments were performed with a cell concentration of 1 x 10^5/dish, nine experiments were performed with a cell concentration of 2.5 x 10^5/dish, and because of the limitation of cell numbers, five experiments were performed with 7.5 x 10^5 cells per dish.

Figures 1A and 1B are representative of experiments examining the effect of lithium on both spontaneous colony formation and that induced with HPCM. As can be seen from these graphs, lithium induced variable enhancement of spontaneous colony formation. For example, the experiment represented by Figure 1A shows enhancement of spontaneous colony formation at higher target cell numbers (5 x 10^5 and 7.5 x 10^5 cells), $P < 0.05$. This difference in spontaneous colony formation induced by lithium, however, was abrogated when HPCM was added to the culture dishes. In the experiment represented by Figure 1B, the lithium-induced enhancement of spontaneous colony formation does not continue to rise with the increasing target cell concentration.

The effect of adherent cell removal on spontaneous colony formation by lithium

In order to determine if the lithium effect may be mediated through an adherent cell population in the marrow and not direct stimulation of CFU-c, adherent cell removal was performed in another three experiments. Cells were cultured at cell concentrations ranging from 2.5 to 7.5 x 10^5 per dish.

Figure 2 is representative of these experiments. In all instances the lithium enhancement of spontaneous colony formation is markedly reduced by the removal of adherent cells. Therefore, it appears that lithium requires adherent cells for enhancement of spontaneous colony formation.

Lithium effect on human marrow colony formation stimulated with varying concentrations of HPCM and its modulation by removal of adherent cells

To determine if the variable effect of lithium on colony formation in HPCM containing cultures may be due to suboptimal amounts of HPCM, lithium at 1 mEq/l was added to cultures containing 0.025 to 0.3 ml of

HPCM. Colony formation was significantly increased in lithium containing cultures at HPCM concentrations of 0.025 ml ($P < 0.05$) and 0.05 ml ($P < 0.025$) as shown in Figure 3A. The enhancing effect of lithium was abolished by prior removal of adherent cells (Figure 3B).

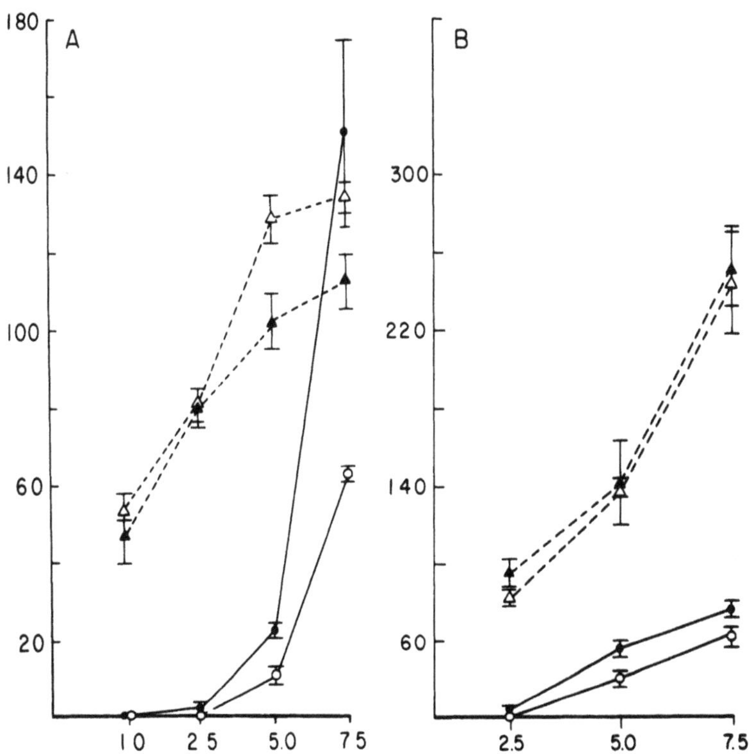

Figures 1A and 1B. Lithium enhancement of spontaneous colony formation. Bone marrow cells were cultured with HPCM without lithium carbonate (open triangles) and with lithium carbonate (closed triangles). Marrow was also cultured without HPCM and without lithium (open circles) and with lithium (closed circles) to see the effect on spontaneous colony formation. Bars represent ± 1 standard deviation. Lithium causes enhancement of spontaneous colony formation but no significant difference in cultures containing HPCM. (Reproduced with the kind permission of Cancer Research).

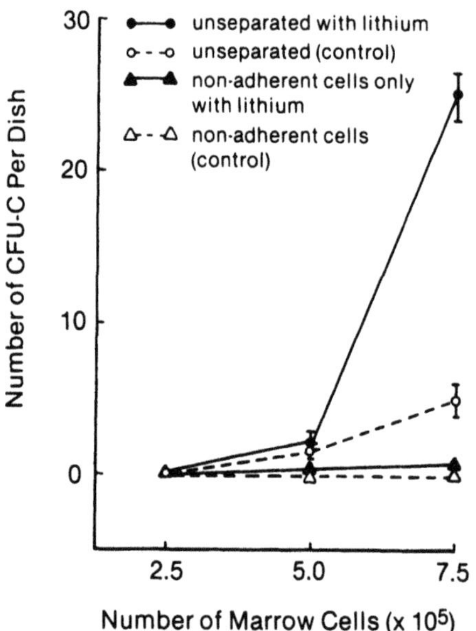

Figure 2. Effect of removal of adherent cells on lithium stimulation of spontaneous colony formation. Bone marrow without adherent cells removed with lithium (closed circles) and without lithium (open circles) was cultured at varying cell concentrations. Without HPCM as described previously, lithium increased spontaneous colony formation. Bone marrow was also cultured after adherent cells had been removed with lithium (closed triangles) and without lithium (open triangles). This procedure abrogated both spontaneous colony formation and lithium induced increases. Bars represent ± 1 standard deviation. (Reproduced with the kind permission of Cancer Research).

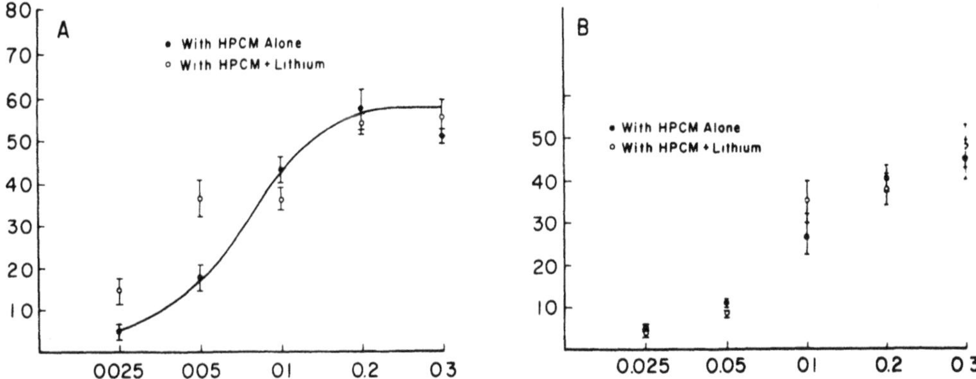

Figure 3. Effect of lithium on colony formation in cultures containing lithium and human placental conditioned media at varying concentrations. (A) Bone marrow was cultured at increasing concentrations of HPCM with HPCM alone (closed circles) and with HPCM and lithium (open circles). Lithium significantly increased colony formation at concentrations of HPCM of 0.025 ml and 0.05 ml in the underlayers. (Reproduced with the kind permission of Cancer Research).

(B) When adherent cells were removed, lithium did not effect colony formation at low concentrations of HPCM.

<u>Lithium-induced elaboration of CSA from light density human marrow cells</u>

To determine if this action is through CSA elaboration, lithium was incubated at varying concentrations (1.0, 2.0 and 4.0 meq/l) with light density ($\leq$ 1.007 g/ml) unfractionated, adherent and non-adherent human marrow cells. The conditioned media were harvested at three days and seven days, filtered through 0.22μ millipore filters and assayed for CSA against light density non-adherent human marrow cells. The data from one such experiment are shown in Table I. The conditioned media from cells incubated without any lithium had poor CSA and stimulated only cluster formation. The unfractionated cell-conditioned media (U-CM) showed increasing CSA with increasing concentrations of lithium and the activity was higher in day three U-CM than day seven. The conditioned media from adherent cells (Ad-CM), on the other hand, stimulated colony formation when prepared incorporating only higher concentrations of lithium (2.0 and 4.0 meq/l). No colony formation was noted using conditioned media from non-adherent cells (NAd-CM) with any of the lithium concentrations. Only cluster formation was observed. Thus, the CSA in U-CM was significantly higher than the arithmetic sum of the activities in Ad-CM and NAd-CM at all concentrations of lithium, suggesting an ongoing interaction between the adherent and non-adherent marrow cells for maximum CSA elaboration.

DISCUSSION

Lithium has been described to release CSA from mouse lung (Harker et al., 1977) and a CSA from human mononuclear cells active against murine and human bone marrow (Joyce and Chervenick, 1975; Spitzer et al., 1979). However, it has been shown that the colony stimulating activities released from human peripheral blood monocytes and lymphocytes are multiple and the CSAs active on human bone marrow are of different molecular weights and released at different time periods than those active on murine bone marrow (Shah et al., 1977). Moreover, Morley and Galbraith (1978) did not confirm that lithium enhanced CSA release from human peripheral blood mononuclear cells. It has been suggested that the colony stimulating cell population in marrow may be of more significance in vivo than peripheral mononuclear cells. We, therefore, decided to examine the possibility that lithium may require a bone marrow adherent cell population for its mechanism of action and that the mechanism of action may be through the release of CSA from that population. When bone marrow adherent cells are removed prior to culture with lithium, there was marked reduction of both spontaneous colony formation and lithium enhancement of spontaneous colony formation.

There have been two previous reports (Morley and Galbratih, 1978; Tisman et al., 1973) of lithium induced augmentation of human myeloid progenitor cell colony formation, either using cultures containing human peripheral blood cells as an underlayer or a human mononuclear cell source of CSA. This could suggest that lithium may have a direct effect on CFU-c as well as an indirect action through release of CSA. When we examined lithium effects in cultures incorporating HPCM, we noticed a variable effect. The significant enhancement was unusual. The concentrations of HPCM used in some of our experiments may not have been those necessary to achieve maximal colony numbers. Therefore, it is conceivable that the target cells in those experiments in which lithium enhanced colony formation despite the simultaneous stimulation with HPCM, may not have been maximally stimulated. We then examined if this variability could be due to suboptimal stimulation by HPCM; lithium did in fact enhance colony formation only at low concentrations of HPCM and this enhancement was abolished by removal of adherent cells. These results suggest that the variability observed in previous experiments (HPCM plus lithium) might have been due to inadequante HPCM concentrations used inadvertently. Previous publications of enhnaced colony formation with leukocyte underlayers may have been due to a similar mechanism; furthermore, the abrogation of this effect by removal of adherent cells suggests the indirect mechanism of lithium action.

The documentation of CSA elaboration from marrow cells may further suggest the myelopoietic augmentation by lithium to be through CSA, although direct action of lithium on myeloid progenitor cells cannot be excluded. The finding of adherent and non-adherent marrow cell interaction in lithium-induced CSA elaboration is of great interest. Recently we have reported adherent and non-adherent cell interaction in CSA elaboration by other myelopoietic augmentors such as BCG, MER (methanol extraction residue of BCG) and Corynebacterium parvum (C. parvum) (Verma et al., 1979a). Further studies by us have revealed

TABLE I

Cell Source of Conditioned Media	Day of Harvest	CSA* in Conditioned Media with Different Lithium Concentrations: 0.0		1.0 meq/l		2.0 meq/l		4.0 meq/l	
		Col**	Clu***	Col	Clu	Col	Clu	Col	Clu
Unfractionated cells	3	0	690	54	580	65	540	70	590
	7	0	250	40	605	43	575	55	360
Adherent Cells	3	0	0	0	0	0	35	0	510
	7	0	0	0	0	2	20	30	530
Non-Adherent Cells	3	0	0	0	0	0	27	0	160
	7	0	0	0	0	0	23	0	435

* Represented as mean colony or cluster incidence per 10^5 non-adherent human marrow cells plated in duplicate

** Colonies of ≥ 40 cell aggregates: scored on day 8 of culture

*** Clusters of 3-39 cell aggregates: scored on day 8 of culture

macrophages and T-lymphocytes to be responsible for this interaction (Verma et al., 1979b). Most recently Gelfand et al. (1979) have demonstrated that lithium may inhibit suppressor T-lymphocyte activity. It is possible, therefore, that the resultant final CSA in response to lithium may be dependent upon the quantitative and qualitative status of various interacting subpopulations of lymphocytes and macrophages. The variable myelopoietic responses described in neutropenic patients may, at least in part, be related to these phenomena.

The comparison of CSA elaborating capacity of various immunoadjuvants, e.g. BCG, MER and C. parvum, with lithium has demonstrated it to be a rather weaker myelopoietic augmentor. The variable myelopoietic affect seen in in vitro experiments has also been noted in patients with chemotherapy induced neutropenia at our institution. These experiments have revealed that while lithium may fail to elaborate CSA from one human marrow specimen, BCG and MER would invariably be successful in doing so. Recently we have encountered such a situation in clinical use of these agents (Figure 4). A 32-year-old patient with a diagnosis of preleukemia manifested by neutropenia and hypercellular marrow (70%) with dyshemopoiesis was admitted to our hospital with bilateral gram-negative pneumonia. While being treated successfully with antibiotics, lithium (900 mg p.o./day) administration failed to increase peripheral blood neutrophil levels. On the other hand, a series of four intravenous injections of MER, given at weekly intervals, induced a prompt rise in the neutrophil counts; this was associated with disappearance of myelopoietic maturational arrest in the marrow. This case illustrates the fact that while one agent may fail to stimulate myelopoiesis the other agent may do so successfully in the same patient.

The experiments described in this paper suggest that lithium augments myelopoiesis at least in part through CSA elaboration by adherent cell population in marrow and this requires an interaction with non-adherent cells for maximum response. The existence of these interactions between different cell populations may be responsible for a variable myelopoietic effect of lithium in different patients and the absence of myelopoietic augmentation in response to one and the presence of myelopoietic augmentation in response to the others.

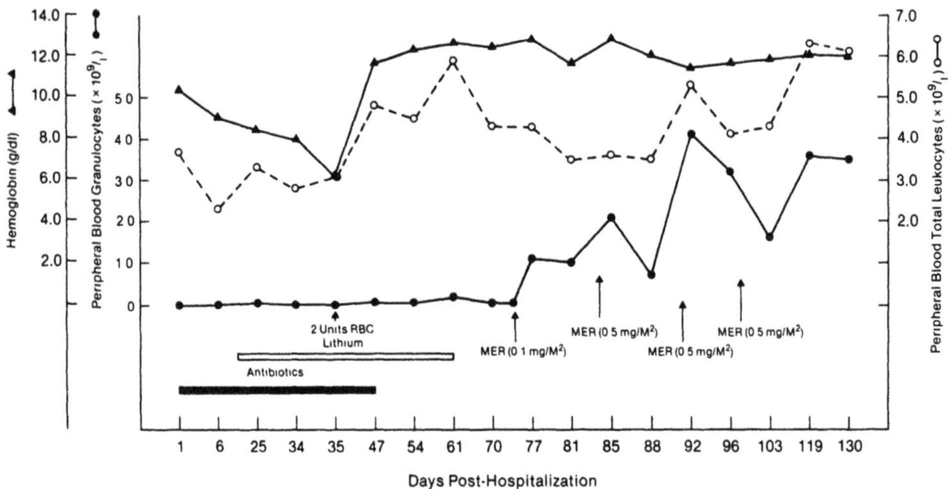

Figure 4. Hematological follow-up of a patient with anemia and leukopenia. The patient did not respond to a 36 day course of oral lithium carbonate (900 mg/day). However, intravenous injections of MER at weekly intervals induced prompt elevation of granulocytes. (Reproduced with the kind permission of Experimental Hematology).

ACKNOWLEDGEMENTS

This research was supported in part by Grants CA 11520, CA 14528, CA 19856 and RR 5511 from NIH, Bethesda, Maryland.

The authors thank Mrs. Ann Ceramer and Ms. Sherrie Smith for their expert technical assistance and Ms. Kathi Orsak for her secretarial assistance in the preparation of the original manuscript.

REFERENCES

Barrett, A.J., Hugh-Jones, K., Newton, K. and Watson, J.G., 1977, Lithium therapy in aplastic anemia, The Lancet 1:202.

Boyum, A., 1977, Separation of lymphocytes, lymphocyte subgroups and monocytes: a review, Lymphology 10:71.

Burgess, A.W., Wilson, E.M.A., and Metcalf, D., 1977, Stimulation by human placental conditioned media of hemopoietic colony formation by human marrow cells, Blood 49:573.

Catane, R., Kaufman, J., Mittelman, A., and Murphy, G.P., 1976, Attenuation of neutropenia from cancer chemotherapy, Proc. Am. Assoc. Clin. Oncol. 17:250.

Charron, D., Barrett, A.J., Faille, A., Alby, N., Schmitt, T., and Degos, L., 1977, Lithium in acute myeloid leukemia, The Lancet 1:1307.

Gelfand, E.W., Dosch, H-M., Hastings, D., and Shore, A., 1979, Lithium: A modulator of cyclic AMP-dependent events in lymphocytes, Science 203:365.

Greco, F.A., Bereton, H.D. and Pomerory, T., 1976, Lithium carbonate attenuation of neutropenia from cancer chemotherapy, Proc. Am. Assoc. Canc. Res. 17:250.

Gupta, R.C., Robinson, W.A. and Smyth, C.J., 1975, Efficacy of lithium in rheumatoid arthritis with granulocytopenia (Felty's syndrome), Arthritis Rheum. 18:179.

Gupta, R.C., Robinson, W.A. and Kurnick, J.D., 1976, Felty's syndrome. Effect of lithium on granulopoiesis, Am. J. Med. 61:29.

Harker, G.W., Rothstein, G., Clarkson, D.W. and Athens, J.W., 1975, Stimulation of neutrophil production by lithium, Clin. Res. 23:103A.

Harker, G.W., Rothstein, G., Clarkson, D.W., Athens, J.W. and McFarlane, T.L, 1977, Enhancement of colony-stimulating activity production by lithium, Blood 49:263.

Joyce, R.A. and Chervenick, P.A., 1975, Effect of lithium on the release of colony stimulating activity (CSA) from blood leukocytes, Proc.Am.Soc.Hematol. 18:126 (Abstract).

Mayfield, D. and Brown, R.G., 1966, The clinical laboratory and electroencephalographic effects of lithium, J. Psychiatr. Res. 4:207.

Morley, D.C., Jr. and Galbraith, P.R., 1978, Effect of lithium on granulopoiesis in culture, Can. Med. Assoc. J. 118:288.

O'Connell, R.A., 1970, Leukocytosis during lithium carbonate treatment, Int. J. Pharmacopsychiatry 4:30.

Rothstein, G., Clarkson, D.R., Larsen, W., Grosser, B.I., and Athens, J.W., 1978, Effect of lithium on neutrophil mass and production, N. Eng. J. Med. 298:178.

Shah, R.A., Caporate, L.H., and Moore, M.A.S., 1977, Characterization of colony stimulating activity produced by human monocytes and phytohemagglutinin-stimulated lymphocytes, Blood 50:811.

Shopsin, S., Friedman, R., and Gershon, S., 1971, Lithium and leukocytosis, Clin. Pharmacol. Ther. 12:923.

Spitzer, G., Dicke, K.A., Gehan, E.A., Smith, T., McCredie, K.B., Barlogie, B., and Freireich, E.J., 1976, A simplified in vitro classification of prognosis in adult acute leukemia: The application of in vitro results in remission-predictive-models, Blood 48:795.

Spitzer, G., Verma, D.S., Barlogie, B., Beran, M., and Dicke, K.A., The augmentation in in vitro spontaneous meyloid colony formation by lithium: in vitro experiments on its mechanism of action, Canc. Res. 1979 (in press).

Stein, R.S., Beaman, C., Ali, M.Y., Hansen, R., Jenkins, D.D. and Jume'an, H.G., 1977, Lithium carbonate attenuation of chemotherapy-induced neutropenia, N. Eng. J. Med. 297:430.

Tisman, G., 1974, Lithium carbonate protection against drug-induced leukopenia in lymphosarcoma patients, ICRS 2:1509.

Tisman, G. and Wu, S.G., 1977, Lithium induced granulocytosis, The Lancet 2:251.

Tisman, G., Herbert, V., and Rosenblatt, S., 1973, Evidence that lithium induces human granulocyte proliferation: Elevated serum vitamin B12 binding capacity in vivo and granulocyte colony proliferation in vitro, Br. J. Haematol. 24:767.

Verma, D.S., Spitzer, G., Zander, A.R., Fisher, R., McCredie, K.B. and Dicke, K.A., 1979a, T-lymphocyte mediated augmentation and suppression of colony stimulating activity elaboration in man, Manuscript submitted.

Verma, D.S., Spitzer, G., Dicke, K.A., Zander, A.R., Vellekoop, L., Beran, M., 1979b, Myelopoietic enhancement by immunoadjuvants: in vitro studies for their rational use in neutropenic patients, Exp. Hematol. 7:228 (Supplement #5).

ORAL LITHIUM CARBONATE INCREASES COLONY STIMULATING ACTIVITY PRODUCTION FROM HUMAN MONONUCLEAR CELLS

Andrew Robert Turner and Mary Joan Allalunis

Experimental Hematology Laboratory
Department of Medicine
Cross Cancer Institute
University of Alberta
Edmonton, Alberta, Canada T6G 1Z2

Oral lithium carbonate therapy produces a reversible neutrophilic leukocytosis (Murphy et al., 1971; Shopsin et al., 1971). What was initially regarded as a medical curiosity in psychiatric patients has been exploited therapeutically in the treatment of neutropenia (Gupta et al., 1976; Schapria et al., 1977; Jacob and Herbert, 1974; Barrett et al., 1977a) and chemotherapy induced bone marrow suppression (Turner and MacDonald, 1979). A true increase in granulocyte mass occurs with lithium ingestion rather than a shift of neutrophils from the marrow reserve or demargination of granulocytes (Rothstein et al., 1978; Stein et al., 1978). Elevated urinary and serum colony stimulating activity (CSA) has been reported in neutropenic patients on lithium (Gupta et al., 1976) and lithium has been shown to augment CSA production *in vitro* from mouse lung (Harker et al., 1977) and mononuclear cells (Joyce and Chervenick, 1975). A major source of CSA in man are the peripheral blood mononuclear cells (Chervenick and LoBuglio, 1972). These studies examined the effects of oral lithium carbonate on human mononuclear cell production of CSA as measured by its capacity to stimulate human granulocyte-macrophage colony formation.

MATERIALS AND METHODS

The subjects of this experiment were eleven hematologically normal individuals who were taking no medication and who were free of clinical evidence of infection throughout the course of the experiment. Written informed consent was obtained prior to initiation of the experiment.

Venous blood was obtained on days 0, 1, 4, 7 and 10 of a 10 day experiment. Total leukocyte counts were determined using a Coulter Counter (Model ZBL). Two hundred cell differential counts were made from Wright's stained preparations. Ten ml of peripheral blood was allowed to clot. The serum was filtered and stored at $-20^{0}C$. A portion of this was used to determine serum lithium levels by flame photometry.

Thirty ml of venous blood (anticoagulated with preservative-free heparin) was applied to Ficoll-Hypaque solution using a modification of the technique described by Boyum (1968) and English and Andersen (1974). Mononuclear cells were aspirated from the 1.077 g/cm^3 interface and washed three times in sterile 0.9% saline. Differential counts were made of smears made using a cytocentrifuge (Shandon Southern Cytospin). The washed mononuclear cells were added to alpha media with 20% fetal calf serum at a concentration of 2×10^6 cells/ml. Each day's cell yield was divided into two aliquots. One half of the cells was incubated for four hours (Baker and Galbraith, 1975) and the other half for seven days (Kurnick et al., 1977). Cells were incubated in a humidified atmosphere containing 8% CO_2. After incubation, the conditioned medium was filtered through a 0.45µ Millipore filter and stored at $-20^{0}C$.

Lithium carbonate was administered orally as 300 mg capsules. The first dose (300 mg) was given twelve hours before the day 1 blood collection was drawn. Thereafter, it was taken three times daily for a total of seven days (21 doses).

Colony stimulating activity (CSA) of the 4 hour and 7 day conditioned media was assayed against normal human bone marrow (Chervenick and Boggs, 1970). The technique was a modification of that described by Pike and Robinson (1970) using methylcellulose in place of agar (Chervenick and Boggs, 1970). One-tenth ml of material to be assayed was added to 0.9 ml of methylcellulose with 20% fetal calf serum and 10^5 non-adherent bone marrow cells. Colonies of more than 40 cells were scored at 12 days using an inverted microscope. Control plates made without a source of CSA yielded no growth.

RESULTS

There was a slight rise in total white cell count in the seven subjects taking lithium for 7 days (Figure 1). No change was noted in the 4 control

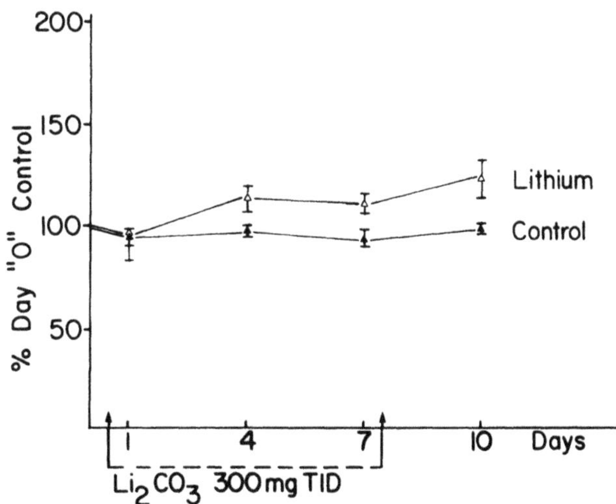

Figure 1. Alteration in total white blood count during course of experiment expressed as a percentage of day 0 levels (mean ± 1 s.e.m.). The differences are significant ($P < 0.05$) at days 4, 7 and 10.

subjects. The increase in WBC in the lithium treated subjects was due primarily to an increase in neutrophils which was maximal at day 7 at 150% of initial neutrophil counts. Six of 7 subjects demonstrated a neutrophilia

(Figure 2). There was no alteration of neutrophil counts in the control subjects. The lymphocyte and monocyte counts did not vary significantly throughout the study (Figure 3).

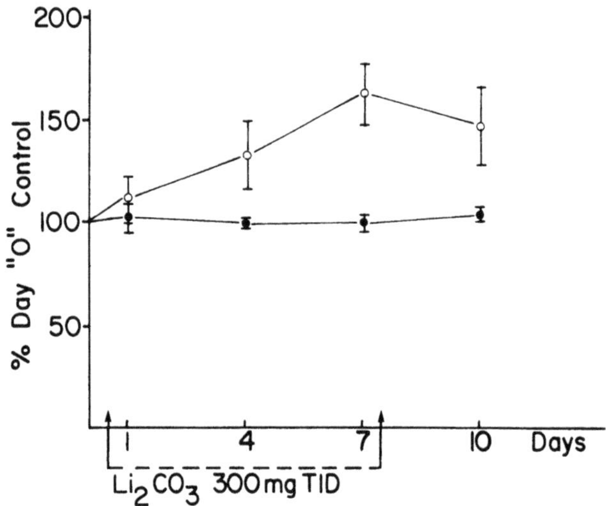

Figure 2. Alteration in absolute neutrophil counts expressed as in Figure 1. The difference between lithium treated subjects (open circles) are significant ($p < 0.05$) on days 4 and 10 and highly significant on day 7 ($p < 0.01$).

Serum lithium levels ranged from 0.5 to 1.0 mM on day 4 and day 7 in the lithium treated group. On days 1 and 10, it was less than 0.2 mM. The pattern of rise and fall of serum lithium levels in both subjects corresponds closely to that reported in pharmacokinetic studies of oral lithium distribution (Amdisen, 1977). The serum levels achieved in this study did not exceed the therapeutic range of lithium in the treatment of psychiatric disorders (0.8 to 1.2 mM) (Baldessarini and Lipinski, 1975). No adverse effects were noted by the subjects.

No alteration in CSA content could be detected in the 4 hour conditioned media. The CSA content of the 7 day mononuclear cell

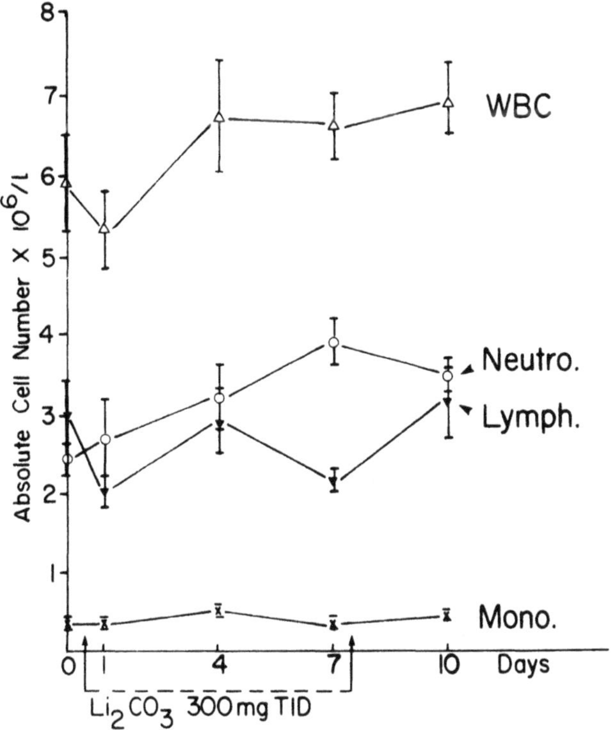

Figure 3. Absolute Differential counts during course of lithium treatment.

conditioned media is presented in Figure 4. A slight increase was noted within twelve hours of initiation of the oral lithium therapy, but was significantly elevated at day 4 and day 7. The peak increase was at day 7, when the CSA content was approximately 1.5 times the baseline and control values. The CSA content of the four controls did not vary during the course of the study. By day 10, CSA content of the 7 day conditioned media from lithium treated subjects approached baseline values.

Differential counts of the mononuclear cell preparations did not vary significantly during the course of the experiment. No sample had more

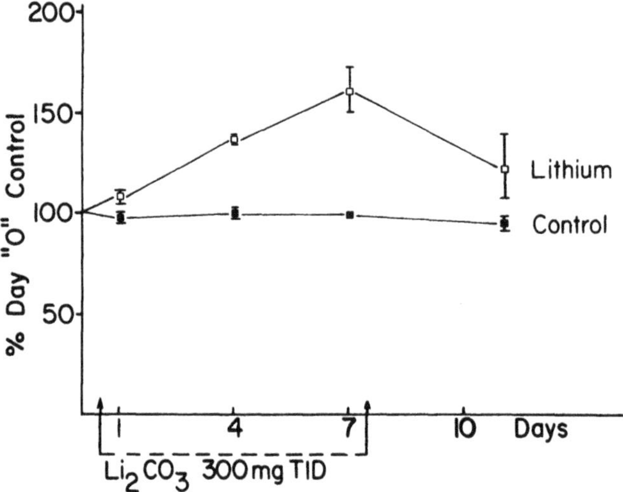

Figure 4. Alteration in CSA content of 7 day conditioned media during course of experiment. The difference between lithium treated subjects and controls is significant at days 4 and 7 ($p < 0.01$).

than 3% contamination with polymorphonuclear cells and most had less than 1% contamination. Lymphoid cells made up two-thirds of the preparation and monocytes the remaining third. Occasional basophils were noted.

DISCUSSION

This study has examined the changes in peripheral blood leukocyte counts and colony stimulating activity (CSA) production in hematologically normal human subjects taking lithium carbonate (300 mg three times daily) for seven days. This particular time period was chosen because a seven day course of lithium carbonate following myelotoxic chemotherapy has been shown to reduce significantly the risk of neutropenic complications (Turner and MacDonald, 1979). In this study, neutrophilia was evident by day 4 of therapy, and there was a coincident rise in CSA production from peripheral blood mononuclear cells.

It is not possible, with the information presently available, to say that the two events are connected. One might expect a delay of several days between the release of CSA and the appearance of mature neutrophils if CSA action on the committed granulocyte-macrophage progenitor is the sole mechanism at work. Neutrophils may be released from the marrow into the blood in increased numbers (cf. neutrophil-inducing activity) (Boggs, 1974). However, no significant shift to the left was noted in differential counts. It has also been suggested that the intravascular life-span of neutrophils may be prolonged when a patient is on lithium carbonate therapy (Mant et al., 1979).

The increase in CSA content of 7 day conditioned media would indicate that synthesis of CSA has been turned on (Harker et al., 1977; Kurnick et al., 1977). The lack of alteration of CSA content in the 4 hour conditioned media supports two conclusions. The first is that the augmentation of colony formation was not due to the presence of lithium or non-specific stimulants in the conditioned media. Secondly, pre-formed CSA was not being released from the mononuclear cells (Baker and Galbraith, 1975).

Previous studies have investigated the mechanism of action of lithium on granulopoiesis. A reversible neutrophilic leukocytosis in lithium treated psychiatric patients has been documented (Murphy et al., 1971; Shopsin et al., 1971). Tisman et al. (1973) suggested that there was an increased granulocyte mass on the basis of an increased vitamin B_{12} binding protein concentration in the sera of patients on lithium. Subsequently, it was shown that small amounts of lithium can cause the release of B_{12} binding protein from mature leukocytes (Scott et al., 1974). However, their conclusions were supported by radioisotope cell labelling studies, which demonstrated an increase in total granulocyte mass (Rothstein et al., 1978). These studies, and others, have shown that the neutrophilia seen in lithium treated patients is not due to demargination (Stein et al., 1978) or emptying of the marrow granulocyte reserve (Rothstein et al., 1978).

Tisman et al. (1973) also reported on augmentation of CFU-c growth when lithium was added to in vitro cultures in therapeutically reasonable concentrations. This increase in CFU-c was not due to a direct stimulation of stem cell proliferation but to an increase in CSA production from the cellular underlayer used. The role of CSA in lithium induced granulocytosis was first proposed by Gupta et al. (1976) who found an increased concentration of CSA in the blood and urine of Felty's syndrome patients treated with lithium. An increase in CSA in urine of lithium treated normal subjects has also been reported (Malloy et al., 1978). The CSA was assayed against murine marrow. Harker et al. (1977) have shown that in vitro incubation of mouse lung tissue with lithium in concentrations achieved in humans, results in increased synthesis of murine CSA. In a study of two neutropenic subjects and one normal control, the addition of 2 mM lithium to blood mononuclear cells resulted in increased CSA production (Barrett et al., 1977b). Morley and Galbraith (1978) have challenged the notion that mononuclear cells will increase CSA production in the presence of lithium. They have suggested that lithium enhances the effect of CSA on the CFU-c stem cell.

The present study has shown a definite increase in CSA production from human mononuclear cells from normal subjects taking oral lithium carbonate. The data suggest that the neutrophilia seen after 7 days therapy was not the maximal level attainable in longer term treatment situations. When such a level is obtained, and a new steady state is established, it may be that the increased CSA production is turned off. In any event, the increased CSA seen in the first few days of lithium therapy may be the reason for the protective effect of a short course of lithium given after chemotherapy (Turner and MacDonald, 1979).

REFERENCES

Amdisen, A., 1977, Serum level monitoring and clinical pharmacokinetics of lithium, Clin. Pharmacokinet. 2:73.

Baker, F.L. and Galbraith, P.R., 1975, Reappraisal of serum colony-stimulating factor, Clin. Res. 22:625A.

Baldessarini, R.J. and Lipinski, J.F., 1975, Lithium salts: 1970-1975, Ann. Intern. Med. 83:527.

Barrett, A.J., Hugh-Jones, K., and Newton, K.A., 1977a, Lithium therapy in aplastic anemia, The Lancet 1:202.

Barrett, A.J., Griscelli, C., and Buriot, D., 1977b, Lithium therapy in congenital neutropenia, The Lancet 2:1357.

Boggs, D.R., 1974, Granulocytes and monocytes, in "Clinical Hematology" (Wintrobe, M.M., ed.), p. 254, Lea and Febiger, Philadelphia.

Boyum, A., 1968, Isolation of mononuclear cells and granulocytes from human blood, Scand. J. Clin. Lab. Invest. 21 (Suppl 97):77.

Chervenick, P.A. and Boggs, D.R., 1970, Bone marrow colonies: Stimulation in vitro by supranatent from incubated human blood cells, Science, 169:691.

Chervenick, P.A. and LoBuglio, A.F., 1972, Human blood monocyte stimulator of granulocyte and mononuclear colony formation in vitro, Science 178:164.

English, D. and Andersen, B.R., 1974, Single step separation of red blood cells, granulocyte and mononuclear leukocytes on discontinuous density gradients of Ficoll-Hypaque, J. Immunol. Methods 5:249.

Gupta, R.C., Robinson, W.A., and Kurnick, J.E., 1976, Felty's syndrome: Effect of lithium on granulopoiesis, Am. J. Med. 61:29.

Harker, W.G., Rothstein, G., Clarkson, D., Athens, J.W., and MacFarlane, J.L., 1977, Enhancement of colony-stimulating activity production by lithium, Blood 49:263.

Jacob, E. and Herbert V., 1974, Lithium therapy for neutropenia, J. Clin. Invest., 53:35a.

Joyce, R.A. and Chervenick, P.A., 1975, Effect of lithium on release of colony-stimulating activity from blood leukocytes, Proc.Am.Soc.Hematol. 18:126a.

Kurnick, J.E., Stonington, O.R., and Robinson, W.A., 1977, Kinetics of colony stimulating factor (CSF) production by mononuclear cells (MNC), Clin. Res. 25:116a.

Malloy, N.L., Zauber, N.P., and Chervenick, P.A., 1978, The effect of lithium on blood and marrow neutrophils, Blood 52:462 (Supplement 1).

Mant, M.J., Herbert, F.A., and Akabutu, J.J., 1979, Successful lithium carbonate therapy in a patient with symptomatic Felty's syndrome, Ann. R. Coll. Physicians Surg. Can. 12:128a.

Morley, D.C. and Galbraith, P.R., 1978, Effect of lithium on granulopoiesis in culture, Can. Med. Assoc. J. 118:288.

Murphy, D.L., Goodwin, F.K., and Bunney, W.E., 1971, Leukocytosis during lithium treatment, Amer. J. Psychiat. 127:1559.

Pike, B.L. and Robinson, W.A., 1970, Human bone marrow colony growth in agar gel, J. Cell. Physiol. 76:77.

Rothstein, G., Clarkson, D.R., Larsen, W., Grosser, B.L., and Athens, J.W., 1978, Effect of lithium on neutrophil mass and production, N. Eng. J. Med. 298:178.

Schapria, D.V., Gordon, P.A., and Herbert, F.A., 1977, Reduction of infections in Felty's syndrome through use of lithium, Arthritis Rheum. 20:1556.

Scott, J.M., Bloomfield, F.J., and Stebbins, R., 1974, Studies on derivation of transcolbalamin III from granulocytes, J. Clin. Invest. 53:228.

Shopsin, B., Friedmann, R., and Gershon, S., 1971, Lithium and leukocytosis, Clin. Pharm. Ther. 12:923.

Stein, R.S., Hanson, G., Koethe, S., and Hansen, R., 1978, Lithium-induced granulopoiesis, Ann. Intern. Med. 88:809.

Tisman, G., Herbert, V., and Rosenblatt, S., 1973, Evidence that lithium induces human granulocyte proliferation: Elevated serum vitamin B12 binding capacity in vivo and granulocyte colony proliferation in vitro, Br. J. Haematol. 24:767.

Turner, A.R. and MacDonald, R.N., 1979, A placebo controlled study of a seven day course of lithium carbonate following myelotoxic chemotherapy, (This volume).

EFFECTS OF LITHIUM CHLORIDE ON HUMAN AND MURINE MARROW MYELOID COLONY FORMATION AND COLONY STIMULATING ACTIVITY

Peter L. Greenberg, Beverly Packard, and Susan M. Steed

Department of Medicine, Veterans Administration Hospital
and Stanford Medical Center
Palo Alto, California 94304

Prior studies have indicated that oral administration of lithium salts causes neutrophilia due to increased granulopoiesis in normal individuals and in some patients with hematologic disorders (Gupta et al., 1976; Malloy et al., 1978; Rothstein et al., 1978). Controversy exists regarding the mechanism whereby lithium exerts this granulopoietic effect. Studies in mice have demonstrated that production of colony stimulating activity (CSA) by extramedullary cell sources (e.g. lung) is enhanced following in vitro exposure to lithium (Harker et al., 1977). Studies with human cells have reported both increased CSA production by peripheral blood leukocytes (Joyce and Chervenick, 1975) and an adjuvant effect on granulopoietic precursor cells (in vitro colony forming cells, CFU-C) (Morley and Galbraith, 1978). Increased urinary and serum CSA levels occur following in vivo administration of lithium (Gupta et al., 1976); however, these sources of CSA are stimulatory for murine but not human marrow CFU-C in vitro.

Recent evidence has suggested that intramedullary production of CSA may be critically related to enhancing granulopoiesis (Chan and Metcalf, 1972; Chan and Metcalf, 1973). Therefore, we have assessed the ability of lithium chloride (LiCl) to augment in vitro production of human and murine marrow cell sources of CSA. In addition, we have evaluated the effects of this agent for altering marrow CFU-C generation in the presence of preformed CSA.

METHODS

Our technique of evaluating CSA production by human marrow cells has previously been described (Greenberg *et al.*, 1978). The physical separation procedure used entails removal of relatively dense cells by Hypaque-Ficoll gradient centrifugation and separation of the remaining cells into mononuclear cell fractions which are either adherent or nonadherent to plastic tissue culture dishes. We have previously shown (Greenberg *et al.*, 1978), and confirmed in this study, that buoyant density adherent cells produce . 90% of the intramedullary CSA, termed CSA_{BM}. Nonadherent buoyant human marrow cells are used as target CFU-C. Colony size and morphology are evaluated at 7-10 days of agar gel culture with medium comprised of McCoy's 5A medium supplemented with fetal calf serum and 0.5 mM 2-mercaptoethanol. Colonies are composed of greater than 50 cells and have been demonstrated cytochemically to be granulocytic and/or monocytic.

To assess the effect of lithium for increasing CSA production, unseparated, adherent and nonadherent cell populations were exposed to LiCl concentrations of 0.5-5 mM for the 7-10 day period of *in vitro* incubation. (Therapeutic serum concentrations of lithium salts are approximately 1 mM). The conditioned media prepared in this manner were assayed for CSA by testing them against nonadherent buoyant human marrow target cells. To evaluate the effect of lithium on CFU-C stimulation, LiCl was added to nonadherent buoyant human marrow cells in the presence of varying concentrations of preformed CSA (human placental conditioned medium). The placental conditioned medium was prepared as previously described (Burgess *et al.*, 1977).

Studies to evaluate mouse endosteal marrow cell production of CSA were performed by adding LiCl to tibias of C57Bl mice. The tibias, depleted of hemopoietic cells by rinsing, were split longitudinally, cultured for 7-10 days to provide conditioned media and assayed for CSA as previously described (Chan and Metcalf, 1972). The effect of lithium on mouse CFU-C was assessed by adding LiCl to mouse marrow target cells in the presence of varying concentrations of preformed CSA (L-cell conditioned medium). The L-cell conditioned medium was prepared as previously described (Greenberg and Mosny, 1977).

Statistical analyses were performed utilizing Student's t test, with p values , 0.05 considered significant.

TABLE I. ALTERATION IN HUMAN CFU-C GENERATION BY LiCl

LiCl (mM)	Dilutions of CSA[a] 1 X	0.5 X	0.25 X	0.06 X
0.5	7.9 ± 5.5[b](4)[c]	10.1 ± 7.7(4)	27.6 ± 4[d] (4)	41.2 ± 7.9[e] (4)
1	13.4 ± 2.4[e](6)	11.7 ± 5.8(4)	24.5 ± 7.1[e](7)	62.0 ± 11.6[e](4)
2	18.9 ± 5.4[e](6)	8.2 ± 7.9 (4)	28.1 ± 10.5[d](7)	73.7 ± 13.2[d](3)
5	-10.5 ± 12.6 (2)	17.9 ± 7.5 (2)	32.4 ± 19.8 (2)	58.9 ± 3.7[d] (2)

a Placental conditioned medium.

b % mean increment in colony number ± SE.

c Number in parenthesis indicates the number of separate experiments performed for the cited value.

d Significantly increased colony number compared to cultures lacking lithium, $p < 0.05$

e Significantly increased colony number compared to cultures lacking lithium, $p < 0.02$

RESULTS

Human Studies

Table I shows the results of experiments demonstrating the ability of LiCl to increase CFU-C generation in the presence of preformed CSA. As indicated, significant peak CFU-C increments occurred (25-74%) at concentrations of 0.5-2 mM LiCl with 0.25 x and 0.06 x dilutions of CSA. At higher CSA concentrations less pronounced CFU-C increments occurred in the presence of LiCl. In contrast, CSA production by human adherent marrow cells (CSA_{BM}) was only minimally and not significantly increased at concentrations of 1 and 5 mM LiCl, the increments being 10 ± 8.1% and 33 ± 14%, respectively. At the higher lithium concentration carry over (i.e. 0.65 mM) of lithium with direct effects on CFU-C generation in the presence of CSA was substantial. LiCl without CSA did not stimulate colony formation.

Murine Studies

No increment in CFU-C generation occurred in six separate experiments using concentrations of 0.1-4 mM LiCl with preformed CSA. Rather, as shown in Table II, dose-related decreases of CFU-C generation occurred, which were significant at LiCl concentrations $\geq$ 2 mM. No increase in endosteal marrow CSA production by mouse tibias was noted at concentrations of 1 and 5 mM (decrements of 9.7 ± 14.3% and 27.5 ± 4.5% respectively, were noted). Again, the carry over of lithium with substantial exposure of marrow target cells to the drug occurred at the higher concentrations.

DISCUSSION

These studies demonstrated that therapeutic concentrations of LiCl (0.5-2 mM) significantly increased *in vitro* myeloid colony formation 25-74% by nonadherent buoyant human marrow cells in the presence of low concentrations of preformed CSA. The low CSA concentrations may be "basal" *in situ* since modulation, dilution and/or depletion of intramedullary CSA levels occurs by nonadherent and dense cells (Broxmeyer *et al.*, 1977;

Greenberg _et al._, 1979; Haskill _et al._, 1972). Our data suggest that lithium may contribute to human granulopoiesis by enhancing CFU-C responsiveness to low/basal levels of CSA. Prior studies by other workers

TABLE II

ALTERATION IN MOUSE CFU-C GENERATION BY LiCl

LiCl (mM)	
0.1	-3.7 ± 13.1[a]
0.5	-11.0 ± 13.5
1.0	-16.4 ± 7.2
1.5	-18.8 ± 6.2
2.0	-29.0 ± 3.9[b]
4.0	-74.7 ± 1.4[b]

a Mean % decrement in colony number ± SE utilizing L-cell conditioned medium as CSA source.

b Significantly decreased colony number compared to cultures lacking lithium, $p < 0.05$

(Morley and Galbraith, 1978) have also indicated that lithium may enhance the effect of CSA on human granulocytic precursor responsiveness. These findings are of interest in view of our prior data demonstrating decreased CSA_{BM} in patients with acute myeloid leukemia who had poor prognoses (Greenberg et al., 1978). The mechanism whereby lithium augments responsiveness to CSA is not known. Prior studies have demonstrated that lithium interferes with cAMP-mediated processes that are regulated by polypeptide hormones (Singer and Rotenberg, 1973). CFU-C proliferation is directly related to intracellular cGMP levels and inversely related to cAMP levels (Kurland et al., 1977; Oshita et al., 1977). Thus, lithium may act by alteration of levels of these reciprocal intracellular cyclic nucleotides.

In mice, CFU-C proliferation was not enhanced following in vitro exposure of these cells to LiCl in the presence of CSA. This lack of murine CFU-C responsiveness to lithium-enhanced stimulation suggests differing in vivo granulopoietic stimulatory mechanisms of lithium in mice and man.

CSA production by human adherent marrow cells and murine marrow endosteal cells (CSA_{BM}) was not significantly increased by in vitro exposure to LiCl. To the contrary, at least in mice, decrements in CSA production were found. At high LiCl concentrations, substantial carry over of lithium occurred in the conditioned media. This likely contributed to the modest increment in human CFU-C proliferation, by lithium's ability to enhance the responsiveness of CFU-C to CSA present in the conditioned media. The low relative amounts of CSA_{BM} production by LiCl does not support the hypothesis that lithium enhances granulopoiesis by increasing CSA production. These findings are in agreement with a prior study utilizing human cells (Morley and Galbraith, 1978) but differ from several others (Harker et al., 1977; Joyce and Chervenick, 1975). Certain differences in technique may explain these disparities, including the cell sources utilized for CSA generation (intra vs. extramedullary cells), the target marrow colony forming cells (nonadherent buoyant vs. unseparated human cells or use of murine cells), differing growth media and lithium concentrations utilized, and, as mentioned above, carry over of lithium in the conditioned media. Further investigations are needed to clarify these issues and should provide a basis for improved understanding of factors involved in granulopoietic regulation.

REFERENCES

Broxmeyer, H., Moore, M., and Ralph, P., 1977, Cell-free granulocyte colony inhibiting activity derived from human polymorphonuclear neutrophils, Exp. Hematol. 5:87.

Burgess, A.W., Wilson, E.M.A., and Metcalf, D., 1977, Stimulation by human placental conditioned medium of hemopoietic colony formation by human marrow cells, Blood 49:573.

Chan, S., and Metcalf, D., 1972, Local production of colony stumulating factor within the bone marrow: Role of nonhemopoietic cells, Blood 40:646.

Chan, S., and Metcalf, D., 1973, Local and systemic control of granulocytic and macrophagic progenitor cell regeneration after irradiation, Cell Tissue Kinet. 6:185.

Greenberg, P.L., and Mosny, S.A., 1977, Inhibitory effects in vitro of interferon on human and murine granulocytic progenitor cells, Cancer Res. 37:1794.

Greenberg, P.L., Mara, B., and Heller, P., 1978, Marrow cell colony stimulating activity in acute myeloid leukemia, Blood 52:362.

Greenberg, P.L., Packard, B., and Steed, S.M., 1979, Granulopoietic effects of lithium on marrow myeloid cells, manuscript in preparation.

Gupta, R., Robinson, W., and Kurnick, J., 1976, Felty's syndrome: Effect of lithium on granulopoiesis, Am. J. Med. 61:29.

Harker, W.G., Rothstein, G., Clarkson, D., and Athens, J., 1977, Enhancement of colony-stimulating activity production by lithium, Blood 49:263.

Haskill, J., McKnight, R., and Galbraith, P., 1972, Cell-cell interaction in vitro: Studied by density separation of colony forming, stimulating, and inhibiting cells from bone marrow, Blood 40:394.

Joyce, R., and Chervenick, P., 1975, Effect of lithium on the release of colony stimulating activity from blood leukocytes, Proc. Am. Soc. Hematol. (December, 1975), p. 126.

Kurland, J., Hadden, J., and Moore, M.A.S., 1977, Role of cyclic nucleotides in the proliferation of committed granulocyte-macrophage progenitor cells, Cancer Res. 37:4534.

Malloy, N., Zauber, N., and Chervenick, P., 1978, The effect of lithium on blood and marrow neutrophils, Proc. Am. Soc. Hematol. (December, 1978), p. 228.

Morley, D., and Galbraith, P., 1978, Effect of lithium on granulopoiesis in culture, Can. Med. Assn. Journal 118:288.

Oshita, A., Rothstein, G., and Lonngi, G., 1977, cGMP stimulation of stem cell proliferation, Blood 49:585.

Rothstein, G., Clarkson, D., Larsen, W., Grosser, B., and Athens, J., 1978, Effect of lithium on neutrophil mass and production, New Eng. J. Med. 298:178.

Singer, I., and Rotenberg, D., 1973, Mechanisms of lithium action, New Eng. J. Med. 289:254.

LITHIUM EFFECTS ON GRANULOPOIESIS IN MICE FOLLOWING CYTOTOXIC CHEMOTHERAPY

Robert A. Joyce, M.D. and Paul A. Chervenick, M.D.

Department of Medicine
University of Pittsburgh School of Medicine
Pittsburgh, PA 15261

Recent clinical studies have suggested that administration of lithium may modify the duration of neutropenia in patients receiving chemotherapy for treatment of acute leukemia (Stein _et al._, 1978) and solid tumors (Stein _et al._, 1977; Lyman _et al._, 1978). Fehir and Rossof (1978) reported similar effects of lithium in dogs following administration of cyclophosphamide. The mechanisms by which lithium increases blood neutrophil concentrations are not completely understood. Neutrophilia is associated with increased marrow neutrophil production (Malloy _et al._, 1978; Rothstein _et al._, 1978), increased neutrophil progenitor cells (CFU-C) (Tisman _et al._, 1973; Joyce and Chervenick, 1979) and enhanced release of colony stimulating activity (CSA) (Joyce and Chervenick, 1975; Harker _et al._, 1977). The present studies describe changes in hematopoiesis during daily administration of lithium chloride (Li) to normal mice and report enhanced recovery of granulopoiesis following administration of cytotoxic drugs.

METHODS

(C_{57} Bl female and DBA male) F_1 male mice bred in our laboratory from stock purchased from the Jackson Laboratory, Bar Harbor, ME, were used in all experiments. Animals were between 10 and 18 weeks of age.

Lithium chloride was diluted in normal saline. When given to mice in a dose of 60 mg/kg, serum Li level 2 hours later was 0.64 meq/L. This dose was used in all subsequent experiments. Vinblastine sulfate (Vbl) and cyclophosphamide (CTX) were diluted in normal saline. Vbl was given in a dose of 4.0 mg/kg; and CTX, 200 mg/kg. Control mice were saline injected. All drugs were administered by intraperitoneal injection. Quantitative marrow counts were measured as described previously (Joyce and Chervenick, 1977). The morphologic features of Wright's stained murine granulocytes and their precursors have been described previously (Chervenick et al., 1968). Concentrations of CFU-C from mouse marrow were determined by measuring colony formation in the soft gel culture system as described by Pluznik and Sacks (1965) and Bradley and Metcalf (1966) using methylcellulose in place of agar (Chervenick and Boggs, 1970) and 10% L-cell conditioned media as a source of CSA.

Serum and lung conditioned media (CM) were tested for CSA by their ability to stimulate colony formation from mouse marrow when added in a volume of 0.1 ml to each 0.9 ml of marrow cell mixture. CM were prepared by incubating lung tissue, 70 mg/ml, in CMRL-1066 tissue culture media containing 15% fetal calf serum. After 7 days at $37^{o}C$ in 7.5 percent CO_2, media were collected, passed through a Millipore filter (pore size, 0.45 μm) and frozen until tested for CSA.

Cell cycle characteristics of mouse CFU-C were measured by determining the degree to which colony forming capacity of the cultured cells was lost following tritiated thymidine (^{3}HTdR) suicide as described previously (Joyce and Chervenick, 1977). Pluripotent hematopoietic stem cells (CFU-S) per humerus were calculated as the product of quantitative marrow counts of donor mice and the number of macroscopic spleen colonies 8 days following intravenous injection of 10^5 marrow cells/mouse into irradiated recipients (900 rads).

RESULTS

Changes in blood neutrophil concentration following daily Li administration to normal mice are shown in Figure 1. There was little change in blood neutrophils by day 4 of Li compared to saline injected controls (2700

± 400/μl vs 2200 ± 200). Thereafter, neutrophil concentration increased, reaching levels nearly 3 fold greater than controls by day 11 (6500 ± 100/μl). With continued Li, neutrophils gradually declined and by day 18 had decreased toward normal.

The effect of Li on marrow granulopoiesis in normal mice is seen in Table I. The number of CFU-C was unchanged from controls by day 2 of Li, but increased nearly 2 fold on days 5 and 8. Similar changes were observed in the mitotic pool on days 5 and 8. In the post-mitotic pool, the maximum increment of cells was detected later, on day 8. By day 11, the concentrations of cells in both the mitotic and post-mitotic pools remained 1.5 to 2 times greater than control values.

Changes in the levels of CSA in the sera of mice given Li are shown in Figure 2. There was no difference in serum CSA during the first several days of Li administration. However, significantly higher levels of CSA were detected on day 5 ($p < 0.001$), at a time when the concentration of blood neutrophils was increasing.

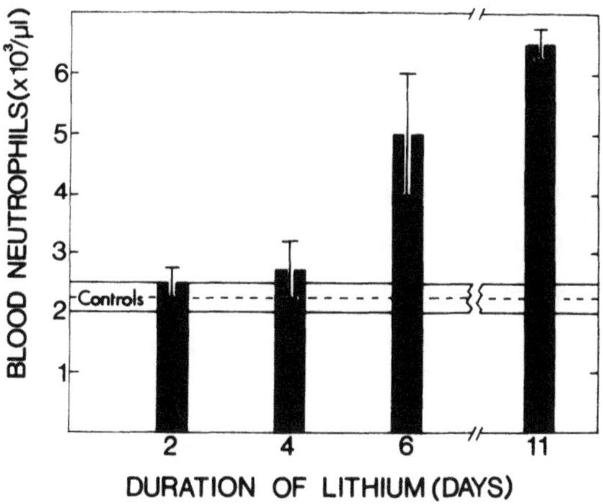

Figure 1. Blood neutrophil concentrations during administration of lithium chloride to normal mice. Data represent the mean ± standard error of groups of 3 to 6 separate mice. Control values are the combined values from saline injected mice during the study.

TABLE I

LITHIUM EFFECT ON MARROW GRANULOPOIESIS[a]

	Cells Per Humerus		
Duration of Lithium (Days)	CFU-C ($x10^3$)	Mitotic Pool ($x10^6$)	Post-Mitotic Pool ($x10^6$)
2	10.6 ± 0.7	1.9 ± 0.1	4.1 ± 0.3
5	19.0 ± 0.9	2.8 ± 0.1	4.2 ± 0.2
8	18.2 ± 0.4	2.9 ± 0.1	6.4 ± 0.1
11	11.9 ± 0.6	2.6 ± 0.1	4.8 ± 0.2
Controls	11.4 ± 0.5	1.4 ± 0.1	3.5 ± 0.1

[a]Data represent values collected from 4 to 6 mice in 2 separate experiments, expressed as mean ± standard error. Controls represent pooled values from saline injected mice during the experiments.

The release of CSA into media conditioned by lung tissue of Li treated mice is seen in Figure 3. A substantial increase in levels of CSA was observed in media conditioned for 7 days by lung tissue of mice after 1 day of Li, reaching levels nearly 3 fold greater than controls (62 ± 2 colonies/10^5 marrow cells vs 26 ± 3 colonies). This increase in release of CSA by lung tissue from mice given Li was sustained through day 10 of Li (53 ± 6 colonies).

The effect of Li on cell cycle characteristics of CFU-C was measured by determining the percent survival of CFU-C after exposure of marrow cells to ^{3}HTdR. No change in CFU-C survival was detected on day 2 of Li compared to untreated controls. However, by day 6 of Li, a significant decrease in survival was observed suggesting that a larger proportion of precursor cells was in replicative cycle.

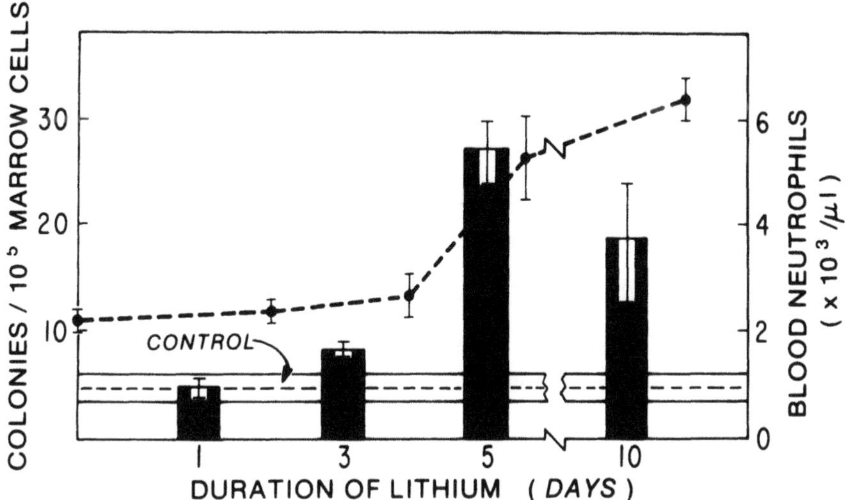

Figure 2. Relationship of blood neutrophil concentration (dashed line) to levels of serum CSA in mice given lithium. Serum was collected from groups of 10 mice on the days indicated in 2 separate experiments. Values represent the number of colonies per 10^5 mouse marrow cells stimulated by 0.1 ml serum, plated in triplicate and expressed as the mean ± standard error. Control values from serum of untreated mice are shown on the horizontal bar as the mean ± standard error.

Changes in marrow CFU-S during Li administration to normal mice were observed earlier than increments of either serum CSA or marrow CFU-C. By day 2 of Li, the number of CFU-S was significantly greater than control values and remained elevated through day 11 of Li administration.

The effects of Li on granulopoietic recovery in mice following cytotoxic chemotherapy was studied using Vbl. Animals were given Vbl, 4 mg/kg, or Vbl plus daily Li starting on the day following Vbl. Changes in blood neutrophil concentrations are seen in Figure 4. During the first 3 days following Vbl, neutrophil concentrations decreased in both groups.

However, blood neutrophils increased to normal levels a day earlier, on day 4, in mice given daily Li (1600 ± 300/μl). Neutrophils then increased in both groups until day 6 and gradually declined thereafter.

The effect of Li on marrow recovery of CFU-C after Vbl is seen in Table II. In mice given Vbl alone, the nadir of marrow CFU-C was reached on day 2 and increased to maximum concentration on day 4 after Vbl. In mice given Li daily following Vbl, CFU-C were significantly greater on day 3 compared with CFU-C from mice given Vbl alone. Maximum increase in CFU-C was also observed on day 3 in mice given Li. It was detected later, on day 4, in mice given Vbl alone.

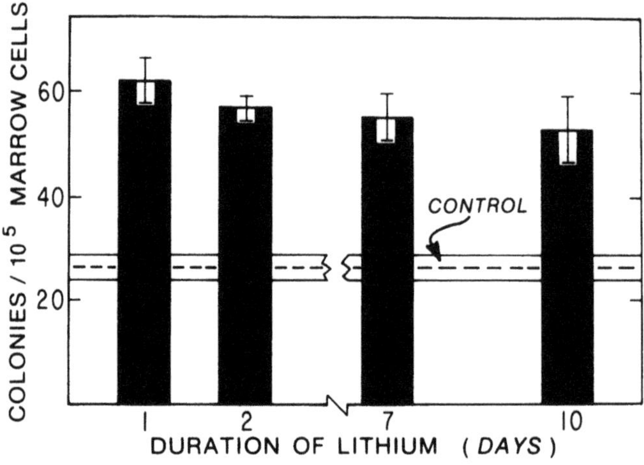

Figure 3. Effect of lithium administration upon CSA release by lung tissue. Values represent the number of colonies per 10^5 mouse marrow cells stimulated by 0.1 ml CM.

Recovery of marrow CFU-C was also measured in mice given Vbl following administration of Li for 2 and 6 days prior to Vbl (Figure 5). In mice given Li for 2 days prior to Vbl, marrow CFU-C reached a nadir on day 1 following Vbl. Thereafter, until day 5, Vbl treated mice given prior Li had significantly greater concentrations of CFU-C than mice given Vbl alone ($p < 0.05$). In mice given Li for 6 days prior to Vbl, the numbers of CFU-C were increased at the time Vbl was given. Following a decrease at day 1, marrow CFU-C increased earlier and reached maximum concentrations sooner compared with mice given Li for 2 days before Vbl or mice given Vbl alone.

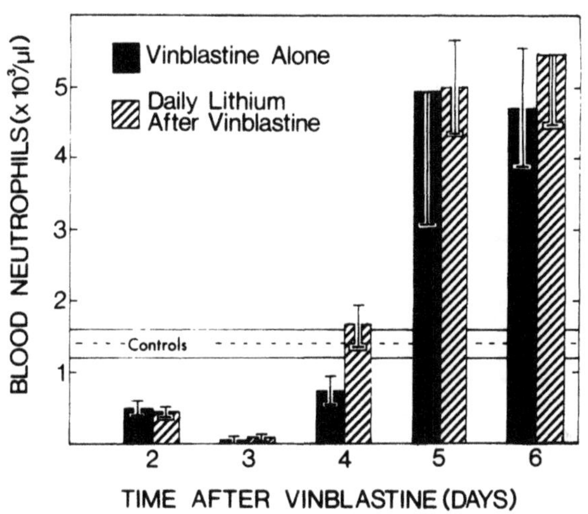

Figure 4. Blood neutrophil concentration after vinblastine, 4 mg/kg, and vinblastine followed by daily lithium, 60 mg/kg. Each value represents the mean ± standard error from 4 to 6 mice.

To determine if Li alters the cytotoxic effect of Vbl on marrow CFU-C, normal marrow cells were incubated in media containing Vbl with and without Li. Cells were then washed and the number of CFU-C measured. No change in the *in vitro* cytotoxic effect of Vbl on CFU-C was noted in the presence of Li.

Similar changes in marrow CFU-C recovery were observed in mice given CTX with and without Li. Administration of Li daily following CTX resulted in a more rapid increment of CFU-C and significantly higher concentrations of marrow CFU-C on days 3 and 4 after CTX ($p < 0.001$). CFU-C declined in both groups on day 5, but remained significantly higher in mice given daily Li compared with mice given CTX without subsequent Li ($29.9 \pm 1.8 \times 10^3$ colonies/humerus vs $17.5 \pm 1.8 \times 10^3$, $p < 0.001$). When Li was given for 6 days before CTX was administered, a more rapid increment in CFU-C was detected on day 3 after CTX compared with CFU-C recovery following CTX alone. Peak levels of CFU-C were reached on day 4 after CTX in both groups, but this was significantly greater in mice given prior Li.

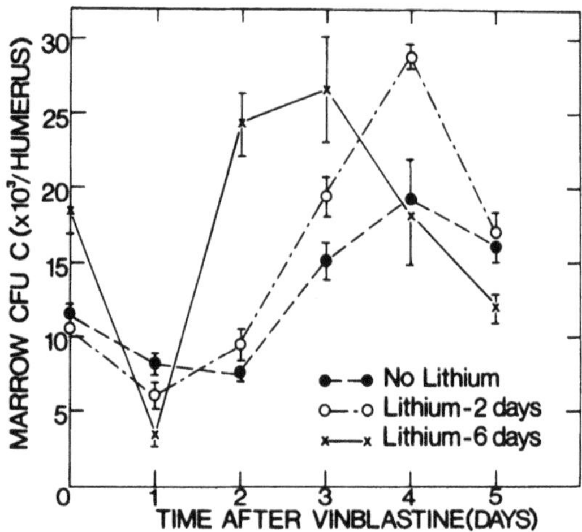

Figure 5. Recovery of marrow CFU-C following vinblastine alone or vinblastine with lithium for 2 and 6 days prior to vinblastine. Data are from two separate experiments plated in triplicate and expressed as the mean ± standard error.

DISCUSSION

These studies demonstrate that the murine hematopoietic system is a useful model to study the effects of Li on neutrophil production. Administration of Li to mice increases blood neutrophil concentration and is associated with increased marrow neutrophil production, increased proliferation of CFU-C and higher levels of serum CSA. In addition, administration of Li enhances the number of CFU-S in normal mice. In mice given cytotoxic chemotherapy, administration of Li enhances the recovery of marrow CFU-C and may lessen the hematotoxicity of these agents on granulocyte progenitor cells.

TABLE II

EFFECT OF LITHIUM ON MARROW CFU-C AFTER VINBLASTINE

Days After Vinblastine	CFU-C ($x10^3$ per humerus)[a]	
	No Lithium	Lithium
2	7.6 ± 0.4	8.5 ± 0.3
3	15.1 ± 1.2	20.0 ± 2.2[b]
4	19.3 ± 2.7	18.4 ± 1.6
5	16.1 ± 1.0	13.1 ± 0.6[b]
6	9.5 ± 0.6	11.4 ± 0.7[b]
Controls	11.4 ± 0.5	

[a]Data represent studies from 4 to 6 mice in separate experiments expressed as mean ± standard error.
[b]$p < 0.05$

REFERENCES

Chervenick, P.A. and Boggs, D.R., 1970, Bone marrow colonies: Stimulati on *in vitro* by supernatant from incubated human blood cells, Science 169:691.

Chervenick, P.A., Boggs, D.R., Marsh, J.C., Cartwright, G.E., and Wintrobe, M.M., 1968, Quantitative studies of blood and bone marrow neutrophils in normal mice, Am. J. Physiol. 215:353.

Fehir, K.M. and Rossof, A.H., 1977, Lithium carbonate protects canine granulopoiesis from damage by cyclophosphamide, Clin. Res. 26:434A.

Harker, W.G., Rothstein, G., Clarkson, D., Athens, J.W., and Macfarlane, J.L., 1977, Enhancement of colony-stimulating activity production by lithium, Blood 49:263.

Joyce, R.A. and Chervenick, P.A., 1975, Effect of lithium on the release of colony-stimulating activity from blood leukocytes, Proc. Am. Soc. Hematol. 18:126.

Joyce, R.A. and Chervenick, P.A., 1977, Corticosteroid effect on granulopoiesis in mice after cyclophosphamide, J. Clin. Invest. 60:277.

Joyce, R.A. and Chervenick, P.A., 1979, Lithium effects on granulopoiesis following vinblastine, Clin. Res. 27:388A.

Lyman, G.H., Williams, C.C., and Preston, D., 1978, A prospective randomized study of the effect of lithium carbonate on the granulocytopenia and incidence of infection associated with intensive chemotherapy and radiation therapy for undifferentiated small cell bronchogenic carcinoma, Blood 52:228 (Supplement 1).

Malloy, E.L., Zauber, N.P., and Chervenick, P.A., 1978, The effect of lithium on blood and marrow neutrophils, Blood 52:228 (Supplement 1).

Rothstein, G., Clarkson, D.R., Larsen, W., Grosser, B.I., and Athens, J.W., 1978, Effect of lithium on neutrophil mass and production, N. Eng. J. Med. 298:178.

Stein, R.S., Beaman, C., Ali, M.Y., Hansen, R., Jenkins, D.D., and Jume'an, H.G., 1977, Lithium carbonate attenuation of chemotherapy-induced neutropenia, N. Eng. J. Med. 297:430.

Stein, R.S., Flexner, J.M., and Graber, S., 1978, Lithium and granulocytopenia during induction therapy of acute myelogenous leukemia, Blood 52:277 (Supplement 1).

Tisman, G., Herbert, V., and Rosenblatt, S., 1973, Evidence that lithium induces human granulocyte proliferation: Elevated serum vitamin B12 binding capacity in vivo and granulocyte colony formation in vitro, Br. J. Hematol. 24:767.

LITHIUM CARBONATE ENHANCES GRANULOPOIESIS AND ATTENUATES CYCLOPHOSPHAMIDE-INDUCED INJURY IN THE DOG

A.H. Rossof, K.M. Fehir, H.S. Budd,
A. Murthy, and S.G.Economou

Departments of Medicine, Therapeutic Radiology, and
General Surgery
Rush-Presbyterian-St. Luke's Medical Center
1753 West Congress Parkway
Chicago, Illinois 60612

When given to manic-depressive psychiatric patients, lithium carbonate (LC) is associated with an increase in the number of circulating neutrophils (PMNs) (Mayfield and Brown, 1966; O'Connell, 1970; Shopsin et al., 1971; Murphy et al., 1971, Watanabe et al., 1974; and Bille et al., 1975). This is an intriguing "side effect" which suggests several potential clinical applications: 1) prevention or attenuation of myelosuppression due to anti-cancer chemotherapy or radiotherapy; 2) treatment of neutropenic disorders not related to cancer therapy; 3) preparation of granulocyte donors prior to leucopheresis; and 4) acceleration of engraftment of bone marrow allografts or autografts. A detailed analysis of LC enhanced granulopoiesis and some prediction of its efficacy in these potential roles would be aided if a suitable animal model were available for comprehensive study. It is the purpose of this report to present our observations on lithium carbonate stimulation of marrow granulocyte-committed colony-forming units (CFU-c) and peripheral blood granulocytes in mongrel dogs and the protection offered these dogs from cyclophosphamide-induced marrow injury.

MATERIALS AND METHODS

Experiment 1

Four mongrel dogs were used in the first experiment. Their stools were free of parasites and they had no eosinophilia of the peripheral blood. Automated blood counts were performed using the Coulter Method S. Differential counts were done on Wright-Giemsa stained air-dried peripheral smears. Absolute granulocyte counts were calculated by multiplying the percent PMNs by the total white blood cell count (WBC).

Marrow granulocyte-committed colony-forming units (CFU-c) in the agar culture system were assayed according to the technique of Marsh et al. (1972). Employing aseptic technique, marrow was aspirated from the iliac crest after anaesthesia with intravenous thiamylal sodium. A standard Limarzi bone marrow aspiration needle was used and 1-2 ml of marrow were aspirated into 1 ml of normal dog serum containing 10-20 units/ml of preservative-free heparin. The bone marrow cells were allowed to sediment by gravity in 15 ml plastic test tubes at room temperature for one to two hours. After washing the buffy coat two times with supplemented tissue culture medium TC-199, a nucleated cell count was performed and so adjusted that 3×10^5 nucleated bone marrow cells were cultured in each 35 mm plastic tissue culture dish. Each dish contained 1 ml of TC-199 supplemented with 1mM sodium pyruvate, 40 mg/ml 1-asparagine, 75 mg/ml DEAE-dextran, 10% fetal calf serum, penicillin-streptomycin mixture, and 0.3% agar. Each dish also contained 0.1 ml of serum from a lethally-irradiated neutropenic dog (Shivey et al., 1958) as a source of colony-stimulating activity (CSA). All specimens were cultured in quadruplicate and incubated at 37°C in a fully-humidified 5% CO_2 atmosphere. Colonies were counted using an inverted tissue culture microscope and were defined as aggregates of $\geq$ 50 cells after seven to ten days incubation.

After baseline peripheral blood studies and marrow CFU-c were obtained on two separate occasions over one week, each dog was given standard commercially available 300 mg capsules of LC by mouth twice daily. The dogs weighed 23-28 kg providing a daily dose of LC equivalent to 21-26 mg/kg body weight or 650-730 mg/m^2 body surface area to each dog. Peripheral blood counts were obtained semi-weekly and marrow CFU-c were obtained weekly after the LC was begun and over the next six weeks.

Experiment 2

Four different mongrel dogs, weighing 26-32 kg each, were selected for this experiment. Two were randomly chosen to receive LC, 300 mg by mouth twice daily. After a minimum of nine days exposure to LC, all four animals were given cyclophosphamide (CPA), 25 mg/kg, by intravenous bolus injection. Thereafter, peripheral blood counts and marrow CFU-c were studied semi-weekly over a period of two weeks.

RESULTS

Experiment 1

The LC treatment of these dogs resulted in prompt increments of the peripheral blood PMNs and marrow CFU-c. The mean data of all four dogs are shown in Table I and selected data are depicted graphically in Figure 1.

When analyzed by the non-parametric Friedman Two-Way Analysis of Variance by Ranks test (Siegel, 1956), the data were found to be highly significant: for the PMN data, $p = 0.003$; and for the CFU-c data, $p = 0.001$. When the hypothesis of no differences was tested against the particular alternate hypothesis that the means after lithium treatment were higher than the baseline means, using a variation of the sign test, the post-treatment means were found to be higher than the pre-treatment means for both sets of data ($p < 0.0001$ for both tests).

Experiment 2

The mean baseline CFU-c were higher in the LC treated dogs (61 and 56 vs 50 and 49) as were the baseline PMNs (11.6 and 13.6 vs 8.2 and 8.4 x $10^3/\mu l$). Prompt reduction of CFU-c and PMNs followed CPA in all four dogs with the nadirs for CFU-c reached at the third post-CPA day: 27 and 29 in the LC treated dogs vs 14 and 18 in the control dogs. Recovery of

TABLE I

HEMATOLOGIC DATA OF DOGS RECEIVING LITHIUM CARBONATE

Day	0	4	7	11	14	18	21	25	28	32	35	39
CFU-c	50		57		61		71		71		66	
PMN/μl x 10^3	5.5	10.7	6.8	9.6	6.2	8.9	10.7	9.3	10.7	8.8	8.4	10.2
WBC/μl x 10^3	10.1	17.7	10.9	15.7	10.1	15.1	14.6	15.4	16.2	14.4	13.7	16.0
Li^+, meq/l	0.06	0.37	0.58	0.84	0.78	0.53	0.80	0.19	1.30	0.35	1.23	0.41

Each CFU-c, PMN, WBC, and Li^+ data point represents the mean value on the given day of LC treatment of all four dogs. Each marrow CFU-c sample was studied in quadruplicate. CFU-c are expressed as colony number per 3 x 10^5 nucleated marrow cells plated. Baseline data ("Day O") were obtained on two separate occasions.

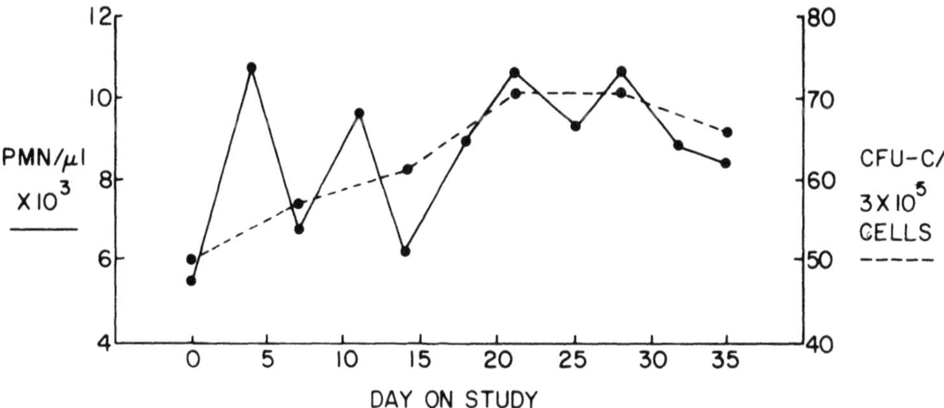

Figure 1. Peripheral blood PMN and marrow CFU-c contents during lithium carbonate treatment of four dogs. See legend to Table I for additional details.

CFU-c was initiated by the sixth post-CPA day in the LC prepared dogs, at a time when CFU-c values remained depressed in the two control dogs. Both control dogs died on the sixth day with no circulating PMNs.

The nadirs for PMNs were reached on the seventh post-CPA day in the LC treated animals with early recovery noted by the eighth day and complete recovery by the tenth day. The data on CFU-c are summarized graphically in Figures 2 and 3.

DISCUSSION

In the mouse, we (1975) and others (Greco, 1978), have been unable to increase the peripheral blood PMNs with lithium. However, our mongrel dogs respond promptly to LC with an increase of peripheral blood PMNs, similar to the effect seen in man. We have also demonstratred that LC increases the population of marrow granulocyte-committed stem cells (CFU-c) which is likely to lead to an expansion of the total body granulocyte population.

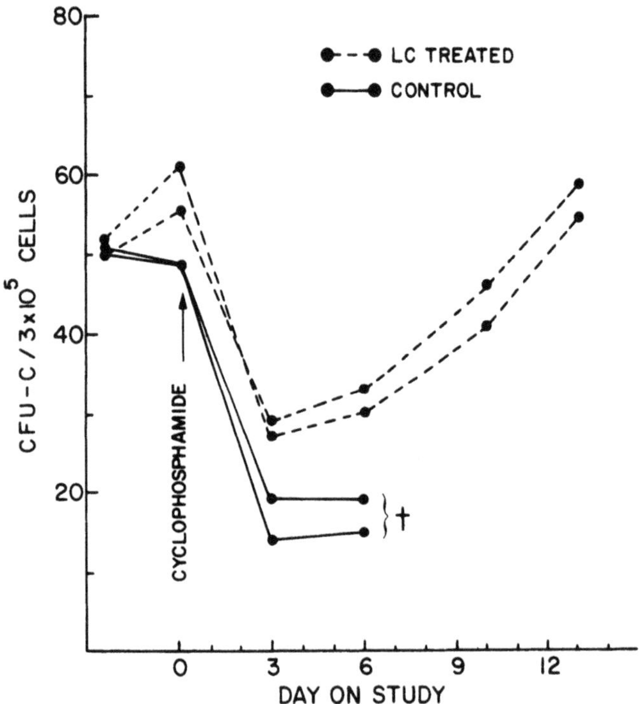

Figure 2. Fluctuations of the absolute marrow CFU-c values/3 x 10^5 nucleated marrow cells in each of the four dogs as a function of the day on study. Day 0 is the day of CPA administration. Dashed lines: LC pretreated animals; solid lines: animals not pretreated with LC. The cross signifies death of the animals.

Consistent with these findings are several related observations made by other investigators. Tisman et al. (1973) demonstrated that the unsaturated vitamin B_{12} binding capacity (UBBC) is elevated in psychiatric patients given LC therapeutically. The UBBC is an indirect assessment of the total body granulocyte pool. Rothstein et al. (1978) have reported their

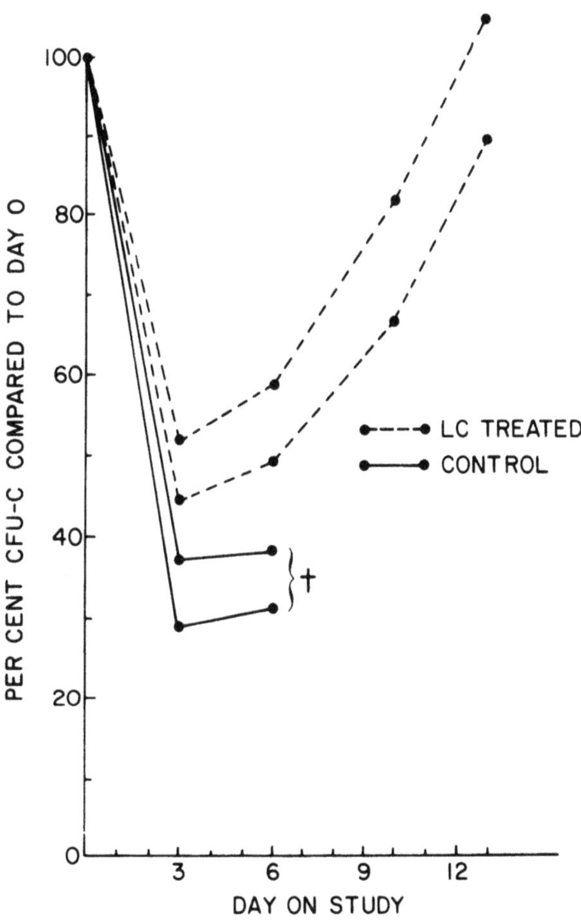

Figure 3. Percent deviations of marrow CFU-c compared to Day 0, the day of CPA administration, as a function of day on study for each of the four dogs. Dashed lines: LC pretreated animals; solid lines: animals not pretreated with LC. The cross signifies death of the animals.

direct measurements of granulocyte pool sizes using $DF^{32}P$-labelled granulocytes in psychiatric patients taking LC. They observed an increase of the total blood granulocyte pool and both of its components, the circulating granulocyte pool and the marginal granulocyte pool. They also observed a prolongation of the half-life of the circulating PMNs of their subjects.

Colony stimulating activity (CSA) is a hormone-like glycoprotein produced by the cells of the mononuclear phagocytic system, the monocytes and macrophages (Robinson and Mangalik, 1975), and by activated T cells (Ruscetti and Chervenick, 1975). This material stimulates granulopoiesis in vitro and possibly contributes to the regulation of granulopoiesis in vivo. In an in vitro system, Harker et al. (1977) have demonstrated that lithium chloride enhances production and elaboration of CSA by mouse lung tissue. This effect depends on de novo protein synthesis since it is inhibited by the addition of puromycin to the tissue culture medium. Enhanced production of CSA apparently also occurs in vivo. Gupta et al. (1976) have shown that the serum and urine levels of CSA can be increased in humans given LC for management of Felty's syndrome.

When considered together, we believe these several observations indicate that the Li^+ stimulates the production of CSA which in turn increases the CFU-c and results in expansion of the total body granulocyte pool. This includes the total blood granulocyte pool and is reflected, in its simplest form, as an increase in the number of circulating granulocytes. The precise subcellular or molecular mechanism(s) by which LC stimulates production of CSA remain unknown at this time (Rossof and Fehir, 1978), although Li^+ inhibition of adenyl cyclase with subsequent lowering of the intracellular cAMP, is a possible mechanism worthy of thorough investigation.

Of the several potential clinical applications of LC enhanced granulopoiesis, the most common and, hence, most important is the prevention or attenuation of myelosuppression due to anti-cancer chemotherapy or radiotherapy. Virtually all patients receiving these forms of treatment sustain damage to the bone marrow organ. This damage is commonly expressed as an acute transient injury with decline and recovery of circulating white blood cells and platelets. Serious acute complications can occur with each course of therapy and chronic complications may be seen after months and years of such therapy. As the tolerance of the bone marrow organ diminishes and doses of myelosuppressive therapy must be reduced accordingly, treatment becomes less effective and patients fail.

What is needed for the adjunctive management of these patients is an inexpensive, easily administered, relatively non-toxic agent that will increase the absolute PMN count without disturbing the PMNs' functional integrity. Several studies indicate that the function of PMNs is preserved in an environment containing Li^+ at concentrations in the therapeutic range (Rossof and Coltman, 1976; Cohen et al., 1979; Siegel et al., 1980). LC has been given to thousands of patients with great safety. For most patients, in the absence of problems of salt and water metabolism, the toxicity of LC is a direct function of serum Li^+ concentration and this can be measured readily in most clinical laboratories allowing careful monitoring of patient dosage.

We conclude from the second experiment that LC modifies the deleterious effect of CPA on granulopoiesis by increasing the baseline values of CFU-c and PMNs and by diminishing the apparent fractional cell kill of CFU-c. This could occur if cells from the totipotential stem cell compartment were shunted into the granulopoietic progenitor pool (CFU-c) or if Li^+ caused an expansion of the totipotential stem cell pool. Unfortunately, methods to evaluate the totipotential stem cell pool do not exist currently for studies in dogs or humans. The PMN nadirs reached were higher in LC prepared dogs, indicating the potential role of LC in attenuating the profound granulocyte nadirs that can occur with aggressive anti-neoplastic chemotherapy. Several pilot studies have recently provided evidence in support of this application of LC in the clinic (Tisman, 1974; Charron et al., 1977; Stein et al., 1977; Greco and Brereton, 1977: Stein et al., 1978; Lyman et al., 1978, Turner et al., 1979; Visca et al., 1979). Our studies provide data concerning the mechanism whereby LC seems effective in these clinical investigations.

ACKNOWLEDGEMENTS

This work was supported by grant CA 17086-03 from the National Cancer Institute, United States Public Health Service, and by the Gail Ann Ditore Hodgkins Fund, The Pearl Shack Memorial Cancer Fund, and the Wadsworth Memorial Research Foundation.

The faithful and careful assistance of Mr. Mike Hacklin and the staff of the Animal Resources Facility is gratefully acknowledged.

REFERENCES

Bille, P.E., Jensen, J.P.K., and Poulsen, J.C., 1975, Studies on the hematologic and cytogenetic effect of lithium, Acta Med. Scand. 198:281.

Charron, D., Barrett, A.J., Faille, A., Alby, N., Schmitt, T., and Degos, L., 1977, Lithium in acute myeloid leukemia, Lancet 1:1307.

Cohen, M.S., Zakhireh, B., Metcalf, J.A., and Root, R.K., 1979, Granulocyte function during lithium therapy, Blood 53:913.

Greco, F.A. and Brereton, H.D., 1977, Effect of lithium carbonate on the neutropenia caused by chemotherapy: a preliminary clinical trial, Oncology 34:153.

Greco, F.A., 1978, Personal communication.

Gupta, R.C., Robinson, W.A., and Kurnick, J.E., 1976, Felty's syndrome: effect of lithium on granulopoiesis, Am. J. Med. 61:29.

Harker, W.G., Rothstein, G., Clarkson, D.R., Athens, J.W., and MacFarlane, J.L., 1977, Enhancement of colony-stimulating activity production by lithium, Blood 49:263.

Lyman, G.H., Williams, C.C., and Preston, D., 1978, A prospective randomized study of the effect of lithium carbonate on the granulocytopenia and incidence of infection associated with intensive chemotherapy and radiation therapy for undifferentiated small cell bronchogenic carcinoma, Blood 52:228 (Supplement 1).

Marsh, J.C., Levitt, M., and Katzenstein, A., 1972, The growth of leukocyte colonies in vitro from dog bone marrow, J. Lab. Clin. Med. 79:1041.

Mayfield, D. and Brown, R.G., 1966, The clinical laboratory and electroencephalographic effects of lithium, J. Psychiat. Res. 4:207.

Murphy, D.L., Goodwin, F.K., and Bunney, W.E., Jr., 1971, Leukocytosis during lithium treatment, Amer. J. Psychiat. 127:1559.

O'Connell, R.A., 1970, Leukocytosis during lithium carbonate treatment, Int. Pharmacopsychiat. 4:30.

Robinson, W.A. and Mangalik, A., 1975, The kinetics and regulation of granulopoiesis, Sem. Hematol. 12:7.

Rossof, A.H., 1975, Unpublished observations.

Rossof, A.H. and Coltman, C.A., Jr., 1976, The effect of lithium carbonate on the granulocyte phagocytic index, Experientia 32:238.

Rossof, A.H. and Fehir, K.M., 1978, Lithium stimulation of granulopoiesis, New Eng. J. Med. 298:280.

Rothstein, G., Clarkson, D.R., Larsen, W., Grosser, B.I., and Athens, J.W., 1978, Effect of lithium on neutrophil mass and production, New Eng. J. Med. 298:178.

Ruscetti, F.W. and Chervenick, P.A., 1975, Release of colony stimulating activity from thymus-derived lymphocytes, J. Clin. Inves. 55:520.

Shively, J.N., Michaelson, S.M., and Howland, J.W., 1958, The response of dogs to bilateral whole body Co60 irradiation, Rad. Res. 9:445.

Shopsin, B., Friedman, R., and Gershon, S., 1971, Lithium and leukocytosis, Clin. Pharm. Ther. 12:923.

Siegel, J., Johnston, R.B., Jr., Lowe, R.S., Epstein, P.S., and Rossof, A.H., 1980, Effects of lithium on neutrophil metabolism in vitro and on neutrophil function during therapy, (This volume).

Siegel, S., 1956, "Non-Parametric Statistics for the Behavioral Sciences," McGraw-Hill, New York.

Stein, R.S., Beaman, C., Ali, M.Y., Hansen, R., Jenkins, D.D., and Jume'an, H.G., 1977, Lithium carbonate attenuation of chemotherapy-induced neutropenia, New Eng. J. Med. 297:430.

Stein, R.S., Flexner, J.M., and Graber, S., 1978, Lithium and granulocytopenia during induction therapy of acute myelogenous leukemia, Blood 52:277 (Supplement 1).

Tisman, G., Herbert, V., and Rosenblatt, S., 1973, Evidence that lithium induces human granulocyte proliferation: elevated serum vitamin B12 binding capacity in vivo and granulocyte proliferation in vitro, Br. J. Haematol. 24:767.

Tisman, G., 1974, Lithium carbonate protection against drug-induced leukopenia in lymphosarcoma patients, IRCS 2:1509.

Turner, A.R., MacDonald, R.N., and McPherson, T.A., 1979, Reduction of chemotherapy-induced neutropenic complications with a short course of lithium carbonate, Clin. Invest. Med., in press.

Visca, U., Mensi, F., Spina, M.P., Bombara, R., Giraldi, B., Massari, A., Rossi, F., and Santi, G., 1979, Prevention of antiblastic neutropenia with lithium carbonate, Lancet 1:779.

Watanabe, S., Taguchi, K., Nakashima, Y., Ebara, T., Iguchi, K., and Otsuki, S., 1974, Leukocytosis during lithium treatment and its correlation to serum lithium level, Folia Psych. Neurol. Japonica 28:161.

LITHIUM TREATMENT OF CYCLIC HEMATOPOIESIS IN THE GRAY COLLIE

William P. Hammond and David C. Dale

Division of Hematology
Department of Medicine
University of Washington
School of Medicine
Seattle, Washington 98195

Cyclic hematopoiesis is a rare human disorder for which a remarkably close analogue exists in collie dogs. This disorder in the dog, variously named the "lethal grey syndrome," the "grey collie syndrome," "canine cyclic neutropenia," and "canine cyclic hematopoiesis" is an autosomal recessive disease characterized by grey coat color, cyclic fluctuations in blood cell counts, recurrent infections, and premature death (Lund et al., 1967). Approximately 50% of these grey collies die from infections before they reach 3 weeks of age. Initial studies showed that the neutrophil counts cycled at 11 to 13 day intervals and that the distribution and survival of neutrophils in the circulation is normal (Dale et al., 1972b). Later studies showed that reticulocytes, platelets, lymphocytes, monocytes, and eosinophils also cycled with the same period length (although not in phase with one another) and suggested that varying marrow production of cells accounted for these fluctuations (Dale et al., 1972a; Patt et al., 1973). In human cyclic hematopoiesis, regular 21 day cycles of neutrophils, monocytes, lymphocytes, eosinophils, platelets, and reticulocytes also occur and the neutropenic periods are accompanied by local infections and considerable morbidity (Dale and Wolff, 1972; Guerry et al., 1973). The human defect likewise appears to reside in a periodic decrease of cell production by the marrow. Thus, we have proposed that a more thorough understanding of this model disease in the dog should provide insights into the mechanisms regulating marrow cell production in man.

Lithium carbonate has been known to cause neutrophilia in patients treated for manic-depressive psychosis for many years (Radomski et al., 1950; Shopsin et al., 1971). Studies of blood neutrophil turnover and marrow neutrophil reserves have suggested that lithium increases neutrophil production, while in vitro experiments have shown an increased growth of human granulocyte-macrophage progenitor cells during lithium therapy (Rothstein et al., 1978; Stein et al., 1978; Malloy et al., 1978). Because of these effects of lithium on neutrophil production, several groups of researchers have given lithium to patients with Felty's syndrome and to patients given chemotherapy for cancer in an attempt to increase their neutrophil counts and thereby reduce the risk of infection (Gupta et al., 1976; Kaplan, 1976; Greco and Brereton, 1977; Stein et al., 1977). These studies have produced variable results, but they strongly suggest that in certain settings lithium may improve circulating neutrophil counts and reduce infections.

Lithium's stimulatory effect upon granulopoiesis in mice and man extends to the dog as well (Fehir and Rossof, 1977). We, therefore, treated three grey collies with lithium carbonate and observed its effect upon their cyclic hematopoiesis.

METHODS

Daily blood counts including hematocrit, reticulocyte, platelet, and differential white cell counts were performed by standard laboratory methods. Bone marrow differential counts of 500 cells were performed on Wright-Giemsa stained smears of freshly aspirated specimens. Estimates of bone marrow neutrophil reserves were made by injecting S. typhosa lipopolysaccharide W (Difco), 0.1 μg/kg intravenously and measuring the increase in blood neutrophil count 6 hours later. Lithium carbonate tablets were given orally to the dogs twice daily, initially at 150 mg, then 300 mg per dose. Serum lithium levels were determined by routine flame photometry and were maintained between 0.5 and 1.5 meq/liter by adjustment of the lithium dosage. During lithium treatment the blood and marrow studies were then repeated.

RESULTS

Changes in the blood neutrophil count cycles developed slowly. During the first 6 weeks of lithium treatment, cycles continued but the neutrophil nadir during cycles gradually rose. After 2 months of therapy, the neutrophil nadir no longer fell below 1,000 cells/mm^3 (Figure 1) and a striking decrease in infections was noted.

Cyclic variation in the monocyte and platelet counts was markedly depressed. Monocyte counts prior to treatment cycled from 50 to over 8,000/mm^3 whereas during lithium treatment, they ranged from 150 to less than 2,000/mm^3 without obvious periodicity. Platelet counts prior to treatment cycled from approximately 300,000 to 1,300,000/mm^3 as opposed to varying between 246,000 to 498,000/mm^3 during lithium.

Before treatment with lithium, the dogs were anemic with hematocrits of 25 to 29 per cent and reticulocytes showed cycling as previously documented. After 2 months of lithium, however, the reticulocyte counts no longer showed apparent cycles and the hematocrits rose to normal levels of 40 to 45 per cent (Figure 2).

Bone marrow differential counts showed elimination of the wide cyclic swings in cell types seen in the untreated grey collie. At no time during lithium treatment did the maturing neutrophil populations reach the very low levels seen in cycling dogs. Marrow neutrophil reserve estimates reflected these changes in the marrow morphology. During lithium treatment bone marrow reserves ranged from 700 to 4,800/mm^3, as opposed to the range from 0 to greater than 25,000/mm^3 in cycling grey collies.

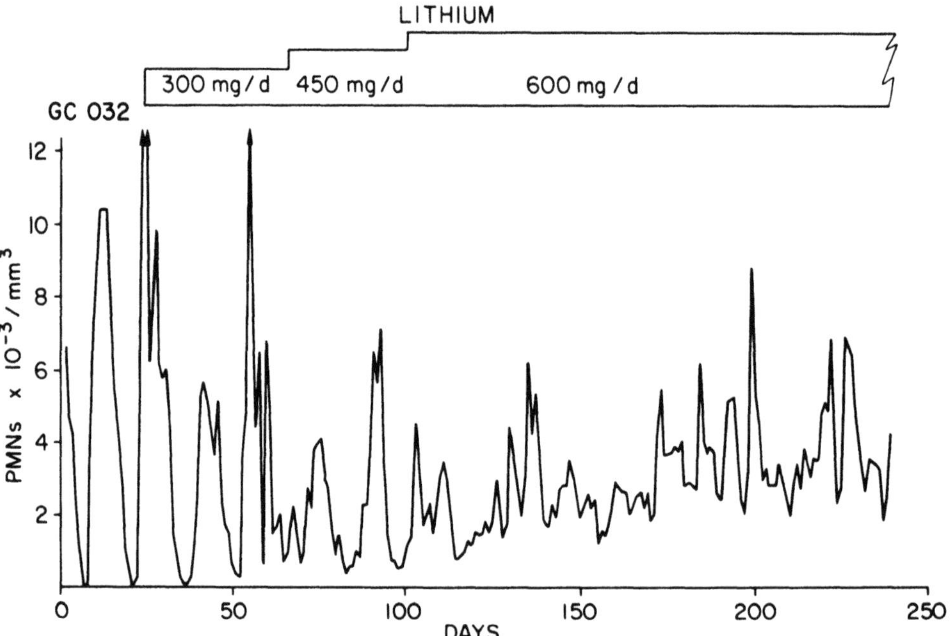

Figure 1. Daily blood neutrophil counts in a grey collie given lithium carbonate up to 600 mg/day.

DISCUSSION

Previous studies of cyclic hematopoiesis in man and dog have demonstrated that this disorder is due to a periodic decrease in cell production. For the canine disease this has been confirmed unequivocally by showing that the defect can be cured by bone marrow transplantation (Dale and Graw, 1974; Jones et al., 1975) and that it can be transmitted to a normal littermate by such transplantation (Weiden et al., 1974). In addition, canine cyclic hematopoiesis can be corrected by chronic endotox-

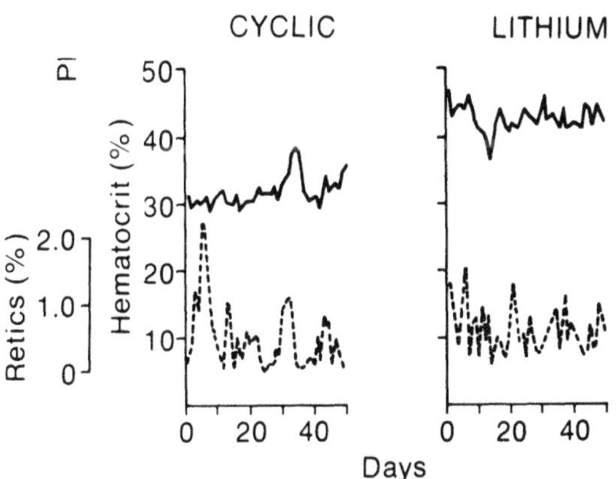

Figure 2. Blood cell counts from representative 50 day periods before and during lithium therapy. Hematocrit is plotted as solid line, reticulocyte count as dashed line.

in treatment, although this leaves the dogs with significant anemia and hepatic abnormalities (Hammond et al., 1978). In view of the impracticalities of these forms of treatment for the relatively benign human disorder, we have examined lithium, as an agent capable of increasing granulocyte production, for its effects upon canine cyclic hematopoiesis prior to initiating trials in patients.

These data demonstrate that lithium carbonate is an effective therapy for canine cyclic hematopoiesis. Not only did neutrophil counts stabilize, but the platelet and monocyte cycles stopped and the reticulocyte variation decreased as the dogs' hematocrits returned to normal. In view of the marked parallels between the human and canine disorders, we would suggest that lithium may be an effective therapy for human cyclic hematopoiesis. Further, the effects of lithium upon this unique stem cell disorder suggest that lithium may have a stimulatory effect upon the proliferation of pluripotent hematopoietic stem cells.

REFERENCES

Dale, D.C. and Graw, R.G., 1974, Transplantation of allogeneic bone marrow in canine cyclic neutropenia, Science 183:83.

Dale, D.C. and Wolff, S.M., 1972, Birth Defects: Original Article Series VIII:59

Dale, D.C., Alling, D.W., and Wolff, S.M., 1972a, Cyclic hematopoiesis: the mechanism of cyclic neutropenia in grey collie dogs, J. Clin. Invest. 51:2197.

Dale, D.C., Ward, S.B., Kimball, H.F., and Wolff, S.M., 1972b, Studies of neutrophil production and turnover in grey collie dogs with cyclic neutropenia, J. Clin. Invest. 51:2190.

Fehir, K.M. and Rossof, A.H., 1977, Lithium carbonate stimulation of marrow colony forming units (CFU-c) and peripheral granulocytes in a canine model, Blood 50:145 (Supplement 1).

Greco, F.A. and Brereton, H.D., 1977, Effect of lithium carbonate on the neutropenia caused by chemotherapy: a preliminary clinical trial, Oncology 34:153.

Guerry, D., Dale, D.C., Omine, M., Perry, S., and Wolff, S.M., 1973, Periodic hematopoiesis in human cyclic neutropenia, J. Clin. Invest. 52:3220.

Gupta, R.C., Robinson, W.A., and Kurnick, J.E., 1976, Felty's syndrome. Effect of lithium on granulopoiesis, Am. J. Med. 61:29.

Hammond, W.P., Price, T.H., and Dale, D.C., 1978, Canine cyclic hematopoiesis: effects of chronic endotoxin administration, Blood 52:1170.

Jones, J.B., Yang, T.J., Dale, J.B., and Lange, R.D., 1975, Canine cyclic hematopoiesis: marrow transplantation between littermates, Br. J. Haematol. 30:215.

Kaplan, R.A., 1976, Lithium in Felty's syndrome, Ann. Int. Med. 84:342.

Lund, J.E., Padgett, G.A., and Ott, R.L., 1967, Cyclic neutropenia in grey collie dogs, Blood 29:452.

Malloy, N.L., Zauber, N.P., and Chervenick, P.A., 1978, The effect of lithium on blood and marrow neutrophils, Blood 52:228 (Supplement 1).

Patt, H.M., Lund, J.E., and Maloney, M.A., 1973, Cyclic hematopoiesis in grey collie dogs: a stem-cell problem, Blood 42:873.

Radomski, J., Fuyat, H.N., Nelson, A.A., and Smith, P.K., 1950, The toxic effects, excretion and distribution of lithium chloride, J. Pharmacol. Exp. Ther. 100:429.

Rothstein, G., Clarkson, D.R., Larson, W., Grosser, B.I., and Athens, J.W., 1978, Effect of lithium on neutrophil mass and production, N. Engl. J. Med. 298:178.

Shopsin, B., Friedmann, R., and Gershon, S., 1971, Lithium and leukocytosis, Clin. Pharmacol. Ther. 12:923.

Stein, R.S., Beaman, C., Ali, M.Y., Hansen, R., Jenkins, D.D., and Jume'an, H.G., 1977, Lithium carbonate attenuation of chemotherapy-induced neutropenia, N. Engl. J. Med. 297:430.

Stein, R.S., Hanson, G., Koethe, S., and Hansen, R., 1978, Lithium-induced granulocytosis, Ann. Int. Med. 88:809.

Weiden, P.L., Robinett, B., Graham, T.C., Adamson, J.W., and Storb, R., 1974, Canine cyclic neutropenia. A stem cell defect, J. Clin. Invest. 53:950.

CLINICAL INVESTIGATION OF LITHIUM THERAPY IN ACUTE LEUKEMIA

Dominique J. Charron, Thierry Schmitt,
and Laurent Degos

Institut de Recherche sur les Maladies du Sang
Hopital Saint-Louis
Paris, France

It has been known for a long time that patients receiving lithium carbonate (Li_2CO_3) for manic-depressive psychosis develop a significant polymorphonuclear leukocytosis (Bille and Plum, 1955; Shopsin et al., 1971). Moreover, in vitro studies have demonstrated a stimulatory effect of Li_2CO_3 on granulopoiesis (Tisman et al., 1973; Harker et al., 1975) and have suggested that Li_2CO_3 acts either by increasing colony stimulating factor (CSF) production by mononuclear cells (Harker et al., 1977) or potentiating the action of CSF (Morley and Galbraith, 1978). The exact mechanism has yet to be clarified by extended in vivo and in vitro studies, although the present data support the evidence for a multilevel action.

We investigated the effect of Li_2CO_3 therapy in the recovery from granulocytopenia induced by intensive chemotherapy in acute leukemia. Patients undergoing chemotherapy for acute leukemia develop a prolonged period of profound neutropenia before the remission is obtained. Any therapeutic regimen designed to shorten this phase would eventually decrease the risk of infection and show some benefit on the remission rate.

The clinical effect of Li_2CO_3 had been assessed previously in Felty's Syndrome (Gupta et al., 1976) and with cancer chemotherapy. No data were available, when we started our study, on the use of Li_2CO_3 in major cytotoxic chemotherapy for acute leukemia.

We report here an extended study on clinical usefulness of Li_2CO_3 in acute leukemia which confirms our preliminary results (Charron et al., 1977) and argues for more use of Li_2CO_3 in hematological disorders.

METHODS AND MATERIALS

Patients

The Li_2CO_3 treated group included 24 patients: 19 with acute myeloblastic leukemia (AML), 3 with acute promyelocytic leukemia (APML), 2 with acute lymphoblastic leukemia (ALL). Six patients were in first relapse, 2 in second relapse. The 2 ALL patients were in third relapse. There were 11 females and 13 males with a median age of onset of 43 and a range from 18-70. The control group included 20 patients (16 AML, 2 APML, 2ALL), 9 females and 11 males with a median age of 42 ranging from 17-65. The diagnosis of acute leukemia was classically made by peripheral blood smears and confirmed by bone marrow aspirate, usually showing over 40% blast cells. The two groups (Li_2CO_3 treated and controls) were seen during the same period of time at the same institutions; they received identical chemotherapy regimens and similar supportive therapy, according to their clinical status. The chemotherapy used in these patients consisted of daunorubicin (2 mg/kg/day for 2 days) and cytosine arabinoside (100 mg/m^2/day for 7 days). The APML patients received platelet transfusions and heparin to prevent and/or stop the development of a disseminated intravascular coagulation (DIC). The 2 ALL patients (in third relapse) were treated with a new anthracyclin derivative (Jacquillat et al., 1978).

Moreover, a protective isolation policy was used for all these patients but no gastrointestinal sterilization was done. The antibiotics and anti-fungal regimens were similar in the two groups.

Dosage of Li_2CO_3

Lithium carbonate was started after confirmation of therapeutic aplasia by bone marrow aspirate. The day for the bone marrow aspirate was decided upon by the kinetics of the blood counts and on previous experience showing the onset of aplasia usually at day 7 to day 10 after the first day of chemotherapy. If the bone marrow still showed numerous blast cells an additional chemotherapy regimen was administered. Li_2CO_3 was given orally 4 times a day in a total dosage of 1g/day. The dose was then adjusted to a serum level of 0.7-0.9 mM/l. Serum lithium levels were measured every other day. Plasma and urine electrolytes were determined every day and plasma sodium levels were maintained over 135 mM/l.

Hematological Surveillance

A hemogram was obtained every day including RBC, WBC and differential, and platelet counts. The biological DIC status in the APML patients was monitored twice a day at the beginning of the treatment and then according to the response to therapy.

Psychological Evaluation

Because of its beneficial effect in psychiatric disorders, we studied the psychological effect of Li_2CO_3 in 8 of our patients. In order to investigate this possibility, we asked a psychologist (N. Alby), working in our department with leukemic patients and their families, to evaluate the level of anxiety and the emotional status of the patients receiving Li_2CO_3. Interviews before treatment, during the therapy, and at the onset of remission were obtained. The Hamilton Scale (Hamilton, 1959) was used to rate the anxiety level.

None of these patients had had a record of psychological disorder before the onset of their hematological disease.

RESULTS

Of 24 patients in whom bone marrow aplasia after chemotherapy was obtained, 20 were evaluated for the effect of lithium. One patient died of bacterial septicemia on the second day after Li_2CO_3 was started. Two patients died from diffuse pulmonary infection respectively at day 4 and 5. Three patients did not achieve a complete remission after aplasia. They were treated again. One died during the second induction treatment. One achieved a complete remission after the second chemotherapy regimen. The third had a partial remission (20% blast cells in the bone marrow aspirate) and survived 5 months with various chemotherapies. Lithium was not discontinued in this patient. None of the patients who died had an Li level over 0.8 mM/l.

Effect on the Polymorphonuclear (PMN) Counts

We selected an absolute granulocyte count of 600/mm^3 to represent the end of the neutropenic period following aplasia for two reasons: 1) In every case but one, a PMN count greater than 600/mm^3 preceded by 24 to 48 hours a PMN count greater than 1000/mm^3. Interestingly, the patient with a delayed (4 days) increase in PMN count developed cytomegalovirus infection; and 2) Most of the severe infections occurred in these patients when PMN counts were less than 500/mm^3. Moreover, none of our patients developed infection or even a febrile episode after they reached a PMN count of 600/mm^3.

We are confident that a PMN count greater than 600/mm^3 represents a clinically significant level in these patients (Li_2CO_3 treated group).

In the control group, out of 20 patients, only 9 reached a "safe" level of 1000 PMN/mm^3 from 600 PMN/mm^3 in less than 48 hours. The delay was 4 days in 4 patients, and 5 days in one patient.

The first noticeable effect of Li_2CO_3 is a more rapid increase in granulocyte count after reaching a level of 600 PMN/mm^3 (Table I). Ninety-five percent of the Li_2CO_3 treated group reached 1000 PMN/mm^3 in less than 48 hours, compared to 45% in the control group.

Duration of the Drug-Induced Neutropenia

The mean duration of the granulocytopenic phase (< 600 PMN/mm^3) was 8 ± 4 days in the Li_2CO_3 treated group with a range from 4 to 17 days. Only two patients showed a prolonged neutropenic phase (15 and 17 days). These two patients had documented viral infection. Ninety percent of the patients (18/20) had a neutropenic phase of less than 12 days.

The mean duration of the granulocytopenic phase was 16 ± 5 days in the control group, with a range from 11 to 24 days. Only 30% (6/20) had a neutropenic phase of less than 12 days (Table II).

The granulocytopenic phase (neutrophils < $1000/mm^3$) had been shown to be 20 ± 5 days in 120 cases of AML previously seen in our institution.

TABLE I

EFFECT OF LI_2CO_3 ON THE DELAY TO REACH 1000 PMN/MM^3 FROM 600 PMN/MM^3 AT THE ONSET OF APLASTIC PHASE

	Delay	No. of Patients	%
Control Patients	< 48 hours	9	(45%)
	> 48 hours, < 4 days	6	(30%)
	4 days	4	(20%)
	5 days	1	(5%)
	Total	20	
Li_2CO_3 Treated Patients	< 48 hours	19	(95%)
	> 48 hours (4 days)	1	(5%)
	Total	20	

Duration of the Thrombocytopenia (Platelets < $50,000/mm^3$)

Only 13 cases were evaluated for this parameter. Seven were excluded because they had received HLA compatible platelet transfusions a few days before the remission. A reduced duration of the thrombocytopenic phase was also observed from 13 ± 5 days in the control group (11 patients evaluated) to 7 ± 4 days in the Li_2CO_3 treated group (Table III).

There was no difference in the delay required to reach 100,000 plateletes/mm^3 from 50,000 platelets/mm^3 in the two groups (usually 3 to 5 days).

TABLE II

EFFECT OF LI_2CO_3 ON THE DURATION OF THE NEUTROPENIC PHASE

	PMN < 600/mm^3	
Controls Group	Mean	Range
20 Patients	16 ± 5 days 30% (6/20) < 12 days	11-24 days
Li_2CO_3 Group		
20 Patients	8 ± 4 days 90% (18/20) < 12 days	4-17 days

The post chemotherapy neutropenic phase starts after proof of aplasia is obtained (7 to 10 days after the beginning of treatment).

TABLE III

EFFECT OF LITHIUM ON THE THROMBOCYTOPENIC PHASE

Platelet Count < 50,000/mm^3

Controls Group	Range
11 Patients	13 ± 5 days
Li_2CO_3 Group	
13 Patients	7 ± 4 days

Transfusion of platelets was decided either because of a very low platelet count (< 15,000/mm^3), DIC, or clinical hemorrhagic symptoms. Moreover, no patient presented additional bleeding after reaching 50,000 platelets/mm^3.

Side Effects

Because of the toxicity of lithium (Schou, 1968; Lee *et al.*, 1971) careful clinical and biological monitoring of our patients was done. Serum lithium levels were determined every other day and the dosage adjusted to a concentration of 0.7-0.9 mM/l even if toxicity is very rarely associated with Li levels below 2 mM/l (Schou, 1968). In every case, the plasma sodium level was maintained over 135 mM/l. Minor or transient side effects were observed. Two transient episodes of diabetes insipidus were seen. Two patients had persistent nausea and occasional vomiting, one of whom developed a documented viral hepatitis. The lithium therapy was, therefore, withheld for 2 and 4 days and reinstated without recurrence of the nausea. Three patients had a minor tremor.

We believe that by selecting patients without heart or kidney disease, by carefully monitoring the serum Li level, and the plasma and urine electrolytes, most toxic episodes can be prevented.

Psychological Studies

The psychological benefit of lithium therapy in 8 of our patients has been assessed by psychological interview. The level of anxiety and the emotional reactivity were both lowered according to the Hamilton Scale (Hamilton, 1959), possibly indicating an additional advantage for the use of lithium in these patients undergoing intense emotional stress because of their unexpected disease and subsequent hospitalization.

Infectious Status

To decrease the incidence of infection is the ultimate goal for using Li_2CO_3 in acute leukemia, as well as in other neutropenic states.

We have observed in the Li_2CO_3 treated group 4 documented septicemias and 6 febrile episodes compared to 8 septicemias and 8 febrile episodes in the control group. The incidence of pulmonary infection was identical. Moreover, the need for leukocyte transfusion was lower in the Li_2CO_3 group than in the control.

However, even with a favorable trend toward reducing the risk of infection, it seems premature to conclude that Li_2CO_3 has a beneficial effect in reducing infectious complications. In this matter, as well as for the remission rate and duration of remission, a large randomized study is needed to be conclusive. This is in progress.

DISCUSSION

As previously mentioned in our preliminary study (Charron et al., 1977), Li_2CO_3 shows a remarkable effect in reducing the neutropenic phase after major cytotoxic therapy in acute leukemia. Moreover, a similar effect is observed for the thrombocytopenic phase. These effects confirm the usefulness of Li_2CO_3 in a hematological disorder. Initially used in Felty's Syndrome (Gupta et al., 1976), lithium carbonate therapy has proven to be of benefit in intensive combination chemotherapy for lymphosarcoma (Tisman et al., 1974), and in attenuating the expected degree of neutropenia in patients with advanced malignancy undergoing cyclic combination chemotherapy (Greco et al., 1976).

Moreover, a randomized study in bronchogenic carcinoma (Lyman et al., 1978) showed that lithium therapy reduced the incidence of infection and the need for dose reduction in patients receiving chemotherapy and radiotherapy.

Other hematological disorders are potential candidates for lithium therapy. A preliminary report has shown some benefit in a patient with congenital neutropenia (Barrett et al., 1977). On the other hand, only transient improvement was obtained in a case of aplastic anemia following hepatitis (Barrett et al., 1976).

Our personal experience shows very little or no effect when an autoimmune mechanism is involved in the development of the neutropenia. We recently observed a case of chronic lymphocytic leukemia (CLL), Stage IV by our classification (Charron, 1977; Binet _et al._, 1977), with profound neutropenia and thrombocytopenia in whom an autoimmune mechanism was suspected. The serum from this patient had an inhibiting effect on colony formation from normal donors. This patient was totally refractory to lithium therapy.

The use of Li_2CO_3 was ineffective in 4 cases of hairy cell leukemia with marked neutropenia (< 1000 PMN/mm^3) (Charron, unpublished observations). This lack of action could be due to either a profound deficit in monocytes (quantitatively and/or qualitatively) (Marie _et al._, 1977) or to an inability of the bone marrow to respond normally to Li. These possibilities and also the role of splenectomy in the response to lithium therapy in hairy cell leukemia are under investigation.

In vitro tests such as urine and serum colony stimulating activity seem to be of value in predicting the _in vivo_ action of Felty's Syndrome. However, there is no proportional correlation between the _in vitro_ effect and the _in vivo_ results (Gupta, 1976). More data are needed on the effect of Li on bone marrow in acute leukemia before treatment, during aplasia, and at the onset of the aplastic phase.

In 3 of 4 patients, lithium induced a modest stimulation of colony and cluster growth in the initial bone marrow sample. In two patients, the number of colonies rose above normal levels 10 days after the onset of the aplastic phase (Charron _et al._, 1977). On the other hand, peripheral blood CFU-C were low, and remained at a very reduced level, before and during lithium therapy, although a transient effect was observed on the granulocyte count in one case of aplastic anemia (Barret, 1977).

This heterogeneity of response to lithium therapy could be due to beginning therapy at different stages of disease. It could also reflect an individual pattern of response, possibly due to a genetic polymorphism as suggested by recent data (Dorus _et al._, 1975).

The action of the lithium ion on the hematopoietic system recently extended to a definitive role on the immune response (Shenkman et al.,

1978). Further in vitro and in vivo studies of its action in the fields of oncology, immunology, and hematology, should be encouraged.

SUMMARY

Lithium carbonate has been used in 24 acute leukemias (19 AML, 3 APML, 2 ALL) to shorten the period of drug induced granulocytopenia and consequently the risk of infection. The lithium therapy was started after confirmation of aplasia by sternal bone marrow aspirate. Initially, the lithium carbonate dosage was 1 g/day. The dosage was then adjusted to a serum lithium level of 0.7-0.9 mM/l. The duration of the granulocytopenic phase (polymorphonuclears < $600/mm^3$) was markedly reduced, from 16 ± 5 days (in control patients), to 8 ± 4 days in the lithium treated patients. The frequency of febrile episodes appeared to be reduced among these patients (4 documented septicemias, 6 febrile episodes) compared to 8 septicemias and 8 febrile episodes in a control treated leukemia population who were not given lithium carbonate. Side effects were very seldom observed and could easily be prevented by daily monitoring of serum lithium and sodium concentrations. Moreover, lithium carbonate seems to have a beneficial psychological effect in these patients. Using the Hamilton Scale, we were able to observe a reduction in the levels of anxiety and emotional reaction. Lithium seems to be a useful adjuvant therapy in leukemia patients by reducing the chemotherapy-induced neutropenia and the consequent risk of infection.

REFERENCES

Barrett, A.J., Longhurst, P.A., Newton, K.A., and Humble, J.B., 1976, Treatment of a patient with aplastic anemia with lithium carbonate, Exp. Hematol. 4:42.

Barrett, A.J., Griscelli, C., Buriot, D., and Faille, A., 1977, Lithium therapy in congenital neutropenia, Lancet 2:1357.

Bille, M., and Plum, C.M., 1955, Komplikationer ved lithium-behandling, Vgeskrift for Laeger 117:293.

Binet, J.L., Leporrier, M., Dighiero, G., Charron, D., D'Athis, Ph., Vaugier, G., Beral, H.M., Natali, J.C., Raphael, M., Nizet, B., and Follezou, J.Y., 1977, A clinical staging system for CLL prognostic significance, Cancer 40:855.

Charron, D., 1977, Classification anatomo-clinique de la leucemie lymphoide chronique. Signification pronostique, Thesis Medicine, Paris University.

Charron, D., Barrett, A.J., Faille, A., Alby, N., Schmitt, T., and Degos, L., 1977, Lithium in acute myeloid leukemia, Lancet 1:1307.

Dorus, E., Pandey, G.N., and Davis, J.M., 1975, Genetic determinant of lithium ion distribution, Arch. Gen. Psychiatry 32:1097.

Greco, F.A. and Brereton, E., 1977, Effect of lithium carbonate on the neutropenia caused by chemotherapy, a clinical trial, Oncology 34:153.

Gupta, R.C., Robinson, W.A., and Kurnick, J.E., 1976, Felty's Syndrome - Effect of lithium on granulopoiesis, Am. Jour. Med. 61:29.

Hamilton, M., 1959, The assessment of anxiety states by rating, Brit. J. Med. Psychol. 32:50

Harker, G.W., Rothstein, G., Clarkson, D.W., and Athens, J.W., 1975, Stimulation of neutrophil production by lithium, Clin. Res. 23:103A.

Harker, G.W., Rothstein, G., Clarkson, D., Athens, J.W. and MacFarlane, J.L., 1977, Enhancement of colony-stimulating activity production by lithium, Blood 49:263.

Jacquillat, D., Weil, M., Auclerc, M.F., Maral, R., Izrael, V., and Bernard, J., 1978, Clinical activity of a new anthracycline derivative in malignant diseases, Proc. Am. Assoc. Cancer Res. 19:362.

Lee, R.V., Jampol, L.M., and Brown, W.V., 1971, Nephrogenic diabetes insipidus and lithium intoxication - complications of lithium carbonate therapy, New Eng. J. Med. 284:93.

Marie, J.P., Degos, L., and Flandrin, G., 1977, Hairy cell leukemia and tuberculosis, New Eng. J. Med. 297:1354.

Morley, D.C. and Galbraith, P.R., 1978, Effect of lithium on granulopoiesis in culture, Canad. Med. Assn. J. 118:288.

Schou, M., 1968, Litnium in psychiatric therapy and prophylaxis, J. Psychiat. Res. 6:67.

Schou, M., Amidsen, A., and Trap-Jensen, J., 1968, Lithium poisoning, Am. J. Psychiatry 125:520.

Shenkman, L., Borkowsky, W., Hulzman, R.S., and Shopsin, B., 1978, Enhancement of lymphocyte and macrophage function in vitro by lithium chloride, Clin. Immunol. Immunopath. 10:187.

Shopsin, B., Friedman, R., and Gershon, S., 1971, Lithium and leukocytosis, Clin. Pharm. and Therapeutics 12:923.

Tisman, G., Herbert, V., and Rosenblatt, S., 1973, Evidence that lithium induces human granulocyte proliferation: Elevated serum vitamin B12 binding capacity in vivo and granulocyte colony proliferation in vitro, Brit. J. Haem. 24:267.

Tisman, G., 1974, Lithium carbonate protection against drug induced leukopenia in lymphosarcoma patients, IRCS 2:1509.

LITHIUM AND GRANULOCYTOPENIA DURING INDUCTION THERAPY OF ACUTE MYELOGENOUS LEUKEMIA: UPDATE OF AN ONGOING TRIAL

Richard S. Stein, John H. Flexner, and Stanley E. Graber

Department of Medicine
Vanderbilt University School of Medicine and
The Veterans Administration Hospital
Nashville, Tennessee 37232

Administration of lithium carbonate to normal subjects and psychiatric patients causes increased production of granulocytes (Rothstein _et al._, 1978; Stein _et al._, 1978b). The administration of lithium carbonate to patients receiving cancer chemotherapy can attenuate neutropenia when regimens of moderate myelotoxicity are employed (Stein _et al._, 1977; Greco and Brereton, 1977). We have previously reported in preliminary form (Stein _et al._, 1978a) that lithium can limit the duration of the severe neutropenia associated with chemotherapy of acute myelogenous leukemia (AML), a situation in which effective therapy is associated with severe neutropenia. This report presents an update of that clinical trial.

METHODS

Forty patients receiving induction therapy for AML between August 1, 1977 and March 1, 1979 were randomly assigned to receive lithium carbonate, 300 mg p.o. t.i.d., or to receive no lithium therapy. All patients received cytosine arabinoside, 100 mg/m^2/day, by continuous intravenous infusion for 7 days, and daunorubicin, 45 mg/m^2/day, intravenously for 3 days. A bone marrow biopsy was performed on day 22. If this marrow did not show either an unequivocal remission or unequivocal persistence of leukemia, a repeat marrow was performed on day 29. If persistent leukemia was present on either biopsy, a second course of chemotherapy was institututed. Patients receiving initial induction therapy and patients receiving induction therapy following relapse were eligible to enter the study. All patients gave informed consent.

Lithium was started within 24 to 48 hours of the institution of chemotherapy, and was continued until remission occurred or for 30 days. The administration of lithium was arbitrarily designed to terminate at 30 days on the grounds that persistent neutropenia at this time would likely mean persistent leukemia and that further evaluation of neutropenia might be confounded by the institution of a second course of chemotherapy.

White blood cells counts, differentials, and platelet counts were obtained at least every other day. Data were linearly interpolated for days on which counts were not done. When granulocytes were transfused, granulocyte counts were performed eight hours following transfusion to avoid the possibility of measuring transfusion related increments of the granulocyte count. Lithium levels were monitored weekly and blood for lithium levels was obtained at least 8 hours after the previous dose. Remission was defined as a marrow with less than 5% blasts (complete remission), or 6 - 25% blasts (partial remission) accompanied by recovery from cytopenias, i.e., granulocytes $> 1000/mm^3$, platelets $> 50{,}000/mm^3$.

All febrile neutropenic patients, temperature $> 100.5^{o}F$, not attributable to transfusions, received antibiotics (a cephalosporin, an aminoglycoside, and carbenicillin or ticarcillin). Initially, patients remaining febrile after 48 hours of antibiotic therapy received 4 days of granulocyte transfusions; granulocytes were then continued only in patients with positive blood cultures or in patients with an obvious source of fever which was responding to granulocyte transfusions. After September, 1978, granulocyte transfusions were given only to febrile patients with a documented source of infection.

The modified Wilcoxon test was used for comparisons of the durations of neutropenia and thrombocytopenia in the treatment groups.

Comparisons of group composition and the number of remissions employed the Chi-squared statistic. One-tailed tests of significance were used.

TABLE I

CHARACTERISTICS OF TREATMENT GROUPS

	No Lithium	Lithium
Patients	22	18
Patients receiving initial therapy	13	11
Patients receiving re-induction therapy	9	7
Age-Median	52	53
Patients with age > 60 years	9	7
Patients with granulocytes > $1000/mm^3$	10	8

RESULTS

Patients

Characteristics of the patient groups are presented in Table I. The groups were not significantly different with respect to the number of patients receiving initial induction therapy as opposed to therapy at the time of relapse, the age of the patients, or the baseline granulocyte counts. Responses to therapy for the 40 patients are presented in Table II. The remission rate was higher in patients not receiving lithium, but this difference was not statistically significant. All patients were considered evaluable. The duration of severe neutropenia and thrombocytopenia was measured directly for the 23 patients in whom recovery of the peripheral blood counts occurred, i.e., patients who achieved a complete or partial remission, and was treated as censored data for purposes of actuarial analysis, in patients in whom marrow recovery did not occur. All patients who achieved a remission achieved at least a partial remission following a single course of chemotherapy, so the re-institution of chemotherapy for consolidation did not affect the measured duration of neutropenia in any patient.

TABLE II

RESPONSE TO THERAPY

	No Lithium	Lithium
Patients	22	18
Remissions with one cycle of therapy	15(68%)	8 (44%) $p = 0.13$
Complete remissions with one cycle	10(45%)	5 (28%) $p = 0.25$
Deaths without remission	7	10

Degree and Duration of Neutropenia

All patients living seven or more days experienced granulocyte nadirs below $100/mm^3$. The median duration of neutropenia, granulocytes $<1000/mm^3$, was significantly shorter in patients receiving lithium than in patients not receiving lithium: 16.7 days vs 25.7 days respectively, $p < 0.02$ (Figure 1). The median duration of neutropenia, granulocytes $< 500/mm^3$, was also shorter in patients receiving lithium although this difference only approached statistical significance: 14.4 days vs 22.0 days, $p = 0.08$. Since the time to the onset of neutropenia was identical for both treatment groups, the shortened duration of neutropenia in patients receiving lithium reflects a more rapid granulocyte recovery in those patients (Table III).

TABLE III

ONSET AND DURATION OF NEUTROPENIA AND THROMBOCYTOPENIA IN TREATMENT GROUPS

	Lithium	No Lithium	
Onset of Neutropenia			
Granulocytes $< 1000/mm^3$	1.0 days	1.9 days	$p > 0.30$
Granulocytes $< 500/mm^3$	2.5 days	4.6 days	$p > 0.30$
Duration of Neutropenia			
Granulocytes $< 1000/mm^3$	16.7 days	25.7 days	$p = 0.019$
Granulocytes $< 500/mm^3$	14.9 days	22.0 days	$p = 0.08$
Duration of Thrombocytopenia			
Platelets $< 50{,}000/mm^3$	20.7 days	22.6 days	$p > 0.30$

Duration of Thrombocytopenia

Because platelet transfusions were used to maintain platelet counts above $20{,}000/mm^3$, we determined the duration of thrombocytopenia, platelets $< 50{,}000/mm^3$, excluding values due to platelet transfusions. The median duration of thrombocytopenia was statistically equivalent (20.7 days vs 22.6 days, $p > 0.30$) in patients receiving lithium as compared to controls.

Lithium Levels and Drug Toxicity

Lithium levels were maintained between 0.5 and 1.0 meq/L without dosage modification in 14 of 18 patients assigned to receive lithium 300 mg t.i.d. Two patients were noted to have levels below 0.5 meq/L following 7 - 14 days on this dosage; these low levels were obtained prior to the institution of ticarcillin. Two patients assigned to lithium died, prior to the institution of lithium. Lithium levels were maintained although all but three patients receiving lithium received a high sodium load in the form of ticarcillin, 18 grams/day, at some time during the trial. Therapeutic lithium levels were also maintained in a patient with an initial blast count of 440,000/mm^3, who developed azotemia, hyperuricemia, hyperphosphatemia, and hypocalcemia. See Table IV.

TABLE IV

LITHIUM LEVELS

N = 18

All Levels 0.5 - 1.0 meq/L	14
1 or More Levels < 0.5 meq/L	2
Early Deaths	2

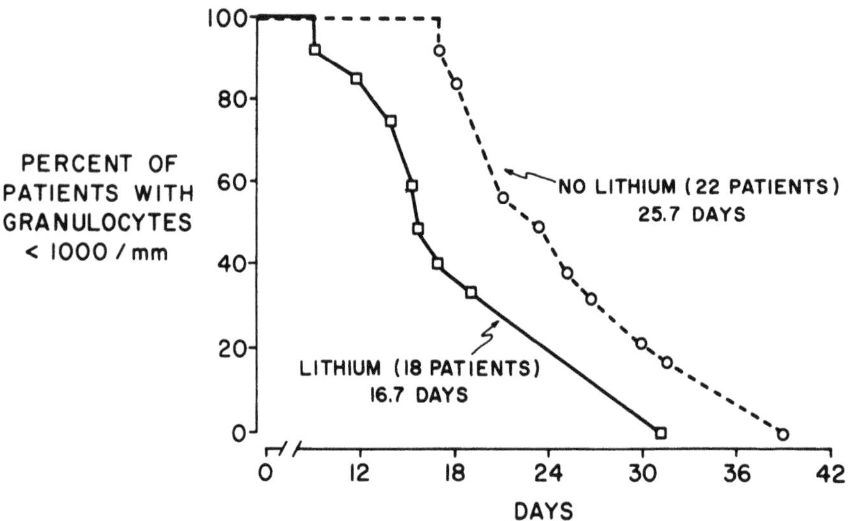

Figure 1. Duration of neutropenia in lithium group and control group, $p < 0.02$.

Toxicity attributable to lithium was not established. All patients in both groups experienced nausea during chemotherapy. One patient with leukemic meningitis discontinued lithium because of nausea, but nausea was not relieved by discontinuing lithium. One patient developed hypokalemia (< 2 meq/L) while on lithium and ticarcillin. Other electrolyte abnormalities were not observed.

Incidence of Fever and Infection

The percentage of days spent with fever was not statistically different in the two treatment groups. Episodes of fever associated with a positive blood culture or documented source occurred 15 times in 15 patients in the no lithium group and 16 times in 14 patients in the lithium group. Granulocyte transfusions were administered to 14 patients in the no lithium group and to 12 patients in the lithium group.

DISCUSSION

Lithium carbonate can limit the degree of neutropenia in patients receiving chemotherapy ordinarily associated with moderate myelotoxicity. A small study (6 patients) employing historical controls has previously suggested that lithium may attenuate neutropenia in patients receiving therapy for AML (Charron et al., 1977). In this randomized study we evaluated whether lithium could attenuate the degree or duration of severe neutropenia in patients receiving induction therapy for acute myelogenous leukemia (AML), patients in whom bone marrow aplasia with life-threatening granulocytopenia must be produced in order to acheive a complete remission.

Forty patients receiving a standard induction regimen for AML were randomized either to receive lithium or no lithium. Lithium did not prevent the development of severe granulocytopenia as granulocyte nadirs below $100/mm^3$ occurred in all patients surviving seven days. However, the median duration of severe granulocytopenia (granulocytes < $1000/mm^3$) was shorter in patients receiving lithium: 16.7 days vs 25.7 days ($p < 0.02$). When the number of days with granulocytes below $500/mm^3$ was considered, the trend favored the lithium group (14.9 days vs 22.0 days) but this difference only approached statistical significance ($p = 0.08$).

In contrast to the ability of lithium to favorably affect granulocyte production, effects of lithium on platelet counts have been variable. Thrombocytopenia was not attenuated in one series of patients receiving cancer chemotherapy (Stein *et al.*, 1977). However, in a series of patients receiving nitrosourea therapy, which is usually severely toxic to platelets, attenuation of thrombocytopenia was noted (Catane *et al.*, 1977). We have observed a small, statistically insignificant increase in the platelet counts of normal volunteers receiving lithium (Stein, unpublished data). In this study, the duration of severe thrombocytopenia, platelets $< 50{,}000/mm^3$, was not significantly shorter in patients receiving lithium as compared to controls: 20.7 days vs 22.6 days, $p > 0.30$.

In this study, lithium did not delay the onset of neutropenia, and the shortened duration of neutropenia reflects an earlier granulocyte recovery in the patients receiving lithium. If, as suggested by previous studies, lithium acts by augmenting the production of colony stimulating activity, CSA (Joyce and Chervenick,1975; Harker *et al.*, 1977), this study suggests that CSA is better able to affect granulocyte production once the marrow has been rendered grossly free of leukemia, or that lithium augmentation of CSA production is clinically relevant only when anti-leukemia therapy has greatly reduced the number of monocytes capable of producing CSA. In this regard, the study is compatible with our unpublished observation that lithium is ineffective in the treatment of neutropenia when neutropenia is secondary to the bone marrow being packed with leukemia.

The incidence of fever and infection during induction therapy of AML is directly related to the degree of neutropenia and the time at risk (Bodey *et al.*, 1966). Studies of granulocyte transfusion have illustrated that recovery from neutropenia is the critical factor affecting survival in septic neutropenic patients (Herzig *et al.*, 1977; Alavi *et al.*, 1977). Protracted neutropenia may necessitate extensive broad spectrum antibiotic therapy with a risk of superinfection with fungi. Thus, shortening the duration of severe neutropenia during induction therapy of AML should decrease morbidity. However, since the administration of lithium did not prevent the development of severe neutropenia (< 100 granulocytes/mm^3), the potential benefits of lithium are limited. Therefore, the failure of lithium to decrease the incidence of infection in this study is not surprising. Larger studies will be necessary to further evaluate this issue. It is also possible that the value of lithium in limiting infection may depend on the circumstances in which therapy is given, i.e., the simultaneous use of protected environments or prophylactic antibiotics, neither of which were used in this study.

In this study, lithium therapy was relatively free of toxicity. Although one patient receiving lithium and ticarcillin became hypokalemic, this toxicity may occur in patients receiving ticarcillin alone. Despite the administration of saline loads in the form of ticarcillin, the administration of lithium carbonate 300 mg t.i.d. was associated with lithium levels between 0.5 and 1.0 meq/L in 14 of 18 patients. No levels above 1.0 meq/L were noted. This dosage of lithium (300 mg t.i.d.) has previously been shown to have a favorable effect on granulocyte production (Gupta et al., 1975; Rothstein et al., 1978; Stein et al., 1978), and this level is associated with an anti-manic effect in psychiatric patients. However, the dosage and blood levels necessary to produce optimal hematologic effects have not been established. It should also be noted that the optimal timing for administering lithium to patients receiving chemotherapy (before therapy, during therapy, and after therapy) is not established.

Despite the favorable effect of lithium on the duration of neutropenia, it is inappropriate to advocate the routine use of lithium during induction therapy of AML as no clinical benefit of lithium has been established. In fact, in this study, the remission rate was slightly lower in patients receiving lithium therapy, although to a statistically insignificant degree. However, since support of the patient with AML during the period of neutropenia is a major clinical problem, this study establishes that further controlled trials of lithium during induction therapy of AML are warranted. Such trials could also determine whether the administration of lithium during induction therapy has any long term effects on either remission duration or on marrow tolerance of further intensification therapy. Since leukemic cells as well as normal cells may respond to colony stimulating activity in vitro (Metcalf et al., 1974), it is possible that lithium might hasten the recovery of leukemic cells as well as the recovery of normal granulocytes. Thus far, however, remission duration does not appear to be affected by lithium. In cases of malignancies other than leukemia, in which lithium would not be expected to increase recovery of the tumor, this study confirms previous reports which have suggested that lithium may be a useful means of limiting the myelotoxicity of chemotherapy (Stein et al., 1977; Greco and Brereton, 1977). If, as suggested in this report, lithium can accelerate the rate of marrow recovery from severe hypoplasia, this study suggests a possible role for lithium in the therapy of marrow transplant patients and other severely neutropenic patients.

ACKNOWLEDGEMENTS

This work was supported by a research Grant 1RO1CA 23971-01 from the National Cancer Institute, the National Institutes of Health and Public Health Service Grant No. 5MO1 RR-95 from the General Clinical Research Centers Branch of the Division of Research Resources, National Institutes of Health.

REFERENCES

Alavi, J.B., Root, R.K., Djerassi, I., Evans, A.E., Gluckman, S.J., Macgregor, R.R., Guerry, D., Schreiber, A.D., Shaw, J.M., Koch, P., and Cooper, R.A., 1977, A randomized clinical trial of granulocyte transfusions for infection in acute leukemia, N. Eng. J. Med. 296:706.

Bodey, G.P., Buckley, M., Sathe, Y.S., and Freireich, E.J., 1966, Quantitative relationships between circulating leukocytes and infection in patients with acute leukemia, Ann. Int. Med. 64:328.

Catane, R., Kaufman, J., Mittelman, A., and Murphy, G.P., 1977, Attenuation of myelosuppression with lithium, N.Eng. J. Med. 297:452.

Charron, D., Barrett, A.J., Faille, A., Alby, N., Schmitt, T., and Degos, L., 1977, Lithium in acute myeloid leukemia, Lancet 1:1307.

Greco, F.A. and Brereton, H.D., 1977, Effect of lithium carbonate on the neutropenia caused by chemotherapy: a preliminary clinical trial, Oncology 34:154.

Gupta, R.C., Robinson, W.A., and Smyth, C.J., 1975, Efficacy of lithium in rheumatoid arthritis with granulocytopenia, Arthritis Rheum., 18:179.

Harker, W.G., Rothstein, G., Clarkson, D., Athens, J.W., and Macfarlane, J.L., 1977, Enhancement of colony stimulating activity production by lithium, Blood 49:263.

Herzig, R.H., Herzig, G.P., Graw, R.G., Bull, M.I., and Ray, K.K., 1977, Successful granulocyte transfusion therapy for gram-negative septicemia, N. Eng. J. Med. 296:701.

Joyce, R.A. and Chervenick, P.A., 1975, Effect of lithium on the release of colony stimulating activity (CSA) from blood leukocytes, Proc. Am. Soc. Hematol. 18:126.

Metcalf, D., Moore, M.A.S., Sheridan, J.W., and Spitzer, G., 1974, Responsiveness of human granulocytic leukemic cells to colony-stimulating factor, Blood 43:847.

Rothstein, G., Clarkson, D., Larsen, W., Grosser, B.I., and Athens, J.W., 1978, Effect of lithium on neutrophil mass and production, N. Eng. J. Med. 298:178.

Stein, R.S., Beaman, C., Ali, M.Y., Hansen, R., Jenkins, D.D., and Jume'an, H.G., 1977, Lithium carbonate attenuation of chemotherapy induced neutropenia, N. Eng. J. Med. 297:430.

Stein, R.S., Flexner, J.M., and Graber, S.E., 1978a, Lithium and granulocytopenia during induction therapy of acute myelogenous leukemia, Blood 52:277 (Supplement 1).

Stein, R.S., Hanson, G., Koethe, S., and Hansen, R., 1978b, Lithium induced granulocytosis, Ann. Int. Med. 88:809.

A PLACEBO CONTROLLED STUDY OF A SEVEN DAY COURSE OF LITHIUM CARBONATE FOLLOWING MYELOTOXIC CHEMOTHERAPY

Andrew Robert Turner and R. Neil MacDonald

Department of Medicine
Cross Cancer Institute
University of Alberta
Edmonton, Alberta, Canada, T6G 1Z2

The administration of myelotoxic cancer chemotherapy is associated with neutropenias which may lead to development of severe infections (Bodey, 1977). Lithium carbonate has been reported to attenuate chemotherapy-induced neutropenia (Stein et al., 1977; Greco and Brereton, 1977; Catane et al., 1977; Lyman et al., 1978; Visca et al., 1979). These studies have shown that the use of lithium carbonate following cytotoxic chemotherapy results in a less severe decrease of neutrophils during chemotherapy cycles and higher nadirs of neutrophil counts during each cycle. This benefit has been obtained using lithium therapy throughout the chemotherapy cycle. Since prolonged lithium therapy may produce deleterious side-effects even when serum levels are carefully monitored (Baldessarini and Lipinski, 1975), a trial of a shortened course of lithium carbonate following chemotherapy was indicated. The lithium carbonate therapy was given with a combination of chemotherapeutic agents which produced a marked neutropenia. The initial studies were done using an alternate cycle cross-over format. Subsequently, a placebo controlled randomized study of a 7 day course of lithium carbonate 300 mg three times daily was done.

METHODS

Patients

The patients were males between the ages of 15 and 51 with metastatic non-seminomatous germ cell tumors without any evidence of bone marrow involvement. They were all treated with a highly effective (MacDonald et al., 1979) but very toxic combination of vinblastine, 0.1 mg/kg I.V. on two successive days, adriamycin, 40 mg/m^2 I.V. on day 2 only, cis-diamminedichloroplatinum, 20 mg/m^2 I.V. on five successive days, beginning on day 2 with agressive hydration and diuresis, and bleomycin, 30 units I.V. on three successive days (Figure 1). The chemotherapeutic cycle was repeated every 21 to 28 days, depending upon WBC and renal function.

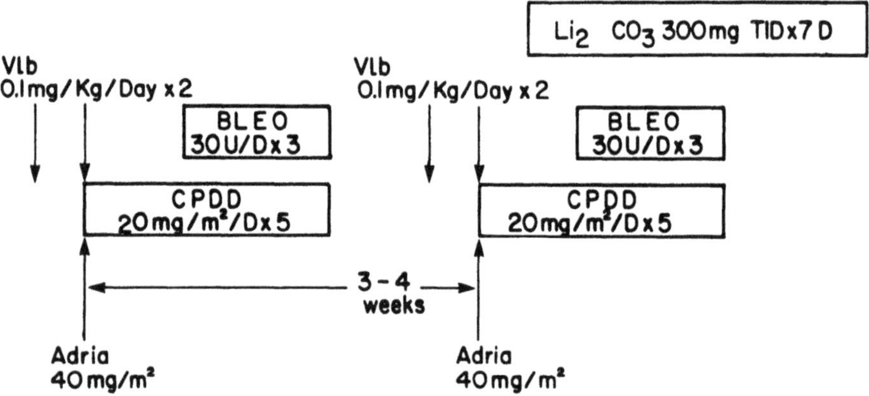

Figure 1. Chemotherapy protocol with lithium carbonate administration noted. For details, see text.

Lithium Carbonate

Lithium carbonate, 300 mg t.i.d. was administered orally for seven days beginning the day following the administration of vinblastine and adriamycin (Figure 1). Serum lithium levels were obtained four days following the start of the lithium carbonate therapy.

Cross-over Study

In the initial study, lithium carbonate was administered on alternate cycles of chemotherapy. A total of 20 cycles (10 paired cycles) in 8 patients were evaluated. Each chemotherapy cycle with lithium was compared to the cycle immediately preceding it. Paired cycles in which there had been an alteration in chemotherapy dosage between cycles were discarded from analysis.

Placebo Controlled Study

For the purposes of this study, a pharmacist prepared gelatin capsules containing either 300 mg of lithium carbonate or a lactose placebo. Twenty-one capsules of lithium carbonate or placebo were packaged by the pharmacist in numerically-coded envelopes and dispensed to the patient. The number on each packet was recorded in the patient's medical record. The patient started taking the study capsules the day following the administration of vinblastine and adriamycin in a manner similar to that above, and continued taking three capsules daily for seven days. Serum was drawn for lithium determination but the clinical laboratory was instructed not to inform the physicians involved of results unless the serum lithium measured was above 1.2 mmole/l. This occurred on only one occasion.

Neutrophil Counts

Each patient had a complete blood count with differential and platelet counts performed prior to each cycle of chemotherapy. These counts were repeated on days 4, 7 and 14 of each cycle. With this combination of chemotherapeutic agents, the nadir of WBC and neutrophil counts occurred around day 7. In a placebo controlled study, the WBC and neutrophil nadirs and the amount of decrease of each during each cycle, was determined before the numerical code, indicating which cycles had included lithium, was broken.

RESULTS

Cross-over Study

During cycles without lithium carbonate, the neutrophil nadir was 610

± 530 (mean ± standard deviation) (Table 1A). During cycles with lithium carbonate, the mean nadir was 1070 ± 290 ($p < 0.05$). The nadirs of platelet counts were not significantly different. None of the cycles given with lithium carbonate resulted in a neutrophil nadir of less than $500/mm^3$, whereas 5 of 10 cycles administered without lithium produced a neutrophil nadir below $500/mm^3$ ($p < 0.01$). The serum lithium levels ranged between 0.4 mM/l and 0.8 mM/l.

Placebo Controlled Study

The mean neutrophil nadir during cycles including lithium carbonate was 1210 ± 990. The cycles which included the placebo control produced a neutrophil nadir of 700 ± 580 (N.S.) (Table 1B). One of 10 cycles with lithium carbonate resulted in a neutrophil nadir below 500, whereas, 6 of 15 cycles including the placebo produced a neutrophil count below $500/mm^3$ ($p < 0.05$). In one case, a serum lithium level of 1.4 mmole/l was reported.

The dosage of chemotherapeutic agents was equivalent in the lithium and placebo cycles. Adriamycin, 54.6 ± 5.3 mg, and 12.1 ± 0.3 mg of vinblastine were administered in the cycles with lithium and 53.3 ± 7.0 mg of adriamycin and 12.8 ± 0.6 mg of vinblastine were given in cycles with the placebo control.

DISCUSSION

Several authors have reported a beneficial effect of lithium carbonate on chemotherapy induced neutropenia (Stein et al., 1977; Greco et al., 1977; Catane et al., 1977; Lyman et al., 1978; Visca et al., 1979). In most of these studies, the amount of myelosuppression induced was purposely minimized to avoid severe neutropenias. Our study was designed to see if lithium would attenuate clinically significant neutropenia. The combination of chemotherapeutic agents being used in this study is very toxic and similar combinations have been reported to cause major infectious morbidity (Einhorn and Donohue, 1977). In both the cross-over study and the placebo-controlled study, there was a significant reduction of serious neutropenic episodes. The routine use of lithium in this context would appear to be justified. A similar conclusion has been made by others using lithium with a combination of high dose chemotherapy and irradiation (Lyman *et al.*, 1978).

The placebo-controlled study has confirmed the initial impression that a prolonged course of lithium treatment is not necessary to produce a beneficial effect on the neutrophil counts. Shortening the treatment time should reduce the risk of adverse effects from lithium therapy and increase patient compliance.

TABLE I

EFFECT OF LI_2CO_3 ON CHEMOTHERAPY-INDUCED NEUTROPENIA

A. Cross-over Study

	Pre-treatment neutrophil count/mm^3	Decrease	Neutrophil nadir/mm^3	No. $< 500/mm^3$
With Li^+ n = 10	3040 ± 680	1970 ± 790	1070 ± 290	0/10
Without Li^+ n = 10	3250 ± 750	2640 ± 730	610 ± 530*	5/10**

B. Placebo-controlled Study

	Pre-treatment neutrophil count/mm^3	Decrease	Neutrophil nadir/mm^3	No. $< 500/mm^3$
With Li^+ n = 10	4310 ± 1550	3100 ± 1970	1210 ± 990	1/10
Placebo n = 15	3940 ± 1660	3220 ± 1510	700 ± 580	6/15*

* $p < 0.05$

** $p < 0.01$

The most frequent side effect ascribed to the lithium was nausea. Nausea occurring shortly after chemotherapy administration may be quite severe. It is difficult to assess what contribution lithium therapy made to this. In addition, it is most probable that a considerable portion of the administered lithium was not absorbed if the patient had frequent emesis. It may be worthwhile examining the use of lithium depot preparations.

The mechanism of lithium induced neutrophilia will be discussed elsewhere (Turner and Allalunis, 1979). Lithium has been shown by others to increase colony stimulating activity (CSA) and we have shown that CSA production from peripheral blood mononuclear cells is increased within 4 days of institution of lithium therapy in hematologically normal subjects. Lithium does not appear to have any direct effect on stem cells. As well, it has not affected the efficiency of the chemotherapeutic regimen on the cancer. All 16 of the patients treated in these trials have achieved a complete remission, and none has relapsed in a median follow-up period of over one year.

REFERENCES

Baldessarini, R.J., and Lipinski, J.F., 1975, Lithium salts: 1970-1975, Ann. Int. Med. 83:527.

Bodey, G.P., 1977, Infectious complications in the cancer patient, Curr. Probl. Cancer 1.

Catane, R., Kaufman, J., and Mittelman, A., 1977, Attenuation of myelosuppression with lithium, N. Eng. J. Med. 297:452.

Einhorn, L.H., and Donohue, J., 1977, Cis-diaminodichloroplatinum, vinblastine and bleomycin combination chemotherapy in disseminated testicular cancer, Ann. Intern. Med. 87:293.

Greco, F.A., and Brereton, H.D., 1977, Effect of lithium carbonate on the neutropenia caused by chemotherapy: A preliminary clinical trial, Oncology 34:153.

Lyman, G.H., Williams, C.C., and Preston, D., 1978, A prospective randomized study of lithium carbonate on the granulocytopenia and incidence of infection associated with intensive chemotherapy and radiation therapy for undifferentiated small cell bronchogenic carcinoma, Blood 52:228 (Supplement 1).

MacDonald, R.N., Turner, A.R., and McPhee, M., 1979, Combination chemotherapy of Stage III testicular cancer, Ann. R. Coll. Physicians Surg. Can. 12:166a.

Stein, R.S., Beaman, C., Ali, M.Y., Hansen, R., Jenkins, D.D., and Jume'an, H.G., 1977, Lithium carbonate attenuation of chemotherapy-induced neutropenia, N. Eng. J. Med. 297:430.

Turner, A.R., and Allalunis, M.J., 1979, Oral lithium carbonate increases colony stimulating activity production from human mononuclear cells, (This volume).

Visca, U., Mensi, F., and Spina, M.P., Bombara, R., Giraldi, B., Massari, A., Rossi, A.F., and Santi, G., 1979, Prevention of antiblastic neutropenia with lithium carbonate, Lancet 1:779.

THE EFFECT OF LITHIUM CARBONATE ADMINISTRATION IN PATIENTS WITH ADVANCED SMALL CELL BRONCHOGENIC CARCINOMA RECEIVING COMBINATION CHEMOTHERAPY AND RADIOTHERAPY

Gary H. Lyman, Charles C. Williams,
William R. Dinwoodie, and Dennis Preston

Department of Internal Medicine
University of South Florida College of Medicine
and the Tampa Veterans Administration Hospital
Tampa, Florida 33612

Undifferentiated small cell bronchogenic carcinoma accounts for 15-20% of all forms of lung cancer. It is characterized by sudden onset of symptoms, evidence of widespread disease at presentation and a rapidly progressive clinical course (Broder et al., 1977). The short tumor doubling time and the large growth fraction found in this histologic type may account for both its characteristic clinical features and its sensitivity to cytotoxic treatments (Muggia et al., 1974).

The marjority of patients with small cell lung cancer are considererd unresectable or inoperable at the time of presentation. Radiation therapy appears to be superior to surgical resection in the management of patients with resectable disease (Fox and Scadding, 1973). Radiation therapy has also been found of value in the palliation of compressive symptoms and in the prevention of disease progression in the cranium (Jackson et al., 1977; Moore et al., 1978).

A number of chemotherapeutic agents used singly will produce an objective response in a significant number of patients with small cell lung cancer. In prospective controlled studies, cyclophosphamide has been shown to produce significantly improved survival in patients with both limited and extensive disease when compared to control patients (Green et al., 1969; Higgins, 1972; Bergsagel et al., 1972).

Further improvement in objective response rate, duration of response, and survival has been observed in this population with combination chemotherapy and combined modality therapy (Broder et al., 1977; Weiss, 1978; Hansen et al., 1978). The combination of cyclophosphamide, adriamycin, and vincristine with or without radiation therapy has been studied extensively (Holoye et al., 1977; Livingston et al., 1978; Lyman et al., 1978a). Higher objective response rates and longer remission durations in small cell bronchogenic carcinoma have been obtained with more intensive regimens of the same agents (Johnson et al., 1976). The dose limiting toxicity associated with such therapy, however, is myelosuppression which also correlates with treatment intensity (Livingston et al., 1978; Lyman et al., 1978a; Johnson et al., 1976).

Lithium has been observed to induce an innocuous leukocytosis in hospitalized psychiatric patients (Shopsin et al., 1971). Lithium has recently been reported to ameliorate the leukopenia associated with systemic chemotherapy (Tisman, 1974; Stein et al., 1977; Catane et al., 1977; Greco and Brereton, 1977).

The prospective randomized clinical trial reported here was undertaken to study the effect of lithium on the response rate, duration of response, survival, and toxicity observed in patients with advanced small cell lung cancer treated with combination chemotherapy and radiation therapy.

METHODS

Fifty-one consecutive patients with undifferentiated small cell bronchogenic carcinoma were entered into a prospective trial after staging evaluation which included history and physical examination, routine hematologic and biochemical studies, chest x-ray, electrocardiogram, bone marrow aspiration and biopsy, and radionuclide scans of liver, bone, and brain. Patients were considered to have limited disease when evident tumor involvement was confined to the chest and supraclavicular lymph nodes while patients with evidence of spread outside of those areas were considered to have extensive disease.

After obtaining an informed consent, patients were stratified on the basis of: 1) age (greater or less than 60 years of age); 2) prior treatment; 3) extent of disease (limited or extensive); and 4) functional status (Karnofsky scale greater or less than 40). Patients were not stratified on the basis of the presence of cardiovascular or other concurrent dieseases.

Patients were randomized to receive one of two treatment arms as shown in Figure 1. Twenty-eight patients were randomized to receive radiation and chemotherapy alone (control group) while 23 patients were randomized to receive identical cytotoxic therapy along with lithium carbonate during the interval between cycles of chemotherapy (lithium group).

All patients were assigned to induction chemotherapy as indicated in Figure 1, consisting of cyclophosphamide, adriamycin, and vincristine. After the completion of nine cycles of induction chemotherapy, all responding patients were started on maintenance chemotherapy consisting of cyclophosphamide, methotrexate, lomustine, and procarbazine. Radiation therapy was routinely administered following the second cycle of induction chemotherapy unless life-threatening symptoms necessitated the immediate initiation of radiation therapy along with chemotherapy at 50% of the calculated doses. Radiation therapy consisted of 3000 rads tumor dose administered as ten 300 rad daily fractions to the primary tumor, mediastinum, and both supraclavicular areas through anterior and posterior portals. Concurrent prophylactic cranial irradiation was administered as 3000 rads in ten 300 rad daily fractions through left and right portals to the mid-plane of the brain.

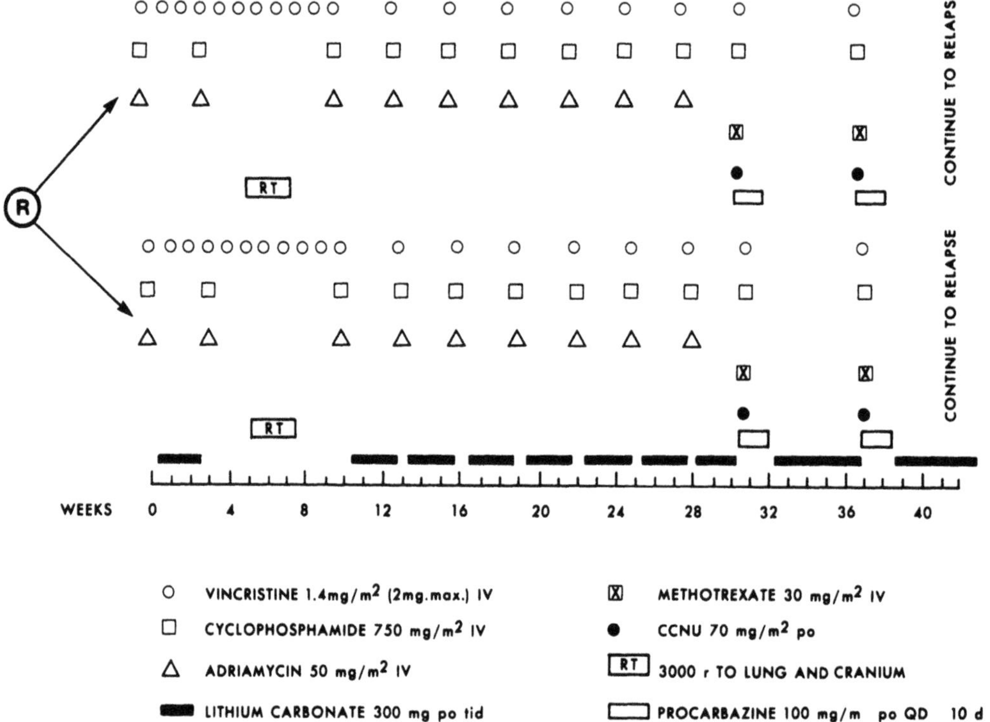

Figure 1. Schema for Protocol USF 7711 for Advanced Small Cell Bronchogenic Carcinoma. Consenting patients were stratified on the basis of age, disease extent, functional status and prior treatment, and were randomized to receive lithium carbonate or not during chemotherapy induction and maintenance. Chemotherapy and lithium carbonate were interrupted after two cycles for chest and prophylactic cranial radiation therapy.

A complete remission was defined as the total disappearance of all objective evidence of tumor at the time of presentation for at least one month without the appearance of any new lesions. A partial remission was defined as at least a 50% reduction in the sum of the products of the two longest perpendicular diameters of all measurable disease at presentation for at least one month without the appearance of any new lesions.

Progressive disease was defined as an increase by more than 25% in the measured product of the two largest perpendicular diameters of any measurable lesion at presentation or the appearance of any new lesions. Survival was determined from the beginning of treatment while response was dated from the time of the first indication of objective response.

Chemotherapy doses were adjusted on the basis of peripheral blood count nadirs, liver function tests, and neurologic toxicity. Patients randomized to receive lithium were given lithium carbonate, 900 mg daily in three divided doses, starting 24 hours after chemotherapy administration and continuing until 48 hours prior to the next treatment cycle (18 days). Lithium carbonate was not administered during the period of radiation therapy. The dose of lithium carbonate was adjusted on the basis of weekly serum lithium levels as well as symptoms of gastrointestinal and central nervous system toxicity. Neither the patient nor the clinician were blinded with regard to lithium carbonate administration.

Response rates were studied using the Chi-squared method while hematologic parameters were assessed using the student's T-test with a pooled variance. Actuarial life table analyses of remission duration and survival were performed using the Wilcoxin-Gehan test (Gehan, 1965).

RESULTS

Patient Population

One patient in each group was found to have histology other than that of small cell carcinoma while two patients in each group died prior to receiving chemotherapy. Of the remaining 45 evaluable patients, 25 were randomized to the control group and 20 to the lithium group.

The mean age of the control group was 59.2 years (range 49-71) and the mean age of the lithium group was 59.1 years (range 37-68). Patients over the age of 60 accounted for 35% and 45% of the control and lithium groups respectively. Five patients were female with four (16%) randomized to the control group and one (5%) to the lithium group. While all patients had a Karnofsky performance status greater than 40 at presentation, 13 patients in each group demonstrated extensive disease, accounting for 52% and 65% of the control and lithium groups respectively. Table I indicates the sites of metastatic involvement at the time of presentation with bone and liver accounting for the majority of extrathoracic sites of spread. There are no significant differences in the pretreatment stratification parameters between the two treatment groups.

TABLE I

ADVANCED SMALL CELL BRONCHOGENIC CARCINOMA

EXTENT OF DISEASE

	TOTAL	LITHIUM	CONTROL
LIMITED DISEASE	19 (42%)	7 (35%)	12 (48%)
EXTENSIVE DISEASE	26 (58%)	13 (65%)	13 (52%)
BONE	16 (36%)	8 (40%)	8 (32%)
BONE MARROW	11 (24%)	4 (20%)	7 (28%)
LIVER	11 (24%)	4 (20%)	7 (28%)
CNS	3 (7%)	2 (10%)	1 (4%)

Hematologic Response

Patients randomized to receive lithium carbonate had significantly higher leukocyte and neutrophil counts at the nadir following chemotherapy compared to control patients (Lyman *et al.*, 1978b). Figure 2 illustrates the change of the mean leukocyte (panel A) and neutrophil (panel B) counts with time following chemotherapy. The significant effects of lithium carbonate were observed regardless of age, pretreatment blood counts, or extent of disease including bone marrow involvement. Patient numbers were too small to determine the effect of lithium carbonate on leukocyte counts in patients receiving prior treatment. Significantly fewer treatment courses were associated with leukocyte counts less than 2000 or 1000 cells/mm^3 and with neutrophil counts less than 500 or 100 cells/mm^3 at the

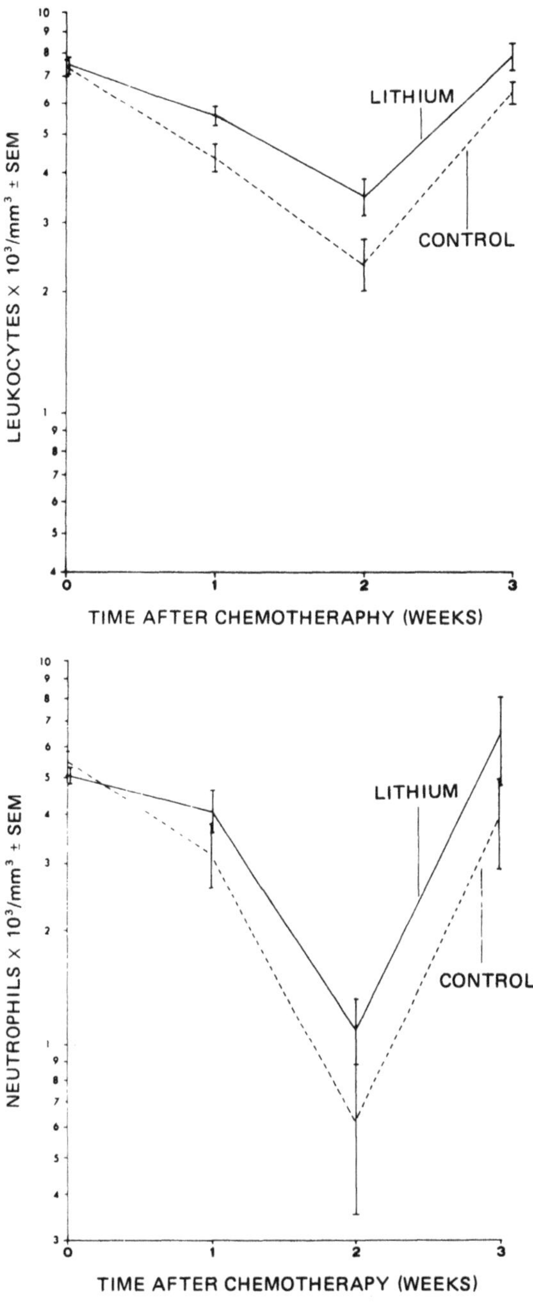

Figure 2. Semilogarithmic plot of the change in mean leukocyte (2A) and neutrophil (2B) counts with time following the administration of systemic chemotherapy in patients with small cell bronchogenic carcinoma randomized to the control group or lithium group. Vertical lines represent standard errors of the means.

nadir in the lithium group than in the control group ($p < 0.01$). Patients randomized to receive lithium carbonate also had significantly higher mean platelet counts at the nadir compared to control patients. While two patients in the control group experienced platelet counts below $100{,}000/mm^3$, none of the patients in the lithium group developed platelet counts below that level.

Significantly fewer protocol determined dose reductions in chemotherapy were necessary in the lithium group compared to the control group. Similarly, fewer protocol required delays in chemotherapy were necessary in the lithium group compared to the control group ($p < 0.01$). Severe febrile episodes requiring hospitalization occurred in eight patients. Seven (88%) of these episodes occurred in the control group as did all six such episodes that developed in the setting of severe neutropenia ($p < 0.05$). No discernible difference between the two treatment groups was observed for hemoglobin or hematocrit determinations and no clinically significant bleeding was encountered.

Tumor Response

Table II summarizes the treatment response information for patients entered on this study. While objective response rates between the two groups are not significantly different, only 4 (20%) of the lithium treated group failed to respond prior to death compared to 9 (36%) of the control group. The overall objective response rates for patients completing two or more cycles of chemotherapy were 88%, 94%, and 91% for the control group, lithium group, and all patients respectively.

Of the 19 patients with limited disease at presentation, nine (47%) experienced a complete remission and 7 (37%) a partial remission. The total objective response rate for patients with limited disease was 75% and 100% for the control and lithium groups respectively. Five patients (71%) with limited disease in the lithium group achieved a complete remission compared to four (33%) with limited disease in the control group ($p < 0.05$). Of the 26 patients with extensive disease at presentation, two (8%) achieved a complete response and 14 (54%) a partial remission. The total objective response rate for extensive disease patients was 54% and 69% for the control and lithium groups respectively.

TABLE II

TREATMENT RESULTS

	TOTAL	GROUP, NO. (%) LITHIUM	CONTROL
COMPLETE RESPONSE	11 (24%)	6 (30%)	5 (20%)
PARTIAL RESPONSE	21 (47%)	10 (50%)	11 (44%)
TOTAL RESPONDERS	32 (71%)	16 (80%)	16 (64%)

The median duration of response of all patients with a complete or partial remission was 41 weeks. As illustrated in Figure 3, the projected duration of response was not significantly different between the two treatment groups with a median duration of response of 37 weeks and 44 weeks in the control and lithium groups respectively. Patients achieving a complete response had a longer duration of remission (median, 37 weeks) than patients achieving a partial response (median, 21 weeks) ($p < 0.10$). The only two patients who have thus far relapsed after achieving a complete response were in the control group. Control group patients achieving a partial response appear to have somewhat longer remission durations (median, 35 weeks) than lithium-treated patients in partial remission (median, 21 weeks).

Fourteen patients have demonstrated evidence of progressive disease after an initial response while four patients have progressed with no evidence of a preceding response. Seven patients (39%) have demonstrated progressive disease in the chest, five (28%) in the liver, and eight (44%) in the central nervous system including four who developed spinal cord compression and one who had not received prophylactic cranial irradiation. Six of the seven patients with progression occurring in the chest were in the control group while other sites of progressive disease did not differ significantly between the two groups.

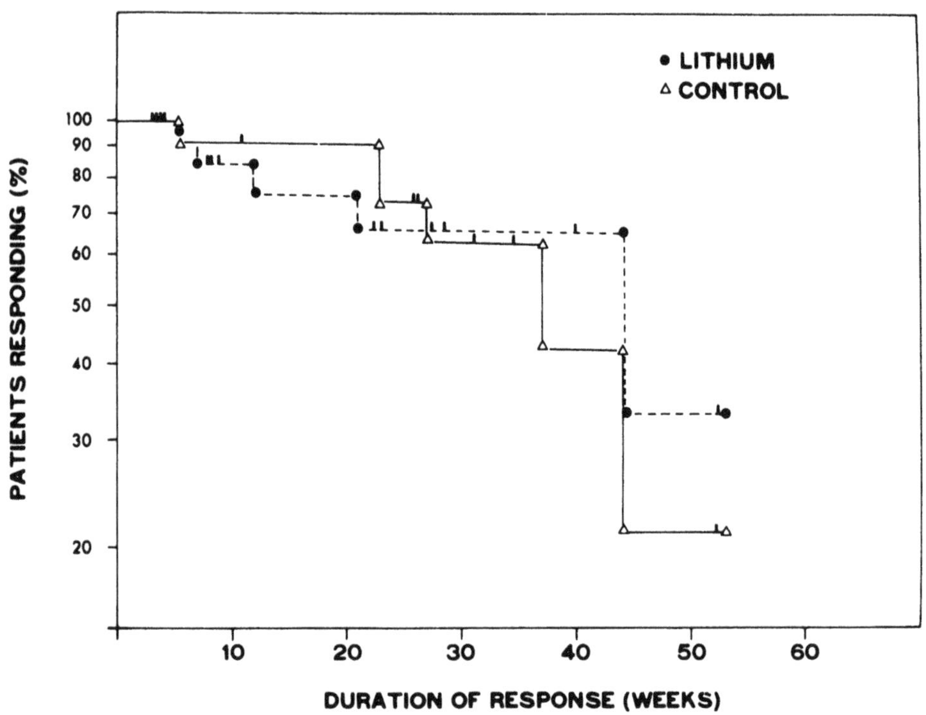

Figure 3. Semilogarithmic actuarial life table plot of the duration of complete or partial response of patients with small cell bronchogenic carcinoma. The ordinate represents the projected percentage of patients in complete or partial remission while the abscissa represents the duration of continuing remission in weeks. Patients were randomly assigned to the control group (N=16) or the lithium group (N=16).

Patient Survival

The projected median survival for the entire group of patients entered on this study is 30 weeks. Patients with limited disease at presentation have significantly longer survival than those with extensive disease with median survivals of 40 weeks and 23 weeks respectively ($p < 0.05$). Figure 4 represents an acturarial life table survival curve for patients entered on the two treatment arms. The projected median survivals for all patients entered on study are 31 weeks and 25 weeks in the control and lithium groups respectively. The greatest difference in survival between the two treatment groups is evident in patients with extensive disease where the projected median survivals are 31 weeks and 16 weeks in the control and lithium groups respectively. The median survival of control patients with limited disease is 40 weeks while the median survival for lithium-treated patients with limited disease has not been reached.

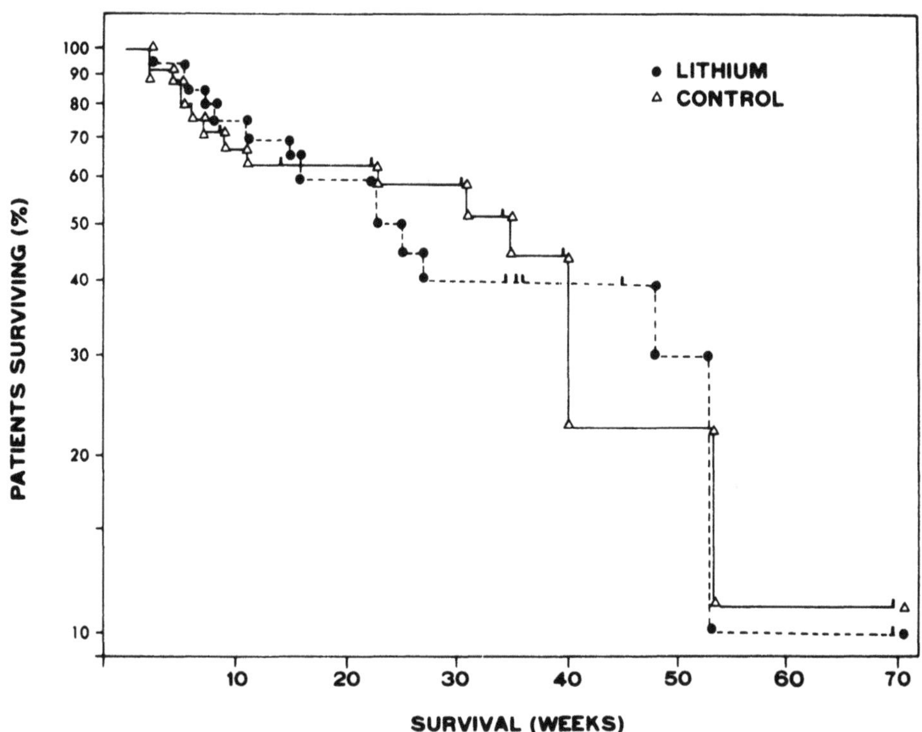

Figure 4. Semilogarithmic actuarial life table plot of the survival of all patients with small cell bronchogenic carcinoma following the initiation of chemotherapy. The ordinate represents the projected percentage of patients surviving while the abscissa represents the time of survival in weeks. Patients were randomly assigned to the control group (N=25) or the lithium group (N=20).

Thirty-two patients (71%) entered on this study have died with nearly equal percentages of deaths occurring in patients with either limited or extensive disease and in patients in each of the two treatment arms. Table III summarizes the causes of death observed to date in this study. Approximately 47% of patients who have died in both treatment arms have died from progressive malignancy while the majority have died of causes unrelated or indirectly related to their malignancy. Six patients have died of presumed infection of which five occurred in the setting of severe leukopenia ($p < 0.05$). All six infection-related deaths occurred in patients in the control group. Five patients have died of known vascular causes and all of these patients were in the lithium group ($p < 0.05$). One patient had a cerebrovascular accident, one had a documented myocardial infarction, and three died in congestive heart failure. If sudden deaths are included as presumed cardiovascular deaths, the later account for 12% and 43% of the deaths in the control and lithium groups respectively ($p < 0.05$).

TABLE III

CAUSES OF DEATH

		GROUP	
	TOTAL	LITHIUM	CONTROL
PROGRESSIVE DISEASE	15	7	8
INFECTION	6	0	6
CARDIOVASCULAR	4	4	0
CEREBROVASCULAR	1	1	0
SUDDEN DEATH	4	2	2
BLEEDING	1	1	0
UNKNOWN	1	0	1
TOTAL	32	15	17

As shown in Table IV, the patient population studied here had a high incidence of previous myocardial infarction and electrocardiographic abnormalities at presentation. Patients with a history of myocardial infarction accounted for 16% and 35% of patients randomized to the control and lithium groups respectively. Deaths have occurred in 73% of patients with a history of previous myocardial infarction and all but one of these deaths occurred suddenly or was of known cardiovascular origin. Patients with an abnormal electrocardiogram accounted for 32% and 60% of the control and lithium groups respectively ($p < 0.05$). Thirty-eight percent of control

TABLE IV

CARDIOVASCULAR RISK FACTORS

	PREVIOUS MI		ABNORMAL EKG	
	NO.	DEATHS	NO.	DEATHS
CONTROL	4	2	9	3
LITHIUM	7	6	12	9
TOTAL	11	8	21	12

patients and 75% of lithium-treated patients with abnormal electrocardiograms at presentation have died ($p < 0.05$). Similarly, 50% of control patients and 85% of lithium-treated patients with a history of a previous myocardial infarction at presentation have died. If patients dying of documented or presumed cardiovascular causes are excluded from analysis, the projected median survivals are 31 weeks and 53 weeks for the control and lithium groups respectively ($p < 0.10$). As shown in Figure 5, if patients presenting with a history of a previous myocardial infarction are excluded from evaluation, the median survivals of the control and lithium groups respectively are 31 weeks and 48 weeks.

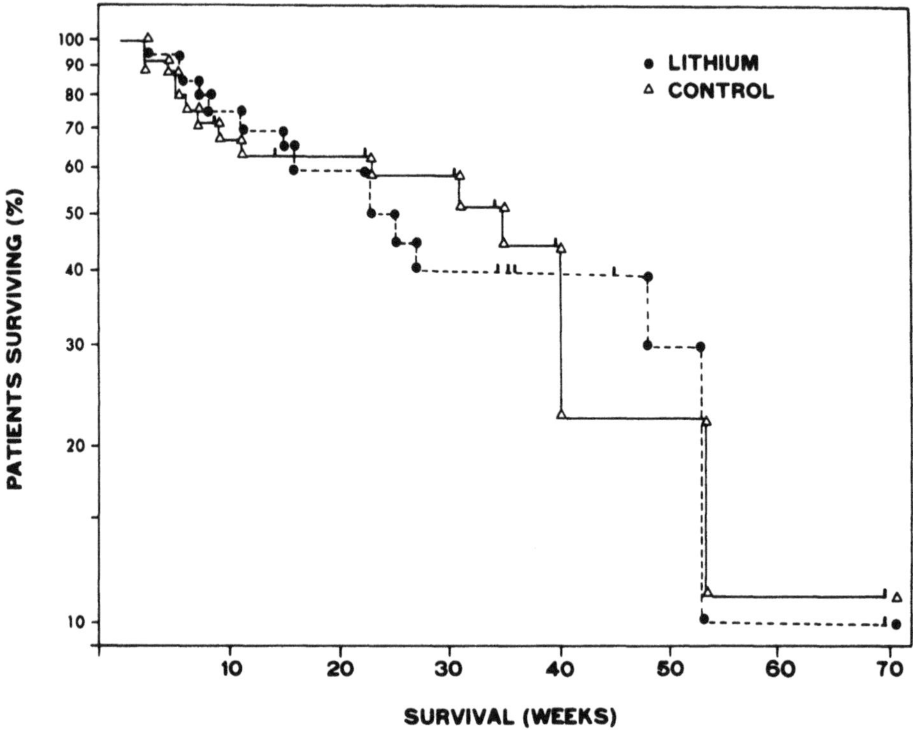

Figure 5. Semilogarithmic actuarial life table plot of the survival of patients with small cell bronchogenic carcinoma following the initiation of chemotherapy exclusive of patients who had sustained a myocardial infarction prior to diagnosis. The ordinate represents the projected percentage of patients surviving while the abscissa represents the time of survival in weeks. Patients were randomly assigned to the control group (N=21) or the lithium group (N=13).

<u>Toxicity</u>

No deaths were directly attributable to lithium administration. One patient developed a serum lithium level in excess of 2 meq/L associated with gastrointestinal symptoms that resolved with discontinuation of the drug. One patient developed clinical diabetes insipidus that resolved with discontinuation of lithium carbonate.

Table V summarizes the toxicity reported for patients on each treatment arm of the study. It was virtually impossible to distinguish the toxicity of lithium carbonate from that of the cytotoxic therapy received. Seven patients (35%) refused further lithium administration primarily due to gastrointestinal symptoms. Eight patients (40%) continued full dose lithium administration while five patients (25%) required minor dose modification based on symptoms attributed to lithium administration.

TABLE V

TOXICITY

	TOTAL	LITHIUM	CONTROL
WEAKNESS	26 (58%)	16 (80%)	10 (40%)
NAUSEA, VOMITING	20 (44%)	14 (70%)	6 (24%)
MUCOSITIS	3 (7%)	2 (10%)	1 (4%)
DYSPHAGIA	13 (29%)	9 (45%)	4 (16%)

DISCUSSION

Undifferentiated small cell carcinoma of the lung is a rapidly progressive malignant disorder with the majority of patients presenting with evidence of metastatic disease. Combination chemotherapy and radiation therapy is capable of producing an objective regression of disease in the majority of patients with a significant prolongation of survival compared to less intensive approaches (Broder *et al.*, 1977; Livingston *et al.*, 1978; Lyman *et al.*, 1978a; Weiss, 1978). Despite such advances in the management of patients with small cell lung cancer, few patients survive beyond two years (Weiss, 1978). Disease relapse, usually in the chest, represents the single most common cause of death in most series (Livingston *et al.*, 1978; McMahon *et al.*, 1979). The study reported here indicates that unselected patients with small cell lung cancer are at considerable risk for death from infection or cardiovascular causes when treated with combination chemotherapy and radiation therapy.

The results reported here confirm our previous experience (Lyman et al., 1978a) and the experience of others (Johnson et al., 1976; Livingston et al., 1978) that patients with small cell bronchogenic carcinoma treated with intensive cytotoxic therapy are at considerable risk for severe neutropenia, neutropenia-related sepsis, and infection-related death. A number of studies have now demonstrated that the sequential administration of lithium between cycles of intensive chemotherapy reduces the leukocyte and neutrophil nadir observed (Tisman, 1974; Stein et al., 1977; Catane et al., 1977; Greco and Brereton, 1977). Our study clearly suggests, in addition, that patients receiving lithium carbonate have a reduced risk of infection and infection-related death in this setting (Lyman et al., 1978b). Similarly, patients receiving lithium carbonate required dose reduction or delay in chemotherapy less frequently than control patients. An interesting but clinically insignificant effect on platelet nadirs was also observed in this study.

While the mechanism of action of lithium in ameliorating the leukopenia associated with chemotherapy in unknown, it can enlarge the total circulating neutrophil cell mass as well as marrow granulocyte reserves (Rothstein et al., 1978; Stein et al., 1978). The enhanced production of leukocytes observed may be the result of lithium stimulation of colony stimulating activity production (Joyce and Chervenick, 1975; Harker et al., 1977). While the effect of lithium on the incidence of sepsis and infection-related death may be entirely related to its effect on leukocyte production, this agent may actually enhance a variety of leukocyte functions (Rothstein et al., 1978; Shenkman et al., 1978; Cohen et al., 1979).

The overall effects of lithium on treatment responsiveness, duration of response, survival and toxicity in this study are difficult to evaluate. Patients in the two treatment groups are virtually identical with regard to the stratification factors of age, functional status, and prior treatment. Patients randomized to the lithium group had a higher frequency of extensive disease at presentation although these differences are not statistically significant. However, significantly more patients with abnormal electrocardiograms at presentation were randomized to the lithium group than to the control group. More patients in the lithium group also presented with a history of a previous myocardial infarction. Adriamycin (Rinehardt et al., 1974; Lenaz and Page, 1976; Bristow et al., 1978), cyclophosphamide (O'Connell and Berenbaum, 1974; Minow et al., 1977), and mediastinal irradiation (Fajardo et al., 1976) have all been associated with an increased risk of cardiovascular complications. Since a greater number of patients with evidence of underlying cardiovascular disease were randomized to the lithium group, these factors may account for the significantly greater risk of death from presumed cardiac origin in this group.

Lithium administration has been associated with a variety of electrocardiographic changes including flattening or inversion of the T-wave, sinoatrial node dysfunction, and premature ventricular contractions (Tilkian, et al., 1976). One episode of acute myocardial infarction and two with fatal myocarditis have been reported in patients receiving lithium (Baldessarini and Stephens, 1970; Tseng, 1971; Swedberg and Winblad, 1974). Associated clinical disorders and the rarity of these complications make it difficult to draw a causal relationship, however. Lithium is capable of altering potassium and other electrolyte concentrations intracellularly, competing with Ca^{++} and Mg^{++} at the neuronal level and altering adenyl cyclase activity (Singer and Rotenberg, 1973). The serum concentration of lithium may be significantly increased in patients with altered hydration and in particular in patients with congestive heart failure or on diuretics (Petersen et al., 1974).

We observed no electrocardiographic changes directly associated with lithium administration. No documented cardiovascular deaths and only one sudden death occurred in patients without evidence of cardiovascular disease at presentation. However, the greater death rates observed in high risk patients randomized to receive lithium, suggests that further intensive study is necessary to assess the potential cardiovascular risk of this agent.

Similarly, it is difficult to assess the contribution of lithium carbonate to the toxic symptoms associated with cytotoxic therapy in this population of patients. Due to overlapping toxicities and the lack of blinding of both physician and patient, it is difficult to legitimately compare toxicities of patients in the two treatment groups. No life threatening toxicity was observed and all toxic symptoms reversed readily with discontinuation of therapy. Serum lithium levels were not predictive of the toxic symptoms observed. In general, symptoms were tolerable and the majority of patients continued lithium administration once initiated.

The objective response rate, duration of response, and patient survival of the 45 patients with small cell bronchogenic carcinoma reported here are comparable to other reports in the literature using similar cytotoxic therapy. In the largest reported series (Livingston et al., 1978), the Southwest Oncology Group observed a complete remission rate of 40% and a partial remission rate of 23% for an overall objective response rate of 63% in 358 patients with small cell carcinoma of the lung. They observed median durations of remission of 42 weeks and 23 weeks in patients achieving complete and partial remissions respectively with an overall median survival of 31 weeks.

In the study reported here, a greater percentage of patients randomized to the lithium group responded than in the control. This difference is not statistically significant, however. There is no significant difference between control patients and those receiving lithium carbonate with regard to duration of response or overall survival. While patients receiving lithium carbonate experienced significantly fewer septic episodes and no deaths attributable to infection, a significantly increased incidence of death due to presumed cardiovascular causes was observed. Similarly, patients with extensive disease at presentation who received lithium carbonate demonstrated shorter remission durations and overall survival than control patients.

While the chest is the most frequent site of progressive disease in our series, the high rate of CNS progression is of concern. Prophylactic cranial irradiation appears to minimize effectively the brain as a site of progression (Jackson et al., 1977; Moore et al., 1978). As treatment regimens continue to improve the survival outlook for patients with small cell lung cancer, however, investigators are reporting with increasing frequency progressive disease in the spinal meninges (Bunn et al., 1978; Brereton et al., 1978). Future studies of the role of prophylactic intrathecal chemotherapy or spinal irradiation will hopefully result in an improved control of disease in this area.

The clearly improved overall survival observed in patients with no history of myocardial infarction receiving lithium carbonate suggests that more careful patient evaluation and selection will be necessary. In patients without significant cardiovascular disease who are receiving cytotoxic therapy for advanced small cell lung cancer, significant benefit may be obtained from the concurrent administration of lithium carbonate. However, further evaluation of the toxic potential of lithium in this setting will be necessary in order to define more clearly its safety when used in conjunction with combined modality cytotoxic therapy in patients with advanced malignancy.

CONCLUSION

Small cell undifferentiated carcinoma of the lung is a rapidly progressive malignancy responsive to radiation therapy and a variety of chemotherapeutic agents. Combination chemotherapy and combined modality approaches have increased response rates and survival while producing significant myelosuppression in the majority of patients. Lithiurn carbonate has been shown to ameliorate the leukopenia associated with systemic chemotherapy. We have summarized the treatment results of 45 evaluable patients entered into a prospective randomized trial of lithium carbonate and combination chemotherapy and radiation therapy for patients with small cell lung cancer. Patients receiving lithium carbonate demonstrated significantly higher leukocyte and neutrophil counts at the nadir following chemotherapy. Treatment was associated with a complete response in 24% and a partial response in 47% of patients with no significant differences between the control group and the lithium group. The median duration of remission was 37 weeks and 44 weeks and the median survival was 35 weeks and 25 weeks in the control and lithium groups respectively. Infection was the cause of death in six patients in the control and in none of the lithium group. Presumed cardiovascular causes accounted for seven deaths in the lithium group and for two deaths in the control group. The risk of cardiovascular death is directly related to a history of pretreatment cardiovascular disease. Further study will be necessary to clarify the safety and utility of lithium carbonate in patients with advanced malignancy.

REFERENCES

Baldessarini, R.J. and Stephens, J.H., 1970, Lithium carbonate for affective disorders: Clinical pharmacology and toxicology, Arch. Gen. Psych. 22:72.

Bergsagel, D.E., Jenkin, R.D., Pringle, J.F., White, D.M., Fetterlay, J.C.M., Klaasen, D.J., and McDermot, R.S.R., 1972, Lung cancer clinical trial of radiotherapy alone plus cyclophosphamide, Cancer 30:621.

Brereton, H.D., O'Donnell, J.F., Kent, C.H., Mathews, M., Dunnick, N.R., and Johnson, R.E., 1978, Spinal meningeal carcinomatosis in small-cell carcinoma of the lung, Ann. Int. Med. 88:517.

Bristow, M.R., Thompson, P.D., Martin, R.P., Mason, J.W., Billingham, M.E., and Harrison, D.C., 1978, Early anthracycline cardiotoxicity, Am. J. Med. 65:823.

Broder, L.E., Cohen, M.H., and Selawry, O.S., 1977, Treatment of bronchogenic carcinoma. II Small cell, Cancer Treat. Rev. 4:219.

Bunn, P.A., Nugent, J.L., and Mathews, M.J., 1978, Central nervous system metastases in small cell bronchogenic carcinoma, Sem. Oncol. 5:314.

Catane, R., Kaufman, J., Mittleman, A., and Murphy, G.P., 1977, Attenuation of myelosuppression with lithium, N. Engl. J. Med. 297:452.

Cohen, M.S. Zakhireh, B., Metcalf, J.A., and Root, R.K., 1979, Granulocyte function during lithium therapy, Blood 53:913.

Fajardo, L.F., Eltringham, J.R., and Steward, J.R., 1976, Combined cardiotoxicity of adriamycin and x-radiation, Lab. Invest. 34:86.

Fox, W. and Scadding, J.G., 1973, Medical research council comparative trial of surgery and radiotherapy for primary treatment of small-celled or oat-celled carcinoma of the bronchus: Ten-year follow-up, The Lancet 2:63.

Gehan, E., 1965, A generalized Wilcoxin test for comparing arbitrarily single-censored samples, Biometrika 52:203.

Greco, E.A. and Brereton, H.D., 1977, Effect of lithium carbonate on the neutropenia caused by chemoterapy: A preliminary clinical trial, Oncology 34:153.

Green, R.A., Humphrey, E., Close, H., and Patnu, M.E., 1969, Alkylating agents in bronchogenic carcinoma, Am. J. Med. 46:516.

Hansen, H.H., Dombernowsky, P., Hansen, M., and Hirsch, F., 1978, Chemotherapy of advanced small cell anaplastic carcinoma. Superiority of a four-drug combination to a three-drug combination, Ann. Int. Med. 89:177.

Harker, W.G., Rothstein, G., Clarkson, D., Athens, J.W., and Macfarlane, J.L., 1977, Enhancement of colony-stimulating activity production by lithium, Blood 49:263.

Higgins, G.A., 1972, Use of chemotherapy as an adjuvant to surgery for bronchogenic carcinoma, Cancer 30:1383.

Holoye, P.Y., Samuels, M.L., Lanzotti, V.J., Smith, T., and Barkley, H.T., 1977, Combination chemotherapy and radiation therapy for small cell carcinoma, JAMA, 237:1221.

Jackson, D.V., Richards, F., II, Cooper, R., Ferree, C., Muss,H.B., White, D.R., and Spurr, C.L., 1977, Prophylactic cranial irradiation in small cell carcinoma of the lung: A randomized study, JAMA 237:2730.

Johnson, R.E., Brereton, H.D., and Kent, H.D., 1976, Small-cell carcinoma of the lung: Attempt to remedy causes of past therapeutic failure, The Lancet 2:289.

Joyce, R.A. and Chervenick, P.A., 1975, Effect of lithium on the release of colony stimulating activity (CSA) from blood leukocytes, Proc. Am. Soc. Hematol. 18:126.

Lenaz, L. and Page, J.A., 1976, Cardiotoxicity of adriamycin and related anthracyclines, Cancer Treat. Rev. 3:111.

Livingston, R.B., Moore, T.N., Heilbrun, L., Bottomley, R., Lehane, D.M., Rivkin, S.E., and Thigpen, T., 1978, Small-cell carcinoma of the lung: Combined chemotherapy and radiation, Ann. Int. Med. 88:194.

Lyman, G.H., Hartmann, R.C., Saba, H.I., Preston, D., Shukovsky, L., Jensen, R., and Knight, M., 1978a, Combination chemotherapy and radiation therapy of undifferentiated small cell bronchogenic carcinoma, South Med. J. 71:519.

Lyman, G.H., Williams, C.C., and Preston, D., 1978b, Prospective randomized study of the effect of lithium carbonate on the granulocytopenia and incidence of infection associated with intensive chemotherapy and radiation therapy for undifferentiated small cell bronchogenic carcinoma, Blood 51:228 (Supplement 1).

McMahon, L.J., Herman, T.S., Manning, M.R., and Dean, J.C., 1979, Patterns of relapse in patients with small cell carcinoma of the lung treated with adriamycin-cyclophosphamide chemotherapy and radiation therapy, Cancer Treat. Rep. 63:359.

Minow, R.A., Benjamin, R.S., and Lee, E.T., 1977, Adriamycin cardiomyopathy-risk factors, Cancer 39:1397.

Moore, T.N., Livingston, R., Heilbrun, L., Eltringham, J., Skinner, O., White, J., and Tesh, D., 1978, The effectiveness of prophylactic brain irradiation in small cell carcinoma of the lung, Cancer 41:2149.

Muggia, F.M., Krezoski, S.K., and Hansen, H.H., 1974, Cell kinetic studies in patients with small cell carcinoma of the lung, Cancer 34:1683.

O'Connell, T.W. and Berenbaum, M.G., 1974, Cardiac and pulmonary effects of high doses of cyclophosphamide and isophosphamide, Cancer Res. 34:1589.

Petersen, V., Hvidt, S., and Thomsen, K., 1974, Effect of prolonged thiazide treatment on renal lithium clearance, Brit. Med. J. 3:143.

Rinehardt, J.J., Lewis, R.P., and Balcerzak, S.P., 1974, Adriamycin cardiotoxicity in man, Ann. Int. Med. 81:475.

Rothstein, G., Clarkson, D.R., Larsen, W., Grosser, B.I., and Athens, J.W., 1978, Effect of lithium on neutrophil mass and production, N. Engl. J. Med. 298:178.

Shenkman, L., Borkowsky, W., Holzman, R.S., and Shopsin, B., 1978, Enhancement of lymphocyte and macrophage function in vitro by lithium chloride, Clin. Immunol. Immunopath. 10:187.

Shopsin, B., Friedman, R., and Gershon, S., 1971, Lithium and leukocytosis, Clin. Pharmacol. Ther. 12:923.

Singer, I. and Rotenberg, D., 1973, Mechanism of lithium action, N. Engl. J. Med. 289:254.

Stein, R., Beaman, C., Ali, M., Hansen, R., Jenkins, D.D., and Jume'an, H.G., 1977, Lithium carbonate attenuation of chemotherapy-induced neutropenia, N. Engl. J. Med. 297:430.

Stein, R.S., Hanson, G., Koethe, S., and Hansen, R., 1978, Lithium-induced granulocytosis, Ann. Int. Med. 88:809.

Swedberg, K. and Winblad, B., 1974, Heart failure as complication of lithium treatment, Acta Med. Scand. 196:279.

Tilkian, A.G., Schroeder, J.S., Kao, J.J., and Hultgren, H.N., 1976, The cardiovascular effects of lithium in man. A review of the literature, Am. J. Med. 61:665.

Tisman, G., 1974, Lithium carbonate protection against drug-induced leukopenia in lymphosarcoma patients, IRCS 2:1509.

Tseng, H.L., 1971, Interstitial myocarditis probably related to lithium carbonate intoxication, Arch. Pathol. 92:444.

Weiss, R.B., 1978, Small-cell carcinoma of the lung: Therapeutic management, Ann. Int. Med. 88:522.

HIGHER LEUKOCYTE NADIRS WITH LITHIUM CARBONATE AFTER CHEMOTHERAPY

Peter G. Steinherz, Gerald Rosen, Fereshteh Ghavimi, Norma Wollner, Ying Wang and Denis R. Miller

Department of Pediatrics
Memorial Sloan-Kettering Cancer Center
New York, New York

Leukocytosis has been observed following lithium carbonate administration in manic-depressive disorders (Mayfield *et al.*; 1966; O'Connell *et al.*, 1970; Murphy *et al.*, 1971). The elevation of the white blood count is modest, reversible, independent of blood lithium concentration, and due to neutrophilia (Murphy *et al.*, 1971; Shopsin *et al.*, 1971; Watanabe *et al.*, 1974; Bille *et al.*, 1975; Perez-Cruet *et al.*, 1978, Yassa *et al.*, 1978). Lithium may stimulate adrenocortical activity (Platman and Fieve, 1968; Shopsin and Gershon, 1971). It enhances marrow proliferation, elevates neutrophil production and increases the granulocyte pool without affecting granulocyte function or inhibiting neutrophil migration into skin lesions (Tisman *et al.*, 1973; Rossof and Coltman, 1976; Malloy *et al.*, 1978; Rothstein *et al.*, 1978; Shenkman *et al.*, 1978; Stein *et al.*, 1978; Cohen *et al.*, 1979; Steinherz and Smithwick, 1979). The mechanism by which lithium exerts its effect *in vivo* is unclear; however, it stimulates the formation of granulocytic colonies in the agar culture system either by stimulating the synthesis of colony stimulating factor (Harker *et al.*, 1977) or by enhancing the action of colony stimulating factor (Morley and

Galbraith, 1978). Increase in leukocyte numbers has also been observed with lithium treatment in patients with neutropenia secondary to Felty's syndrome or aplastic anemia, and in congenital and acquired neutropenia (Gupta et al., 1975; Gupta et al., 1976; Barrett et al., 1977; Blum et al., 1979; Chan et al., 1979; deAlarcon et al., 1979). Reports of improved counts after cancer chemotherapy in small trials (Tisman, 1974; Greco and Brereton, 1977; Charron et al., 1977; Catane et al., 1977; Stein et al., 1977; Tiefenbach et al., 1977; Steinherz et al., 1979a) prompted us to evaluate lithium carbonate after chemotherapy in a randomized, paired, prospective study (Steinherz et al., 1979b.).

MATERIALS AND METHODS

Patients: Eighty-six cycles (43 paired cycles) of chemotherapy in patients with various solid tumors with minimal or no bone marrow invasion by the malignancy, who were on cyclic chemotherapeutic protocols that produce neutropenia $\leq 1000/mm^3$ 40-50% of the time were studied. A patient could be studied more than once if he received pairs of different therapies. For each pair he would be considered as a separate patient in the analysis of the data. The patients were attending the Pediatric Day Hospital of Memorial Sloan-Kettering Cancer Center. They were seen during their regular visits for chemotherapy. Each pulse of chemotherapy lasted 3-7 days. On the last day of treatment, after informed consent was obtained, the patients were randomized to receive lithium carbonate or no treatment. When a patient received the initial chemotherapy again during the next cycle of treatment with no dose reduction, lithium was given to those who received no lithium the first time. Four patients in whom the chemotherapy dose was reduced after the first course and would have received a lower dose before lithium than in the control period were excluded from analysis. The chemotherapy delivered to seven patients before lithium was higher than in the control period. They were included in the analysis. Four patients could not take the drug because of nausea or emesis and were excluded from analysis. The remaining 35 pairs (in 21 patients) served as their own controls. The diagnoses of the patients are listed on Table I. Twenty received lithium after the first chemotherapeutic course. Patients with fever or on antibiotic treatment were not entered on the study. The patients' ages ranged from 3-23 years (median 16). There were 24 males and 11 females.

TABLE I

DIAGNOSES OF THE PATIENTS

Ewing's Sarcoma	21
Rhabdomyosarcoma	7
Neuroblastoma	3
Wilms' Tumor	2
Nasopharyngeal carcinoma	1
Teratoma	1
	35

Chemotherapy: Twenty-one patients received a seven drug chemotherapy regimen (Figure 1). They were studied after the first or the second five day treatment of this protocol. Eleven patients received the same drugs but the same total drug dose was given over three days instead of five (Figure 2). Three recieved a seven day treatment for neuroblastoma with high dose cyclophosphamide (> 40mg/kg X 2), vincristine, papaverine, hydroxyurea, cytosine arabinoside, and triflouro-thymidine. No patient received radiotherapy or corticosteroids during the study period.

Lithium: Lithium is not approved for use in children. An investigational exemption for a new drug (IND) was obtained from the Food and Drug Administration. Lithium carbonate (300 mg capsules) was obtained from Smith, Kline and French Laboratories. The drug was given orally according to the patient's size: surface area $< 0.5\ m^2$ = 150 mg daily; 0.5 - 1.0 m^2 = 300 mg daily; 1.0 - 1.5 m^2 = 300 mg B.I.D.; $> 1.5\ m^2$ = 300 mg T.I.D. The serum level achieved was 0.2 - 1.2 meq/liter (median 0.7). In an occasional patient with low blood levels, the initial dose was increased. Lithium levels were measured weekly by flame spectrophotometry. The drug was continued until the white count began to rise again after the nadir. This occurred after approximately 14 days of lithium administration.

White Blood Count: White blood counts were done weekly on an automated Coulter counter. Differential counts were done manually. More frequent counts were obtained when low counts or fever occurred. The person performing the counts had no knowledge of the study status of the patient.

Statistical Methods: The Wilcoxon paired rank test (Snedecar and Cochran, 1976) or the t-test on the square-root transformation of the white blood counts were used to evaluate the differences observed.

RESULTS

The initial white blood count (WBC) was similar in both groups. The median nadir of the WBC after lithium was $1900/mm^3$ while it was $1200/mm^3$ in the control period ± 340 ($p < 0.05$) (Table II). The polymorphonuclear leukocyte counts paralleled the WBC. Their range was 4-76% of the WBC at the nadir (median 34%). They are not reported because a differential count was not done with every WBC count. There were nine patients with WBC nadirs under $1000/mm^3$ in the treated group for a total of 39 patient days, while in the control group 13 patients spent 69 patient days with WBC $\leq 1000/mm^3$ ($p < 0.01$) (Table III). Comparing the number of days the WBC was under $1000/mm^3$ within each patient the Wilcoxon paried rank test showed a difference ($p < 0.01$). In 11 of the 14 patients whose WBC fell $\leq 1000/mm^3$, the number of days the WBC was $\leq 1000/mm^3$ with lithium treatment was less than without treatment, and the WBC nadir of the treated period was greater or equal to that of the control period. Four patients (11%) required hospitalization for 37 patient days for fever while neutropenic after lithium, while eight patients (23%) spent 104 days in the hospital in the control period ($p < 0.01$) (Table III). No amelioration of anemia or thrombocytopenia was observed.

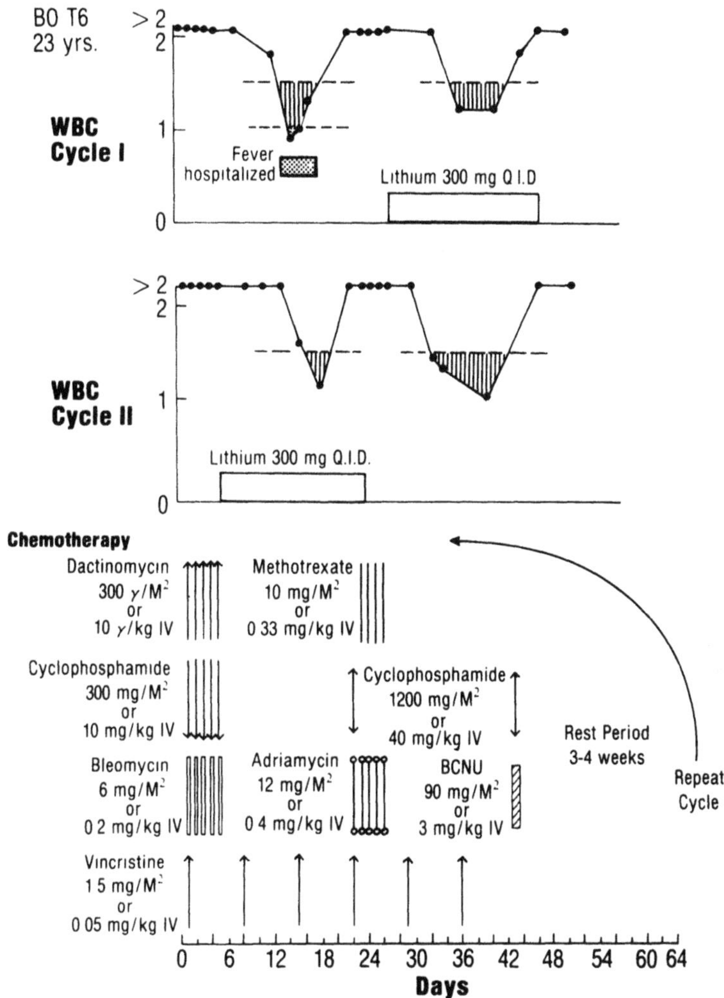

Figure 1. Course of patient B.O. on the T_6 protocol. After the first five days of chemotherapy the WBC fell to 900/mm^3 and the patient needed to be hospitalized for antibiotic treatment because of fever. When he received the same chemotherapy in the second cycle with lithium, the WBC nadir was 1300/mm^3. With the second five day chemotherapy the WBC nadir was 1200/mm^3 with lithium and 1000/mm^3 in the control period.

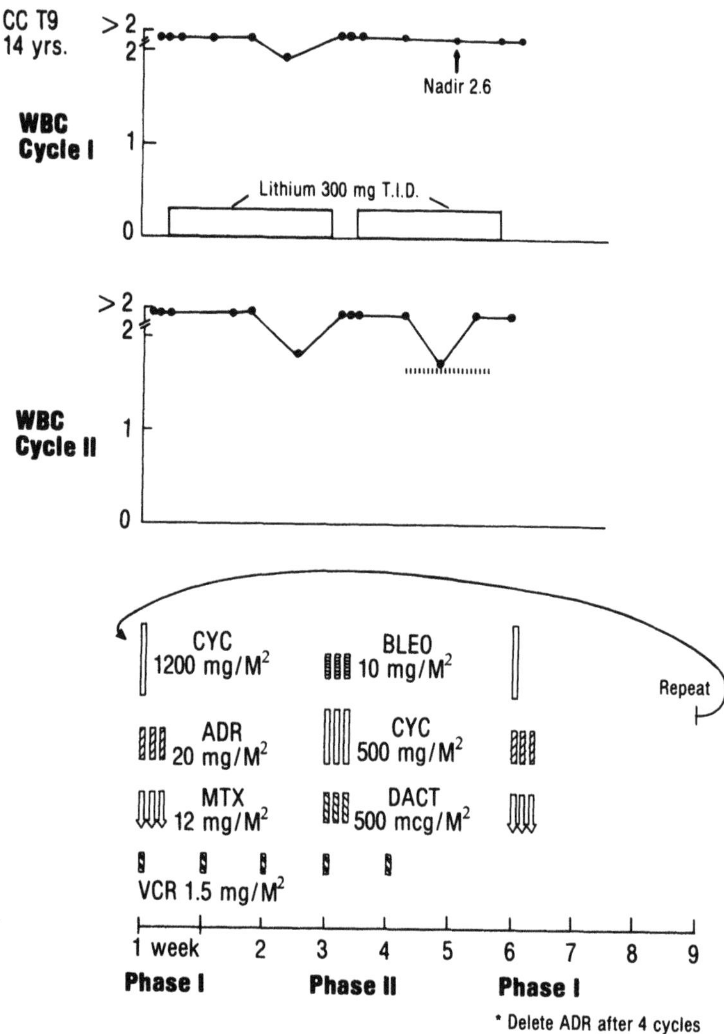

Figure 2. Course of patient C.C. on the T_9 protocol. During the first cycle with lithium the WBC nadir was $1900/mm^3$ and $2600/mm^3$ after the first and second pulse of chemotherapy, while in the second cycle the WBC fell to $1800/mm^3$ and $1700/mm^3$ respectively.

TABLE II

EFFECT OF LITHIUM ON THE WHITE BLOOD COUNT NADIR

	White Blood Count - Median (Range)		
	Lithium	No Lithium	P*
Initial Count	5000 (2600-11400)	5500 (2200-11500)	NS
Nadir	1900 (100-2900)	1200 (100-4600)	< 0.05
Decrease % of Initial count	65% (26-98%)	71% (11-97%)	NS

* One sided paired t-test. NS: not significant.

TABLE III

REDUCTION IN THE INCIDENCE OF SEVERE NEUTROPENIA BY LITHIUM

	Lithium	No Lithium	P*
Number of patients	35	35	
Number with WBC ≤ 1000	9 (27.5%)	13 (37.1%)	
Total patient days ≤ 1000	39	69	< 0.01
Average days WBC ≤ 1000	1.1	2.0	
Number of patients hospitalized	4 (11%)	8 (23%)	
Total patient days in hospital	37	104	< 0.01
Average days hospitalized	1.1	3.0	

* One sided Wilcoxon test

The nadir counts are summarized in Figure 3.

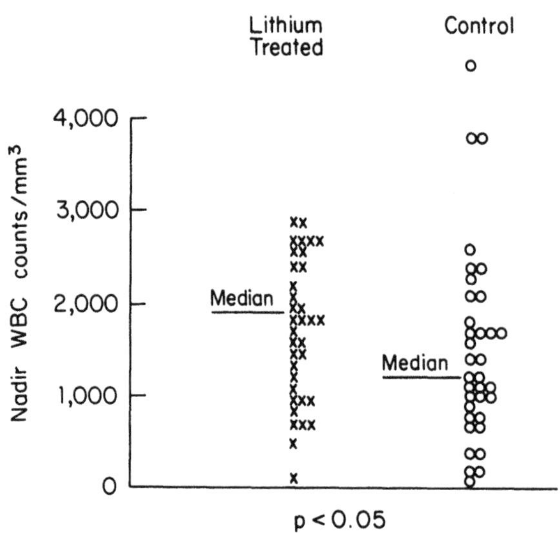

Figure 3. Nadir of the white blood counts after chemotherapy with and without lithium carbonate.

Toxicity: Four patients could not swallow the lithium capsules because of their size. One developed diarrhea on the first day of treatment and the mother discontinued treatment before a serum level was obtained. Two patients had nausea or emesis and discontinued the drug; one had no serum level obtained while the other had 0.7 meq/liter. One patient, at a serum level of 0.8 meq/liter, developed lethargy and depression. A six year old child had a transient episode of slurred speech when his blood level was 1.2 meq/liter. His neurological examination and electroencephalogram were normal. He had a subsequent course of lithium without difficulty. All the side effects observed disappeared with drug discontinuation.

DISCUSSION

The myelosuppressive effects of chemotherapy are very inconsistent. Not only are they influenced by the drug and dosage delivered, but by the patient's marrow reserve, nutritional status, other medications given, presence or absence of intercurrent infection and by other unknown factors. Under these conditions it is very difficult to evaluate the effect an agent has on the neutropenia caused by chemotherapy. Previous reports on the effect of lithium were either in non-randomized studies; or when the patient served as his own control, various chemotherapies and dosages were used; or the treatment included corticosteroids; or patients with bone marrow involvement, where the bone marrow recovery was more a function of the tumor cells being cleared from the marrow by chemotherapy than of myelosuppression, were included (Charron et al., 1977; Greco and Brereton, 1977; Lyman et al., 1978; Stein et al., 1977; Stein et al., 1978a; Stein et al., 1978b).

In our study, the patients were randomized after the first chemotherapy. They were evaluated only if the same chemotherapy was delivered twice and only if the cytotoxic therapy dose before lithium was equal or greater than before the control period. Thirty-two of 35 trials involved only two very similar protocols. No patients with leukemia or with bone marrow involvement were studied. Patients taking steroids or antibiotics or with infection were not entered.

The study showed that the median granulocyte nadir was significantly higher in cycles where lithium was administered after chemotherapy. Fewer patient days were spent with significant neutropenia ($\leq 1000/mm^3$) and consequently fewer patients developed fever while neutropenic, reducing the number of days spent in the hospital for intravenous antibiotic treatment from 104 days to 37 days.

Lithium administration can be toxic and serum levels must be monitored. The most common side effect is nausea and there is the potential for electrolyte abnormalities in dehydrated patients. Therefore, we do not administer lithium concurrently with chemotherapy when most of the patients have nausea and emesis from the chemotherapeutic agents. We begin treatment the day after chemotherapy. This eliminates another potential problem. If lithium works by promoting stem cell differentiation, one would not want to cycle normal cells before chemotherapy when these cells would be susceptible to the toxic effects of the cytotoxic drugs. We discontinue lithium treatment before the next course of chemotherapy, after the granulocytes have regenerated. We have seen no decrease in the ability of lithium treated patients to tolerate subsequent chemotherapy. Because of better counts they actually receive the therapy on time with fewer delays and fewer dose reductions. However, the possibility of long term stem cell depletion needs to be evaluated over a longer period of time. There is no evidence that lithium enhances tumor growth; however, the cycling of tumor cells which would not stop dividing before the next chemotherapy, from the resting state to the growth phase would enhance the cytotoxic effect of the chemotherapy on the tumor.

The improved granulocyte counts associated with lithium administration in this study appeared significant and clinically useful. However, because lithium may be teratogenic (Fredrich and Nielsen, 1969; Nora et al., 1974) we do not recommend its widespread use before further studies are conducted, except for patients on chemotherapeutic protocols where the incidence of severe neutropenia and infectious complications is high. Its use in patients with bone marrow replacement remains to be elucidated.

ACKNOWLEDGEMENTS

This work was supported by NCI Grant # 057 538 and the Smith, Kline and French Laboratories. The authors wish to thank Mr. M. Kelick for technical assistance and Ms. L. Kelly for typing the original manuscript.

REFERENCES

Barrett, A., Hugh-Jones, K., Newton, K. and Watson, J.G., 1977, Lithium therapy in aplastic anemia Lancet 1:202.

Bille, P.E., Jensen, M.K., Jensen, J.P.K., and Paulsen, J.C., 1975, Studies on the haematologic and cytogenic effects of lithium, Acta. Med. Scand. 198:281.

Blum, S.F., 1979, Lithium therapy of aplastic anemia, N. Eng. J. Med. 300:677.

Chan, H.S.L., Saunders, E.F. and Freeman, M.H., 1979, Lithium therapy in childhood neutropenia: Correlation between clinical response and in vitro studies, Ped. Res. 13:429.

Catane, R., Kaufman, J., Mittelman, A. and Murphy, G.P., 1977, Attenuation of myelosuppression with lithium, N. Eng. J. Med. 297:452.

Charron, D., Barrett, A.J., Faille, A., Alby, N., Schmitt, T. and Degos, L., 1977, Lithium in myeloid leukemia, Lancet 1:1307.

Cohen, M.S., Zakhireh, B., Metcalf, J.A. and Root, R.K., 1979, Granulocyte function during lithium treatment, Blood 53:913.

deAlarcon, P.A., Goldberg, J., Nelson, D., Tice, D. and Stockman, J.A., 1979, Beneficial effects of lithium in a child with normal colony stimulating activity and congenital neutropenia, Ped. Res. 13:431.

Freidrich, U. and Nielsen, J., 1969, Lithium and chromosome abnormalities, Lancet 2:435.

Greco, F.A. and Brereton, H.D., 1977, Effect of lithium carbonate on the neutropenia caused by chemotherapy: A preliminary clinical trial, Oncology 34:153.

Gupta, R.C., Robinson, W.A. and Smyth, C.J., 1975, Efficacy of lithium in rheumatoid arthritis with granulocytopenia (Felty's syndrome), Arthritis Rheum. 18:179.

Gupta, R.C., Robinson, W.A. and Kurnick, J.E., 1976, Felty syndrome: Effect of lithium on granulopoiesis, Am. J. Med. 61:29.

Harker, W.G., Rothstein, G., Clarkson, D., Athends, J.W. and MacFarlane, J.L., 1977, Enhancement of colony-stimulating activity production by lithium, Blood 49:263.

Lyman, G.H., Williams, C.C. and Preston, D., 1978, A prospective randomized study of the effect of lithium carbonate on the granulocytopenia and incidence of infection associated with intensive chemotherapy and radiation therapy for undifferentiated small cell bronchogenic carcinoma, Blood 52:228 (Supplement 1).

Malloy, N.L., Zauber, N.P. and Chervenick, P.A., 1978, The effect of lithium on blood and marrow neutrophils, Blood 52:228 (Supplement 1).

Mayfield, D. and Brown, R.G., 1966, The clinical laboratory and electro-encephalographic effects of lithium, J. Psychiat. Res. 4:207.

Morley, D.C. and Galbraith, P.R., 1978, Effect of lithium on granulopoiesis in culture, Canad. Med. Assn. Jour. 118:228.

Murphy, D.L., Goodwin, F.K. and Bunney, W.E., 1971, Leukocytosis during lithium treatment, Amer. J. Psychiat. 127:135.

Nora, J.J., Nora, A.H.and Towes, W.H., 1974, Lithium, Ebstein's anomaly, and other congenital heart defects, Lancet 2:594.

O'Connell, R.A., 1970, Leukocytosis during lithium carbonate treatment, Int. Pharmacopsychiat. 4:30.

Perez-Cruet, J., Dancey, J.T. and Waite, J., 1978, Lithium effects on leukocytosis and lymphopenia, in "Lithium in Medical Practice" (Johnson, F.N. and Johnson, E., eds.) pp. 271-277, MTP Press, Lancaster, England.

Platman, S.R. and Fieve, R.R., 1968, Lithium carbonate and plasma cortisol response in the affective disorders, Arch. Gen. Psychiat. 18:591.

Rossof, A.H. and Coltman, C.A., 1976, The effect of lithium carbonate on the granulocyte phagocytic index, Experientia 32:238.

Rothstein, G., Clarkson, D.R., Larsen, W., Grosser, B.I. and Athens, J.W., 1978, Effect of lithium on neutrophil mass and production, N. Eng. J. Med. 298:178.

Shenkman, L., Borkowsky, W., Holzman, R.S. and Shopsin, B., 1978, Enhancement of lymphocyte and macrophage function in vitro by lithium carbonate, Clin. Immun. Immunopath. 10:187.

Shopsin, B. and Gershon, S., 1971, Plasma cortisol response to dexamethasone suppression in depressed and control patients, Arch. Gen. Psychiat. 24:320.

Shopsin, B., Friedman, R. and Gershon, S., 1971, Lithium and leukocytosis, Clin. Pharm. Ther. 12:923.

Snedecor, G.W. and Cochran, W.G., 1976, "Statistical Methods," p. 128, Iowa State University Press, Ames, Iowa.

Stein, R.S., Beaman, C., Ali, M.Y., Hansen, R., Jenkins, D.D. and Jum'ean, H.G., 1977, Lithium carbonate attenuation of chemotherapy-induced neutropenia, N. Eng. J. Med. 297:430.

Stein, R.S., Flexner, J.M. and Graber, S., 1978a, Lithium and granulocytopenia during induction therapy for acute myelogenous leukemia, Blood 52:277 (Supplement 1).

Stein, S., Hanson, G., Koethe, S. and Hansen, R., 1978b, Lithium-induced granulocytosis, Ann. Int. Med. 88:809.

Steinherz, P., Rosen, G., Ghavimi, F., Wang, Y. and Miller, D., 1979a, Randomized trial of lithium carbonate after chemotherapy, Proc.Am.Assoc.Cancer Res. 20:106.

Steinherz, P., Rosen, G., Ghavimi, F., Wollner, N., Wang, Y. and Miller, D., 1979b, Improved leukocyte counts after chemotherapy with lithium carbonate, Proc.Am.Assoc.Cancer Res. 20:439.

Steinherz, P.G. and Smithwick, E., Unpublished data.

Tiefenbach, A., Kanja, J., Potkonjak-Seska, M. and Mestrovic, B., 1977, Effect of Li_2CO_3 on leukopenia in children during the treatment of acute leukemia, Lij. Vjes. 99:163.

Tisman, G., 1974, Lithium carbonate protection against drug-induced leukopenia in lymphosarcoma patients, IRCS 2:1509.

Tisman, G., 1977, Lithium induced granulocytosis, Lancet 2:251.

Tisman, G., Herbert, V. and Rosenblatt, S., 1973, Evidence that lithium induces human granulocyte proliferation: Elevated serum vitamin B12 binding capacity in vivo, and granulocyte colony proliferation in vitro Brit. J. Haemat. 24:767.

Watanabe, S., Taguchi, L., Nakashima, Y., Ebara, T., Iguchi, K. and Otsuki, S., 1974, Leukocytosis during lithium treatment and its correlation to serum lithium level, Folia. Psych. Neuro. Jap. 28:161.

Yassa, R., Nair, W. and Schwartz, G., 1978, Treatment of leukopenia with lithium carbonate: A preliminary report, Am. J. Psychiatry 135:1423.

PREVENTION BY USING LITHIUM CARBONATE OF NEUTROPENIA DUE TO ANTIBLASTICS

U. Visca, F. Mensi, M.P. Spina,
R. Bombara, B. Giraldi, A. Massari,
F. Rossi, and G. Santi

Second Division of Medicine
Predabissi Provincial Hospital
Melegnano (Milano), Italy

For about two and a half years, since Gupta's 1975 paper on the use of lithium in the Felty syndrome, we have made lithium therapy a part of our oncolytic regimes (Gupta et al., 1975). Incidentally, our first case was in fact a patient with the Felty syndrome and failed to respond, possibly because of poor patient compliance.

We have now treated a total of 70 patients, of whom 55 are available for assessment. They include 40 with solid tumors, 10 with Hodgkin's and non-Hodgkin's lymphomas, two with acute myelogenous leukemia (AML), two with acute lymphoblastic leukemia (ALL), and one with bone marrow aplasia.

We conducted two separate studies. In the first we compared patients treated with lithium with suitable untreated controls. In the second we compared results within individual patients receiving lithium concurrently with alternate cycles of antitumoral therapy, for instance, in the first and third cycle and not in the second and fourth, or vice versa.

The lithium dosage was 900 mg daily in three divided doses taken at 8-hour intervals. Whenever possible, we started lithium therapy about one week ahead of antiblastic medication, this being the time usually needed for lithium-induced leukocytosis to appear, or else simultaneously, and continuing in all cases for three weeks or more. With the exception of lymphoma and acute leukemia cases we avoided the concurrent administration of costicosteroids in order to keep our results clean. Blood lithium levels were checked initially twice a week, later every 15-20 days, not to exceed 1.6 meq/liter. Each WBC count was the mean of two independent counts, and each neutrophil count was likewise the mean from two different smears; both counts were done before treatment and repeated several times afterwards; the post-treatment value was the lowest count elicited in the first 3 weeks after completion of the antiblastic cycle.

In two previous reports (Visca et al., 1978; Visca et al., 1979) we assessed our results in a limited number of cases from our first group, selected to constitute as homogeneous a series as possible, in the hope of minimizing the influence of uncontrollable variables such as age, the number of previous treatments received, the nature of the malignancy, and the patient's general deterioration at the time of treatment, all of which are known to weigh on the degree of neutropenia that is likely to occur with antiblastic therapy. Right now we are collecting data from our second trial for statistical processing.

Eighteen patients were included in our first study. They were of either sex, between 50 and 65 years of age, all having solid tumors of various organs and all receiving antiblastic therapy for the first time. Of these, nine were treated concurrently with lithium and nine were not (the treatment group also includes one case of AML because the result was interesting); the nine untreated controls constituted a fairly matching group in terms of the criteria just mentioned, with about the same tumor locations, and treated with the same antiblastic drugs that were used in the lithium-treated group (see Tables I-III).

TABLE I

PATIENTS TREATED WITH LITHIUM WHILE UNDER CHEMOTHERAPY

	Sites	Antiblastic therapy			
		Before		After	
		Leucocytes	Neutrophils	Leucocytes	Neutrophils
1	Stomach	4,400	2,800	6,500	3,900
2	Breast	5,800	3,300	7,200	5,000
3	Stomach	6,400	3,900	7,600	5,300
4	Breast	4,800	3,700	3,900	3,100
5	Stomach	11,000	5,500	12,000	8,100
6	Lung	4,400	2,000	4,100	2,800
7	Stomach	3,700	1,850	5,600	4,200
8	Lung	4,100	2,500	4,300	3,000
9	Acute meyloid leukemia	6,300	4,700	8,500	3,800

Value per mm^3 of leucocytes and neutrophils before and after therapeutic treatment. The results for each patient refer to the first antiblastic cycle.

TABLE II

PATIENTS NOT TREATED WITH LITHIUM WHILE UNDER CHEMOTHERAPY

	Sites	Antiblastic therapy			
		Before		After	
		Leucocytes	Neutrophils	Leucocytes	Neutrophils
1	Stomach	8,100	5,200	5,000	3,300
2	Stomach	6,000	4,100	3,400	2,200
3	Breast	6,700	3,700	6,000	3,700
4	Ovary	6,400	3,700	3,300	1,800
5	Breast	5,900	3,800	3,200	2,000
6	Breast	8,100	6,100	7,100	5,100
7	Sigmoid	6,000	3,100	5,700	3,100
8	Sigmoid	8,700	3,500	7,700	4,400
9	Lung	4,600	2,700	3,800	3,000

Value per mm^3 of leucocytes and neutrophils before and after therapeutic treatment. The results for each patient refer to the first antiblastic cycle.

TABLE III

WBC AND NEUTROPHIL COUNTS BEFORE AND AFTER CHEMOTHERAPY IN PATIENTS WITH OR WITHOUT LITHIUM PROPHYLAXIS

	Lithium (n=9)		No lithium (n=9)	
Count	Before	After	Before	After
WBC ($p < 0.05$)	5656 ($\pm$2227)	6633 ($\pm$2597)	6722 ($\pm$1325)	5022 ($\pm$1707)
Neutrophils ($p < 0.01$)	3361 ($\pm$1223)	4356 ($\pm$1647)	3989 ($\pm$1051)	3178 ($\pm$1104)

The tumors were (lithium/controls): stomach 4/2; lung 2/1; breast 2/3; sigmoid 0/2; ovary 0/1; and AML 1/0. WBC and neutrophil counts recorded are concentrations per mm^3.

None of the patients listed in this study, except the single case of AML, developed adverse or toxic effects attributable to lithium severe enough to warrant discontinuation.

Table I depicts the patients treated with lithium listing the variations of WBC and neutrophil counts observed. All of these patients were having their first cycles of antiblastic therapy. As can be seen from Table I, all patients responded with variable increases of WBC and neutrophil counts except case 4 who experienced reduced counts and case 6 who had no change. The mean variation of overall WBC count was + $850/mm^3$, representing 15% of the mean pretreatment value ($P < 0.05$); and the mean variation of neutrophil count was + $980/mm^3$, representing 29% of the mean pretreatment value ($P < 0.01$).

The patients not treated with lithium are summarized in Table II. With the single exception of case 3, all patients showed a fall of WBC and neutrophil counts, most quite marked. The mean variation of overall WBC count was - $1700/mm^3$, representing 25% of the mean pretreatment value; and the mean variation of neutrophil count was - $800/mm^3$, representing 20% of the mean pretreatment value.

Figures 1 and 2 summarize the data of the first two tables in graph form. Full dots and solid lines represent lithium-treated cases; circles and broken lines represent the untreated. Table III summarizes the different responses of these two groups in terms of mean values and standard deviations.

In all lithium-treated cases in which we examined the bone marrow, we found evidence of stimulation and increased maturative activity of the granulocytopoietic line.

We have also noted a very frequent increase of the monocyte count, and a less constant increase of the eosinophil count. So far we have seen no notable changes of platelet counts. Right now we are particularly interested in the increase of monocyte counts, which, if confirmed, may tell us something valuable about the action of lithium.

In one case each of AML and ALL, at a certain point during induction antiblastic therapy, we administered lithium in order to alleviate granulocytopenia. In both patients, lithium therapy brought about an increase of neutrophils, prompt and marked in the first case, more gradual and less pronounced in the second, along with reduction or disappearance of circulating and (in the first case only) bone marrow blast cells. Today both these patients are in a stage of clinical and hematologic remission on a maintenance regime of 6-mercaptopurine and methotrexate plus lithium therapy. We do not yet know the role of lithium carbonate in the favorable courses of these patients, but the fact remains that the addition of lithium to the antiblastic treatment seemed to be of benefit. Is this mere happenstance? Or could lithium have a modulating action on cell differentiation beside proliferation, or perhaps work as an immunological adjuvant? The mechanism of action of lithium is still unknown; all we have is a number of working hypotheses currently being investigated. As stated above, lithium-induced leukocytosis occurs after about one week of treatment; it usually lasts throughout administration, and abates thereafter in a matter of 4 or 5 days.

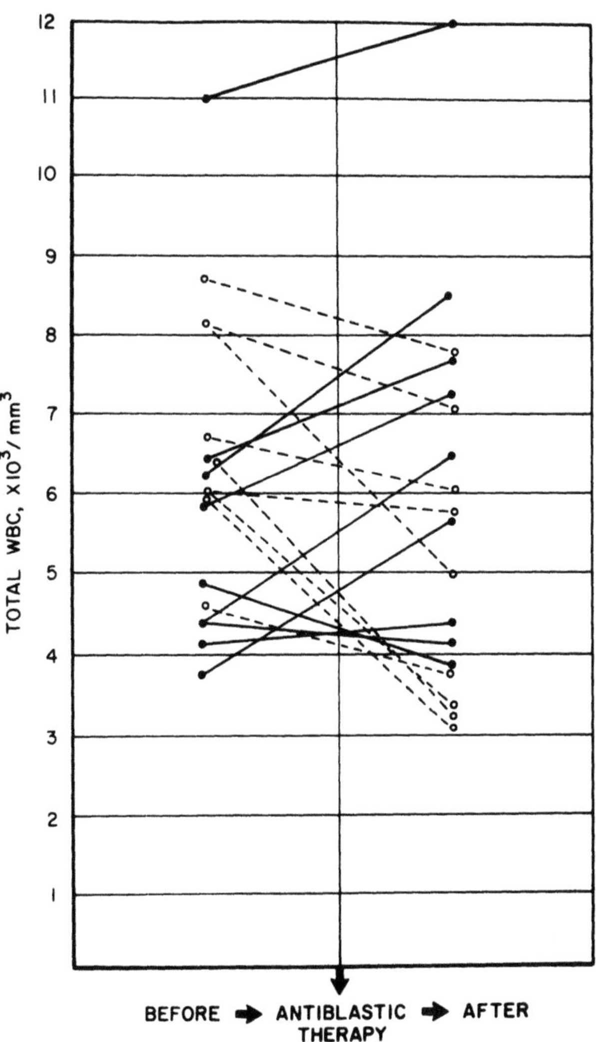

Figure 1. Total WBC counts of 18 patients reported. Patients represented by closed dots and solid lines were treated with lithium carbonate while those represented by open circles and dashed lines were not so treated.

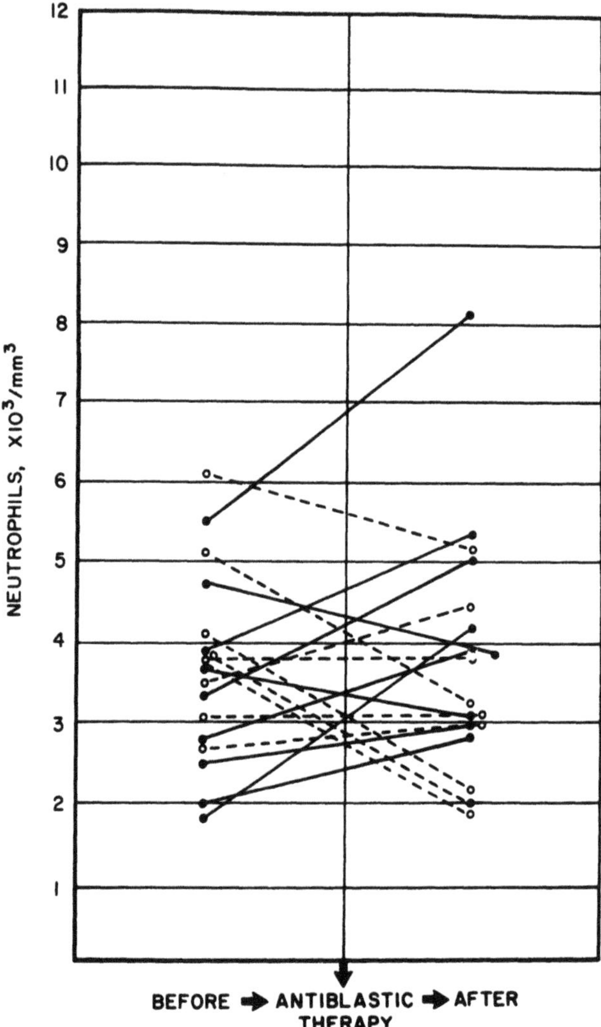

Figure 2. Total neutrophil counts of 18 patients reported. Patients represented by closed dots and solid lines were treated with lithium carbonate while those represented by open circles and dashed lines were not so treated.

One should also recall that lithium is not the only agent that produces neutrophil leukocytosis in man; so do, for instance, hydrocortisone, prednisone, various endotoxins, etiocholanolone, and epinephrine, though by different mechanisms and dynamics. The hypothesis of liberation of bone marrow reserves and/or the marginal quota of neutrophils found no confirmation in the studies of Stein and his associates (Stein et al., 1978) in human volunteers; these authors believe that this effect is a real increase of granulocyte production. Right now the most widely accepted hypothesis is based on the in vitro studies of Tisman et al. (1973), and Harker et al. (1977), who found that lithium would increase the production of CSA (colony stimulating activity) in agar cultures of mouse bone marrow. According to Harker et al. (1977), the CSA factor might originate in vivo in certain tissues, such as the lung; the fact that this action is inhibited by puromycin suggests that lithium acts by way of promoting active protein synthesis.

The increase of monocyte counts noted in our patients seems to corroborate the hypothesis that lithium causes a real proliferation of granulocytes, it being generally known that granulocytes and monocytes originate in a common progenitor cell. In man, too, along with macrophages and mitogen-stimulated lymphocytes, the peripheral blood monocytes are producers of CSA, which in turn stimulates the production of CFU-c. Also Harker et al. (1977) believe that lithium increases the production of CSA starting from human mononuclear cells. In summary, therefore, we submit that the increased monocyte counts observed in our patients might at the same time represent an effect of lithium therapy and constitute the triggering factor of CSA stimulation. Figure 3 attempts a recapitulation of current hypotheses on the mechanism of action of lithium.

We noted no therapeutic results in our one case of bone marrow aplasia treated with lithium. This is at variance with a recent report by Barrett and his colleagues (1977), who claimed good results with lithium in two cases of post-hepatitis aplastic anemia. This discrepancy may be explained tentatively by assuming a marked and stable reduction of CFU-c in our patient, precluding therapeutic responsiveness. If this hypothesis is correct, we might envisage lithium therapy as a diagnostic aid to discover whether a given case of pancytopenia is due to altered production of CSA or of CFU-c, the latter as a result of intrinsic damage or of failure of CFU-S (the totipotential stem cell) replenishment.

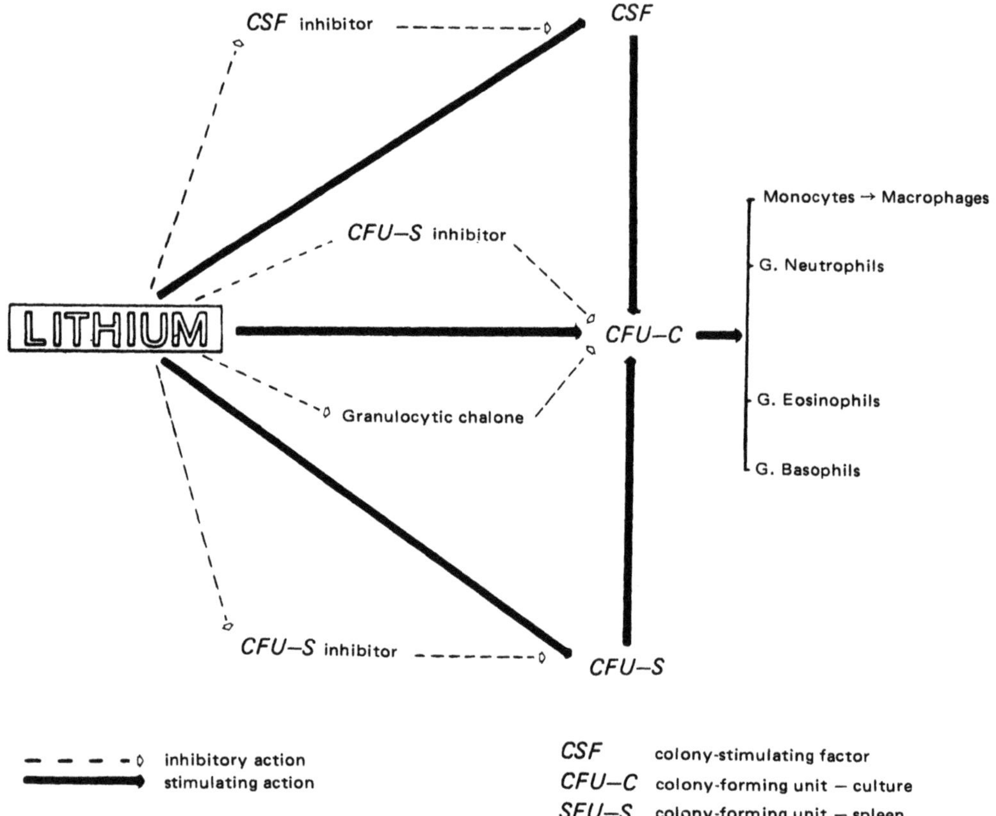

Figure 3. Diagrammatic representation reviewing the currently accepted hypotheses concerning the mechanism of action of lithium.

Obviously, the whole problem of lithium action is open to considerable speculation with many hypotheses standing in need of verification. In addition to those already discussed, a new and fascinating facet of lithium physiology seems to emerge from the 1976 studies of Shenkman and his associates, namely that of an immunological adjuvant (Shenkman et al., 1976).

Quite recently, in a meeting with Dr. A. Robert Turner in Rome, we had a chance to compare our thoughts on the possible role of lymphokinins in the mechanism of action of lithium, for which we hypothesize the following sequence of events: Lithium liberates lymphokinins through stimulation of T lymphocytes; this causes an increase of neutrophils and monocytes; the monocytes, in turn, stimulate the production of CSA, thereby maintaining the proliferation of the myelo-monocytic pool.

REFERENCES

Barrett, A.J., Hugh-Jones K., Newton, K., and Watson, J.G., 1977, Lithium therapy in aplastic anemia, Lancet 1:202.

Gupta, R., Robinson, W.A., and Albrecht, D., 1975, Granulopoietic activity in Felty's syndrome, Ann. Rheum. Dis. 34:156.

Harker, W.G., Rothstein, G., Clarkson, D., Athens, J.W., and Macfarlane, J.L., 1977, Enhancement of colony stimulating activity production by lithium, Blood 49:263.

Shenkman, L., Borkowsky, W., Holzman, R.S., and Shopsin, B., 1978, Enhancement of lymphocyte and macrophage function in vitro by lithium chloride, Clin. Immunol. Immunopathol. 10:187.

Stein, R.S., Hanson, G., Koethe, S., and Hansen, R., 1978, Lithium induced granulocytosis, Ann. Int. Med. 88:809.

Tisman, G., Herbert, V., and Rosenblatt, S., 1973, Evidence that lithium induces vitamin B12-binding capacity in vivo and granulocyte colony proliferation in vitro, Br. J. Haematol. 24:767

Visca, U., Mensi, F., Spina, M.P., Bombara, R., Giraldi, B., Massari, A., Rossi, F., and Santi, G., 1978, Prevenzione della neutropenia da antiblastici con litio carbonato, Gazz. Med. Ital. 137:595.

Visca, U., Mensi, F., Spina, M.P., Bombara, R., Giraldi, B., Massari, A., Rossi, F., and Santi, G., 1979, Prevention of antiblastic neutropenia with lithium carbonate, Lancet 1:779.

A SEVEN YEAR LABORATORY AND CLINICAL EXPERIENCE WITH LITHIUM CARBONATE AS AN ADJUVANT TO CANCER CHEMOTHERAPY

Glenn Tisman and Show Jen Grace Wu

USC School of Medicine and
Whittier Cancer Research Laboratory
13025 East Bailey
Whittier, California 90601

Early studies of lithium treated patients suggested that ingestion of this drug causes granulocytosis (Shopsin _et al._, 1971; Murphy _et al._, 1971). Later, both _in vitro_ granulocyte culture (Tisman _et al._, 1973) and _in vivo_ granulocyte pool measurements (Stein _et al._, 1977; Rothstein _et al._, 1978) demonstrated that the lithium associated granulocytosis was most likely due to an increase in granulocyte production. Most cancer patients undergoing combination chemotherapy will eventually experience drug limiting, and in some, life-threatening leukopenia and it was postulated that lithium carbonate ingestion might help as an adjuvant in the treatment of patients receiving myelosuppressive chemotherapy.

In a preliminary study, we were able to show a definite leukocyte sparing effect from lithium ingestion for lymphosarcoma patients undergoing intensive combination chemotherapy (see Table I) (Tisman, 1974; Tisman _et al._, 1975). Interestingly, however, patients with myeloproliferative syndrome and various untreated acute leukemias did not demonstrate granulocytosis in response to lithium ingestion (Table II) (Tisman _et al._, 1975; Tisman _et al._, 1976). Others have now confirmed that lithium induced granulocytosis provides apparent therapeutic advantages

TABLE I

PATIENT	DIAGNOSIS	WBC Count After 4 Separate Courses Of CVP				WBC Count After 5th Course of CVP While Receiving Li_2CO_3*
1	Lymphosarcoma	4500	5200	4000	4200	6500
2	Lymphosarcoma	5500	5800	9500	3600	6200
3	Lymphosarcoma	5000	6500	6500	3000	4950
4	Lymphosarcoma	4600	4800	4200	2050	5600
5	Lymphosarcoma	6500	6700	8000	4800	7200
6	Lymphosarcoma	4150	4100	4200	3800	6200

*The mean difference between the last WBC count before the administration of lithium carbonate and the WBC count after the administration of lithium carbonate was $2533/mm^3$ with a standard error of ± 221. This represents a significant difference, $p < 0.001$.

CVP is the combination of cyclophosphamide, vincristine, and prednisone.

for patients with other malignancies, including cancer of the prostate, testicle, breast, lung, acute myelogenous leukemia and lymphoma (see Table III) (Catane et al., 1977; Turner et al., 1978; Stein et al., 1977; Greco and Brereton, 1977; Charron et al., 1977).

TABLE II

	Patients	WBC Pre-Li_2CO_3	WBC 2 Weeks Post Li_2CO_3
1.	Normal	7,600	11,200
2.	Normal	8,000	12,600
3.	Normal	7,000	10,000
4.	Normal	6,300	9,300
5.	Normal	4,900	10,600
6.	Acute granulocytic leukemia	2,600	1,800
7.	Acute granulocytic leukemia	1,200	1,400
8.	Acute granulocytic leukemia	4,200	3,600
9.	Myelofibrosis	3,600	3,700
10.	Myelofibrosis	4,400	4,200
11.	Myelofibrosis	80,000	75,000
12.	Myelofibrosis	1,400	1,500
13.	Myelofibrosis	1,500	1,500
14.	Myelofibrosis	19,600	10,700
15.	Idiopathic pancytopenia	2,100	2,600

Responses to lithium carbonate among 5 normal volunteers and 10 patients with various hematologic disorders.

TABLE III

AUTHORS FINDING ADMINISTRATION OF LITHIUM CARBONATE AS AN ADJUVANT TO CANCER CHEMOTHERAPY ASSOCIATED WITH A BENEFICIAL GRANULOCYTE RESPONSE

Authors	Year	Type of Cancer
1. Tisman, G.	1974	Lymphoma
2. Jacob, E., et al.	1974	Various Neutropenias
3. Tisman, G., et al.	1975	Breast Cancer
4. Catane, R., et al.	1977	Prostate Cancer
5. Charron, D., et al.	1977	AGL
6. Stein, R.S., et al.	1977	Breast Cancer
7. Greco, F.A., et al.	1977	Lung Cancer
8. Turner, R.A.	1978	Testicle
9. Visca, U., et al.	1979	G.I., Breast, Lung, and AGL
10. Williams, C.C., et al.	1979	Small Cell Lung Cancer
11. Steinherz, P., et al.	1979	Not Mentioned

Lithium ingestion under certain circumstances can affect *in vivo* mammalian cell RNA and DNA synthesis (Hsu and Rider, 1978). Lithium has also been reported to be an inhibitor of adenyl cyclase (Geisler *et al.*, 1978), DNA polymerase (Lazarus and Kitron, 1974) and of at least three magnesium requiring enzymes of glycolysis (Birch, 1978). Since DNA and RNA synthesis are targets of many cancer chemotherapy medications, it was decided to study the interaction, if any, of lithium with standard cancer chemotherapy drugs.

A short term (4 hour) *in vitro* cell culture technique was employed both for human bone marrow and murine L1210 leukemia cells to study biochemical interactions between lithium and standard cancer chemotherapy drugs. In addition, radioautography was employed in an attempt to study directly the effects of lithium on human bone marrow red blood cell precursors.

MATERIALS AND METHODS

All of the radioactive materials were purchased from Amersham/Searle Corporation (Arlington Heights, Illinois) and the specific activities are as follows: thymidine (6-^{3}HTdR), 27 Ci/mM; deoxyuridine (1',2'-^{3}HdU), 42 Ci/mM; 5-fluorouracil (6-^{3}HFU), 3 Ci/mM. RPMI 1640 medium and Hank's balance salt solution were purchased from Grand Island Biological Company (Grand Island, New York).

Bone Marrow Cell Culture

Short term bone marrow culture was carried out essentially as previously descibed (Tisman et al., 1972; Tisman and Herbert, 1973). Approximately 10 ml of human bone marrow was aspirated into a 30 ml syringe containing 10 ml of tris-buffered (0.06 M, pH 7.4) Hank's balance salt solution plus 100 mg of heparin. After aspiration, the bone marrow suspension was washed and the resuspension cells were immediately passed through a 21 gauge hypodermic needle for a total of four passes. The cells were then centrifuged at room temperature at 500 g for 10 minutes. The supernatant fluid was discarded and a sufficient quantity of tris-Hank's balance salt solution (THBSS) - autologous serum (ratio 3:1) was added to yield a concentration of 1 - 12 x 10^{6} nucleated cells per 0.3 ml aliquots of cell suspension needed for each culture tube.

Bone marrow cells were cultured in 10 ml vacutainer tubes. All experiments were done in triplicate. Each tube contained 0.3 ml of marrow cell suspension. Except for controls, 0.1 ml of freshly prepared stock solutions (drugs were dissolved in THBSS) of either methotrexate (MTX) (Lederle; Pearl River, New York), 5-fluorouracil (5-FU) (Roche; Nutley, N.J.), 5-azacytidine (Ben Venue Laboratories; Bedford, Ohio), cis-diamminedichloroplatinum (II) (Ben Venue), daunorubicin hydrochloride (Ben Venue), vinblastine (Velban) (Lilly; Indianapolis, Indiana) or cytosine arabinoside (Cytosar) (Upjohn; Kalamazoo, Michigan) were added to appropriate culture tubes in the presence or absence of various concentrations of lithium chloride (J.T. Baker; Philipsburg, N.J.). The concentration of each chemotherapeutic agent used in the incubation medium was an estimate to that which would be present in the patient's body fluid after administering the drug as an intravenous bolus, assuming the drug would be distributed in approximately 40,000 ml of body fluid.

After the drugs were added to the culture tubes, the final volume of each tube was adjusted to 0.9 ml with THBSS. Cultures were incubated in triplicate for 4 hours at 37° in a 7.5% CO_2 in air atmosphere. One hour before incubation was ended, 0.1 ml of either ^{3}HTdR (10 μCi/ml), or ^{3}HdU (10 μCi/ml) or ^{3}H5FU (20 μCi/ml) was added. At the end of the 4 hour incubation, the culture was terminated by adding 2 ml of cold THBSS. The washed cells were then subjected to shock lysis, TCA precipitation or PCA extraction. The desired portions of either precipitates or extracts were then prepared for scintillation counting as previously described.

L1210 Cell Cultures

All of the media and chemicals used to maintain murine L1210 leukemia cell growth were purchased from Grand Island Biological Company (Grand Island, New York). Mouse leukemia L1210 cells were adapted to grow and were maintained routinely in RPMI 1640 medium supplemented with 14% heat inactivated (56°C for one hour) dialyzed fetal bovine serum, glutamine (0.29 mg/ml), penicillin (100 units/ml), nystatin (0.25 μg/ml), and streptomycin (100 μg/ml).

The cells were transplanted every 3 or 4 days and only log phase (approximately two days after cell transplantation) L1210 leukemia cells were used for short term culture experiments. The short term leukemia cultures were carried out exactly as short term bone marrow cultures, except that: 1) RPMI 1640 was used in place of THBSS, 2) autologous human serum was replaced by fetal calf serum, and 3) the two shock lysis steps (to remove hemoglobin from human bone marrow cells) were omitted when dealing with L1210 cells.

Radioautography

After incubation, cells to be used for radioautography were washed in 2 ml of cold THBSS and centrifuged as in short term human bone marrow culture experiments. The cell button was resuspended in 1 ml of fetal calf serum and centrifuged at 500 g for 5 min. The supernatant fluid was discarded. The cells were resuspended in approximately 0.05 ml of fresh fetal calf serum and slide-over-slide smears were prepared on previously cleaned routine hematology laboratory slides. The slide so prepared were fixed in methanol for 5 to 10 min., dipped into Kodak NT-2 liquid emulsion, transferred into desiccant-containing slide boxes, and incubated at $4^{o}C$ for 24 hours in the dark. After development, the slides were stained with a mixture of 5 ml of Giemsa, 3 ml of ethanol and 92 ml of buffer (pH 5.75) (85 ml of 0.1 M citric acid, plus 150 ml of 0.2 M Na_2HPO_4 in 1 liter). After staining, the slides were covered with a buffer for 5 min. and then they were dried. After short term *in vitro* culture, cell morphology was easily interpreted and appeared normal. Background grain counts were less than 1 per 5 red blood cell areas. In each case, 1000 cells were counted and the labelling index and grains per labelled cell were calculated. Only red blood cell precursors capable of incorporating label into DNA were counted (the pronormoblasts through polychromatophilic normoblasts).

RESULTS

Clinical Studies

The clinical results of administration of lithium to various patients are shown in Tables I and II. Table I reveals distinct and statistically significant ($p < 0.001$) lithium induced leukocytosis afforded to lymphosarcoma patients undergoing myelosuppressive combination chemotherapy. Table II, however, reveals a population of patients, most with a malignant proliferation of marrow cells, who did not respond to lithium treatment with the expected granulocytosis.

Laboratory Investigations

Figure 1 reveals the data obtained from five short term human bone marrow cell cultures. Note that lithium at 1 meq/L in five separate samples had no significant effect on the incorporation of ^{3}HdU into bone marrow DNA. Also, this figure shows that in two separate bone marrow samples, the concomitant incubation of lithium (1 meq/L) and cytosine arabinoside (2 x 10^{-5}M), daunomycin (2.4 x 10^{-6}M), methotrexate (1 x 10^{-6}M), and 5-FU (1 x 10^{-7}M), did not alter drug inhibitory effects on the

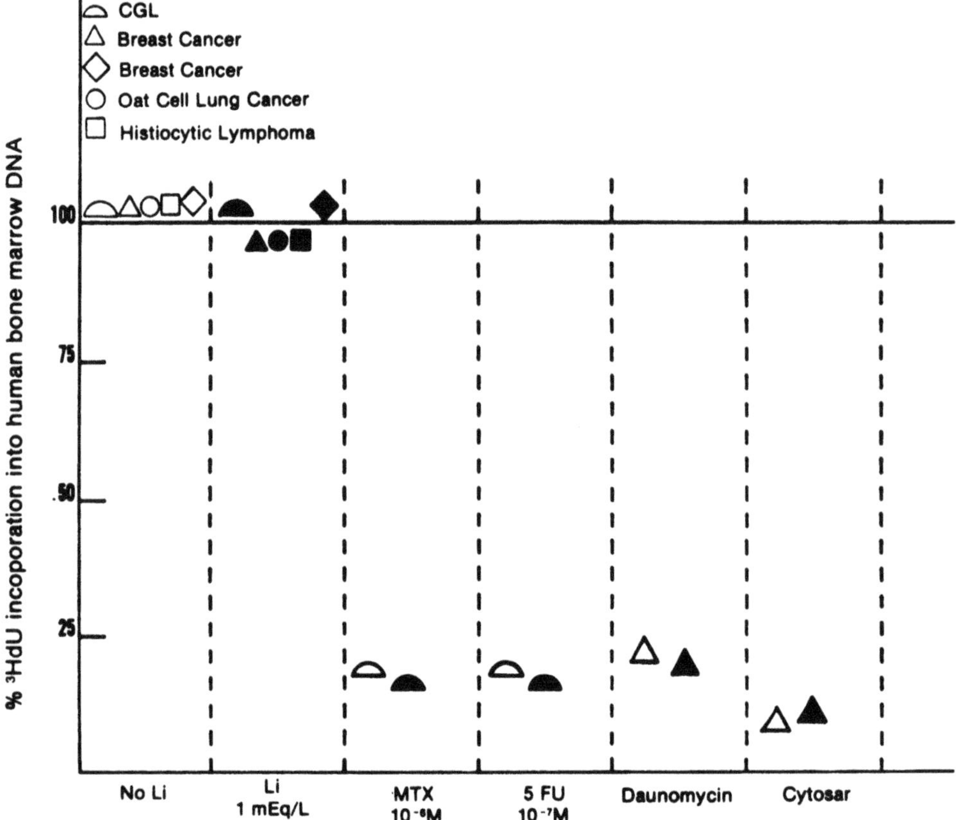

Figure 1. Results of 5 short term human bone marrow cultures in 5 patients. Note the activity of the cancer chemotherapy drugs and the absence of any lithium effect versus bone marrow cells alone or versus drug effects. MTX = methotrexate; 5-FU = 5-fluorouracil; daunomycin concentration = 2.4 x 10^{-6}M; cytosine arabinoside concentration = 2 x 10^{-5}M.

TABLE IV

SHORT TERM CULTURE OF AUER ROD POSITIVE ACUTE GRANULOCYTIC LEUKEMIA PERIPHERAL BLOOD CELLS (95% BLASTS)

Preincubation With	Without Li	Li 0.5 meq/1	Li 1.0 meq/1	Li 1.5 meq/1	Li 3 meq/1	Li 5 meq/1	Radioactive Label
No Drug	100 ± 4*	96 ± 7	106 ± 6	100 ± 9	98 ± 6	100 ± 12	^{3}H dU
Daunomycin (2.4 x 10^{-6}M)	68 ± 9		68 ± 4				^{3}H dU
No Drug	100 ± 3		95 ± 8				^{3}H 5FU
MTX (10^{-4}M)	98 ± 4		102 ± 3				^{3}H 5FU
MTX (10^{-5}M)	95 ± 5		100 ± 7				^{3}H 5FU

*Numbers represent percent of a control ± 1 S.D. not containing drugs or lithium

TABLE V

Additives to L1210 Cultures	Hours of Culture	
	69 Hours	113 hours
Control (No Drugs)	100*	100
Li^+, 0.88 meq/L	106	97
MTX $(1.6 \times 10^{-8}M)$	30	17
MTX $(1.6 \times 10^{-8}M^+)$ + Li^+, 0.88 meq/L	29	19
5FU $(8.8 \times 10^{-8}M)$	19	29
5FU $(8.8 \times 10^{-8}M^+)$ + Li^+, 0.88 meq/L	17	29

*L1210 cell counts reported as percent of control not containing drugs or lithium

incorporation of ^{3}HdU into DNA. Table IV reveals the effects of varying concentrations of lithium chloride on the short term culture of Auer rod positive acute granulocytic leukemia peripheral blood cells (95% blast forms). Note that lithium, in concentration as high as 5 meq/L, in short term culture (4 hours' incubation), did not show any significant activity versus the incorporation of ^{3}HdU into leukemia blast cell DNA. In addition, daunomycin inhibited to 68% of control values both in the absence and presence of 1 meq/L of lithium chloride, suggesting that lithium does not interfere with daunomycin activity versus ^{3}HdU. This patient was subsequently treated with daunomycin plus cytosine arabinoside and had a dramatic *in vivo* lysis of leukemia cells (WBC dropped from 146,000 to 4,300/mm^3 in 4 days). In the lower panel of Table IV one notes that by preincubation with either 1 meq/L of lithium chloride alone or concomitant preicubation of lithium chloride and methotrexate, the ^{3}H5FU incorporation into blast cell RNA was not changed suggesting absence of lithium effect on RNA synthesis. Table V demonstrates the results of a long term incubation of L1210 cells with methotrexate and 5FU alone and in the presence of 0.88 meq/L of lithium chloride. Note that lithium itself does not significantly affect the cell count at both 69 and 113 hours of continuous culture. In addition, the concomitant incubation of lithium with methotrexate or 5-fluorouracil did not enhance nor inhibit the suppression of cell growth produced by these two antimetabolites. Table VI reveals the results of two different experiments (A and B) utilizing a short term (4 hour) culture of L1210 cells. In experiment A, one notes that preincubation for 3 hours with varying concentrations of lithium chloride from 0.5 to 2 meq/L (within the usual therapeutic range) did not significantly affect the incorporation of ^{3}HdU into L1210 cell DNA. In addition, the predicted inhibition of ^{3}HdU incorporation into DNA produced by 5FU or methotrexate was not affected by co-incubation with lithium in concentrations ranging from 0.5 to 2 meq/L. In experiment B, the effect of lithium on a complex inter-relationship between methotrexate and 5-fluorouracil was explored. It is known that methotrexate demonstrates an anti-purine effect in L1210 cells. One result of this effect is to increase intracellular levels of phosphoribosylpyrophosphate (PRPP) which results in enhancement of ^{3}H5FU incorporation into L1210 cell RNA (Cadman et al., 1979). This enhancement of ^{3}H5FU uptake can be seen by preincubation of L1210 cells with methotrexate concentrations between 10^{-7} and 10^{-5}M. Note that co-incubation with lithium at a concentration of 1 meq/L did not interfere with this complex interaction which requires many magnesium dependent enzyme systems. This experiment also demonstrates that lithium at 1 meq/L does not affect L1210 cell RNA synthesis measured by the incorporation of ^{3}H5FU in RNA. That ^{3}H5FU is incorporated almost exclusively into L1210 RNA as opposed to DNA or protein was demonstrated by fractionation experiments (Tisman et al., 1972) not shown here. Table VII displays the effects of preincubation for 3 hours with either chemotherapy drugs alone or drugs plus 1 meq/L of lithium chloride on the subsequent incorporation of ^{3}HdU into L1210 cell DNA. Notice that even though cis-diamminedichloroplatinum, vinblastine, methotrexate, 5-fluorouracil, 5-azacytidine, mitomycin C, cytosine arabinoside and

TABLE VI

SHORT TERM CULTURES OF L1210: EXPERIMENTS A + B

Preincubation With	Without Li	Li 0.5 meq/l	Li 1 meq/l	Li 1.2 meq/l	Li 2 meq/l	Radioactive Label
A.						
No Drug	100 ± 1*	110 ± 3		106 ± 5	106 ± 3	^{3}H dU
5-FU (10^{-6}M)	62 ± 2	62 ± 4		71 ± 5	69 ± 7	^{3}H dU
MTX (10^{-7}M	60 ± 5	65 ± 2		67 ± 5	69 ± 6	^{3}H dU
B.						
No Drug	100 ± 4		108 ± 11			^{3}H 5FU
MTX (10^{-5}M)	152 ± 7		154 ± 14			^{3}H 5FU
MTX (10^{-6}M)	149 ± 8		143 ± 10			^{3}H 5FU
MTX (10^{-7}M)	132 ± 9		130 ± 12			^{3}H 5FU

*Values represent percent of a control ± 1 S.D. not containing drugs or lithium.

daunomycin all demonstrated significant inhibition of ^{3}HdU incorporation into L1210 cell DNA, that concomitant incubation with lithium chloride (1 meq/L) did not interfere with apparent drug activity with respect to the incorporation of ^{3}HdU into the acid precipitate.

TABLE VII

SHORT TERM CULTURE OF L1210 CELLS

	^{3}H dU INCORPORATION INTO DNA % of Control	
Preincubation With	Without Li	With Li (1 meq/l)
Control (No Drug)	100*	102
Cis-diamminedichloroplatinum (2 x 10^{-5}M)	69	71
Vinblastine (4 x 10^{-7}M)	89	92
Methotrexate (10^{-7}M)	29	30
5-Fluorouracil (10^{-6}M)	49	50
5-Azacytidine (4 x 10^{-5}M)	68	70
Mitomycin C (2.2 x 10^{-6}M)	80	83
Cytosine arabinoside (1 x 10^{-5}M)	0.3	0.3
Daunomycin (2.4 X 10^{-6}M)	2	2

Values represent percent of a control not containing drugs or lithium

TABLE VIII
BONE MARROW RADIOAUTOGRAPH

	Control (No Li)*	Li, 2.5 meq/L*
Labelling Index ± 2 S.D.	0.13 ± 0.03	0.15 ± 0.02
Average Grains Per Labelled cell ± 2 S.D.	19.9 ± 1.8	19.0 ± 1.4

*1000 red cells counted (polychromatophilic through pronormoblast)

Table VIII reveals the absence of a significant effect of preincubation for 3 hours with 2.5 meq/L LiCl on bone marrow red blood cell precursor (polychromatophilic through pronormoblast) labelling index and grain count/labelled cell. In addition, the short term cultures from which these cells were harvested revealed no Li effect on ^{3}HdU or ^{3}HTdR incorporation into acid precipitable DNA of both red and white blood cell precursors. The marrow cells were from a breast cancer patient with erythroid hyperplasia secondary to bleeding and only red blood cell precursors were abundant enough for radioautographic data collection. Radioautographs were made only from the ^{3}HdU cells.

DISCUSSION

Many groups have demonstrated granulocytosis in lithium treated psychiatric and normal patients and cancer patients undergoing cancer chemotherapy. We have, however, found a group of hematologically abnormal patients who do not respond to lithium ingestion with a predictable elevation of the white blood cell count (Table II). Though the meaning of this abnormal response to lithium ingestion (lithium stimulation test, Tisman *et al.*, 1975; Jochimsen and Corder, 1979) is not yet clearly defined, it may be of use in evaluating the presence of an underlying hematological disorder. However, much more work on this point remains to be done.

Many reports have confirmed the effectiveness of lithium carbonate as an adjuvant to cancer chemotherapy. It was therefore imperative to explore possible interfering effects of lithium on commonly used cancer chemotherapy drugs. Many biological processes, including glycolysis, nucleotide metabolism and antimetabolite activation are known to be magnesium dependent. Prior work had already demonstrated lithium inhibition of many key enzyme systems. Some of the reported effects of lithium included:

1) *in vivo* inhibition of mammalian RNA and DNA synthesis,
2) inhibition of hormone stimulated adenyl cyclase activity,
3) both stimulation and inhibition of ATPase activity (Glen, 1978),
4) inhibition of DNA polymerase, and
5) interference with energy production and phosphoribosyl-pyrophosphate (PRPP) generating glycolysis.

That magnesium-lithium interference might exist was suggested because the value of the charge-to-radius ratio of lithium is similar to that of magnesium (Williams, 1973).

In spite of all of the above, in our experiments we were unable to demonstrate a significant interaction between therapeutic concentrations of lithium and the cancer chemotherapy drugs tested in our short term cultures. Not only did lithium not affect the antimetabolic activity of the drugs added to human bone marrow cell cultures, there was also no lithium effect noted on human acute granulocytic leukemia and murine L1210 cell cultures. Additionally, in long term murine L1210 cell cultures, lithium did not enhance L1210 cell proliferation nor alter antimetabolite inhibition of L1210 cell growth.

Although lithium may induce granulocytosis in long term *in vivo* cultures with feeder layers (Tisman *et al.*, 1973), there appears to be no detectable effect on human bone marrow cell DNA (as measued by ^{3}HdU incorporation into acid precipitable material) or RNA synthesis (as measured by by ^{3}H5FU incorporation into acid precipitable material) in short term suspension maintenance cultures. Radioautography results in a human short term bone marrow cell culture also suggested the absence of a lithium stimulatory or inhibitory effect on red blood cell precursors. However, as with white blood cell cultures, lithium effects on red blood cell precursors, if present, may only be recognizable in long term cultures.

From our very preliminary reports employing short term culture techniques, we are unable to demonstrate lithium interference with cancer chemotherapy antimetabolic activity. Since all the drugs tested in short term culture had a demonstrable metabolic effect, we feel that if lithium were to interfere with such an effect, it would be apparent even during the short term incubation (4 hour) experiments here employed. However, only a well controlled propsective study will be able to confirm whether or not lithium actually has any clinically significant synergistic or antagonistic effects on cancer chemotherapy drug activity.

REFERENCES

Birch, N.J., 1978, Metabolic effects of lithium, in "Lithium in Medical Practice" (F.N. Johnson and S. Johnson, eds.), pp.89-114, University Park Press, Baltimore.

Cadman, E., Benz, C., and Heimer, R., 1979, Enhanced 5-fluorouracil (5FU) nucleotide formation following methotrexate (MTX) is the consequence of increased intracellular phorphoribosylpyrophosphate (PRPP), Proc. Amer. Assn. Cancer Res. 20:258.

Catane, R., Kaufman, J., Mittelman, A., and Murphy, G.P., 1977, Attenuation of myelosuppression with lithium, New Eng. J. Med. 297:452.

Charron, D., Barrett, A.J., Faille, A., Alby, N., Schmitt, T., and Degos, L., 1977, Lithium in acute myeloid leukemia, Lancet 1:1307.

Geisler, A., Klysner, R., and Thams, P., 1978, Influence of lithium on hormonal stimulation of adenylate cyclase, in "Lithium in Medical Practice" (F.N. Johnson and S. Johnson, eds.), University Park Press, Baltimore.

Glen, A.I.M., 1978, Lithium regulation of membrane ATPases in "Lithium in Medical Practice" (F.N. Johnson and S. Johnson, eds.), University Park Press, Baltimore.

Greco, F.A. and Brereton, H.D., 1977, Effect of lithium carbonate on neutropenia caused by chemotherapy: A preliminary clinical trial, Oncology 34:153.

Hsu, J.M. and Rider, A.A., 1978, Effect of maternal lithium ingestion on biochemical and behavioral characteristics of rat pups, in "Lithium in Medical Practice" (F.N. Johnson and S. Johnson, eds.), University Park Press, Baltimore.

Jochimsen, P.R. and Corder, M.P., 1979, Demonstration of prolonged bone marrow dysfunction in mastectomy patients who received adjuvant chemotherapy, Proc. Amer. Assn. Cancer Res. 20:368.

Lazarus, L.H. and Kitron, M., 1974, Depression of DNA polymerase activity by lithium, Lancet 2:225.

Murphy, D.L., Goodwin, F.K., and Bunney, W.E., Jr., 1971, Leukocytosis during lithium treatment, Am. J. Psychiat. 127:1559.

Rothstein, G., Clarkson, D.R., Larsen, W., Grosser, B.I., and Athens, J.W., 1978, Effect of lithium on neutrophil mass and production, New Eng. J. Med. 298:178.

Shopsin, B., Freidman, R., and Gershon, S., 1971, Lithium and leukocytosis, Clin. Pharm. and Ther. 12:923.

Stein, R.S., Beamann, C., Ali, M.Y., Hansen, R., Jenkins, D.D., and Jume'an, H.G., 1977, Lithium carbonate attenuation of chemotherapy-induced neutropenia, New Eng. J. Med. 297:430.

Stein, R.S., Hanson, G., Koethe, S., and Hansen, R., 1977, An in vivo evaluation of lithium-induced granulocytosis, Blood 50:161 (Supplement 1).

Tisman, G., 1974, Lithium carbonate protection against drug-induced leukopenia in lymphosarcoma patients, IRCS 2:1509.

Tisman, G. and Herbert, V., 1973, Studies of effects of cyclic adenosine 3', 5'-monophosphate in regulation of human hemopoiesis in vitro, In Vitro 2:86.

Tisman, G., Herbert, V., Go, L.T., and Brenner, L., 1972, Inhibition by penicillamine of DNA and protein synthesis by human bone marrow, Proc. Soc. Exp. Biol. Med. 139:355.

Tisman, G., Herbert, V., and Rosenblatt, S., 1973, Evidence that lithium induces human granulocyte proliferation: Elevated serum vitamin B12 binding capacity in vivo and granulocyte colony proliferation in vitro, Brit. J. Hema. 24:767.

Tisman, G., Safire, G., and Wu, G., 1975a, Lithium carbonate protection against cancer chemotherapy induced leukopenia, Clin. Res., 23:115A.

Tisman, G., Safire, G., and Wu, G., 1975b, Lithium carbonate stimulation test in blood disorders, Clin. Res. 23:103A.

Tisman, G., Kellon, D.B., Wu, S., and Safire, G.E., 1976, Failure of lithium to induce leukocytosis in a patient with granulocytic leukemia in complete remission, Clin. Res. 24:322A.

Turner, R.A., Alalunis, M.J., MacDonald, R.N., and McPherson, T.A., 1978, Effects of a short term course of lithium carbonate on granulopoiesis, Clin. Res. 26:856A.

Williams, R.J.P., 1973, The chemistry and biochemistry of lithium, in "Lithium - Its Role in Psychiatric Research and Treatment"(S. Gershon and B. Shopsin, eds.), Plenum Publishing Corporation, New York.

LITHIUM ATTENUATION OF CHEMOTHERAPY-INDUCED GRANULOCYTOPENIA: STATISTICAL AND CLINICAL SIGNIFICANCE?

F. Anthony Greco

Division of Oncology, Department of Medicine
Vanderbilt University Medical Center
Nashville, Tennessee 37232

Does lithium significantly attenuate the degree and/or duration of chemotherapy-induced granulocytopenia? Several studies have addressed this question (Tisman, 1974; Greco, *et al.*, 1976; Greco and Brereton, 1977; Stein *et al.*, 1977; Catane *et al.*, 1977; Lyman *et al.*, 1978), and all have reported that the mean granulocyte nadir is significantly higher, or the mean or median duration of granulocytopenia is significantly shorter, following chemotherapy plus lithium (P values ranging between 0.01 and 0.05). There is not a single "negative" study reported. When these data are considered with the fact that lithium increases granulocyte production (Rothstein *et al.*, 1978), one can easily conclude that the statistically significant attenuation of chemotherapy-induced granulocytopenia by lithium is a real effect. Further clarification of this significant effect requires detailed inspection of these data. It was obvious during our initial studies of lithium in patients receiving chemotherapy (Greco *et al.*, 1976; Greco and Brereton, 1977) that the ability of lithium to limit the nadir of granulocytopenia was at best marginal except in a few patients. We were also uncertain, as were Stein and co-workers (Stein *et al.*, 1977) if our "statistically significant" observations were biologically important. Therefore, I have again looked at the study of Stein and co-workers and carefully reviewed our own data (Greco and Brereton, 1977) in an attempt to gain a better appreciation of the observed "lithium effect." At this writing, these two studies are the only detailed reports available. Both these studies report significant ($P \leq 0.05$) lithium attenuation of granulocytopenia induced by chemotherapy.

The basic design of these studies was similar in that each patient served as his own control, and lithium carbonate was given orally during alternate cycles of combination chemotherapy. The mean granulocyte values during the cycles containing lithium were compared to the mean granulocyte values during the cycles not containing lithium. In both studies the mean granulocyte nadir during the chemotherapy cycle was significantly higher for cycles given with lithium ($P = 0.05$ and $P < 0.05$). The actual serial granulocyte numbers for each patient were not given in either study, although we depicted in graphic form the percentage change of the granulocyte nadir in each patient. In the Stein et al. study, 14 of 18 paired comparisons (lithium versus no lithium) showed that the decrease in the number of granulocytes was less in the cycle on lithium. However, how much less in each patient was not stated. In addition, the standard deviations of the granulocyte means and ranges were not reported. By examination of the actual granulocyte counts in each patient in our study, it became clear that the elevated counts of a few patients were making the mean counts for the entire group higher. Since the individual patient granulocyte counts, standard deviations of the means, or ranges are not reported in the study of Stein et al., it is impossible to determine if the elevated counts of a minority of patients were substantially elevating the mean counts for the entire group.

In our study, the mean counts were indeed substantially increased by elevated counts in only a few patients. Table I illustrates the actual granulocyte nadirs of 15 patients during three sequential cycles of combination chemotherapy. Only during the second cycle was lithium administered with chemotherapy. The mean granulocyte nadir during the lithium (second cycle) is 26% and 46% higher than the cycle before lithium (first cycle) and cycle after lithium (third cycle) respectively. When the counts are evaluated in each patient by the Wilcoxon matched-pairs signed-

TABLE I

GRANULOCYTE NADIRS ($CELLS/MM^3$)

Patient No.	First Cycle Without Li_2CO_3	Second Cycle With Li_2CO_3	Third Cycle Without Li_2CO_3
1	1820	2000	2240
2	660	750	20
3	76	70	120
4	90	90	258
5	180	160	240
6	2195	3920	2015
7	1800	6480	1785
8	270	2200	270
9	1600	1870	2090
10	450	200	85
11	5440	2880	1610
12	130	160	192
13	90	400	55
14	1900	2000	324
15	1350	1416	588

The actual granulocyte nadir counts ($cells/mm^3$) during three consecutive chemotherapy cycles given without lithium (first and third cycles) and with lithium (second cycle).

ranks test (Beyer, 1968), the granulocyte nadir is significantly higher during the chemotherapy cycle with lithium than the cycle before (P = 0.05) or after (P = 0.05) not containing lithium. By inspecting the actual nadir in each patient (Table I), one sees that patients 6, 7, and 8, made the results "significant." Deletion of any one of these three patients from consideration renders the mean nadirs "not significantly" different (P > 0.05). Obviously, this is not appropriate and the results remain "significant."

Clinicians and statisticians are usually aware that "statistically significantly different" should not be equated with "important" or "different." The determination of importance, unfortunately, can not be based upon a formula, statistical table or signed-rank tests, particularly when an observed "effect" is not dramatic. Certainly, the lithium effect is not dramatic, but marginal and observable in only a minority of patients. Only a few patients appear to be partially protected from chemotherapy-induced granulocytopenia by lithium and the effect in these few makes the result statistically significant. Subgroups of patients may benefit clinically, and further work is necessary to identify these patients and adequately document the benefit. The information to date does not support the routine use of lithium in patients receiving cancer chemotherapy.

REFERENCES

Beyer, W.H., 1968, Non-Parametric Statistics, in: "Handbook of Tables for Probability and Statistics," 2nd edition, p. 399, Chemical Rubber Company, Cleveland.

Catane, R., Kaufman, J., Mittleman, A., Murphy, G.P., 1977, Attenuation myelosuppression with lithium, N. Eng. J. Med. 297:452.

Greco, F.A., Brereton, H.D., Pomeroy, T., 1976, Lithium carbonate attenuation of neutropenia, Pro. Amer. Soc. of Clin. Oncol. 17:250.

Greco, F.A., Brereton, H.D., 1977, Effect of lithium carbonate on the neutropenia caused by chemotherapy: A preliminary clinical trial, Oncology 34:153.

Lyman, G.H., Williams, C.C., Preston, D., 1978, A prospective randomized study of the effect of lithium carbonate on the granulocytopenia and incidence of infection associated with intensive chemotherapy and radiation therapy for undifferentiated small cell bronchogenic carcinoma. Blood 52:228, (Supplement 1).

Rothstein, G., Clarkson, D., Larsen, W., Grosser, B.I., Athens, J.W., 1978, Effect of lithium on neutrophil mass and production, N. Eng. J. Med. 298:178.

Stein, R.S., Beaman, C., Ali, M.Y., Hansen, R., Jenkins, D.D., Jume'an, H.G., 1977, Lithium carbonate attenuation of chemotherapy-induced neutropenia, N. Eng. J. Med. 297:430.

Tisman, G., 1978, Lithium carbonate protection against drug-induced leukopenia in lymphosarcoma patients, IRCS 2:1509.

IN VIVO AND IN VITRO EFFECTS OF LITHIUM ON GRANULOPOIESIS IN HUMAN NEUTROPENIC DISORDERS

William A. Robinson, Maureen A. Entringer,
James Huber, and Ramesh Gupta

Divisions of Medical Oncology and Rheumatic Diseases
Department of Medicine
University of Colorado Medical Center
Denver, Colorado 80262

Administration of lithium salts to humans increases peripheral blood neutrophil counts (O'Connell, 1970; Shopsin *et al*., 1971). It has been shown that this is due to a true increase in neutrophil mass, rather than a shift in peripheral blood neutrophil pools (Tisman *et al*., 1973; Rothstein *et al*., 1978). The mechanism of action of lithium in this regard has been studied by a number of investigators using *in vitro* techniques (Joyce and Chervenick, 1975; Harker *et al*., 1977; Morley and Galbraith, 1978; Spitzer *et al*., in press). It has been shown that lithium leads to increased production of the granulocyte colony stimulating factor (CSF) by adherent peripheral blood and bone marrow cells. CSF is the presumed humoral regulator of granulocyte production and has been partially characterized as a glycoprotein with a molecular weight of approximately 35,000 daltons (Robinson and Mangalik, 1975; Metcalf, 1977). Further, it has been shown that lithium does not alter the functional capacity of neutrophils, suggesting that it may be useful as a therapeutic agent in human neutropenic disorders (Rossof and Coltman, Jr., 1976; Cohen et al., 1979).

Administration of lithium salts to humans with neutropenia of various etiologies has also been shown to increase peripheral blood neutrophil levels (Tisman et al., 1974; Gupta et al., 1975; Gupta et al., 1976; Catane et al., 1977; Stein et al., 1977; Charron et al., 1977; Barrett et al., 1977). These include Felty's syndrome and the neutropenia occurring following cancer chemotherapy. The presumed mechanism of action of lithium in this regard is through increased CSF production. The spectrum of clinical usefulness of lithium in the treatment of human neutropenias has not, however, been fully established. The following studies were undertaken in an attempt to further delineate, using in vitro and in vivo techniques, in what situations lithium might be beneficial.

In these studies the effect of lithium salts on granulocyte colony formation by bone marrow from patients with a variety of neutropenic disorders and acute non-lymphocytic leukemia (ANLL) has been studied. All of these patients had normal or increased serum colony stimulating activity (CSA). No significant effect of lithium carbonate on granulocyte colony numbers was noted in any of the neutropenias or ANLL cells studied when an adequate source of colony stimulating factor was present. In contrast, administration of lithium salts to patients with Felty's syndrome, a condition in which CSA production appears to be low, has been shown to increase peripheral blood neutrophil levels. Rises in peripheral blood neutrophil levels were accompanied by concomitant rises in serum CSA values in the patients. These data suggest that lithium may be most beneficial in neutropenic disorders associated with low CSA levels.

METHODS AND MATERIALS

Seven patients with idiopathic neutropenia of varying types were studied. The nature of the neutropenia is noted in Table I. All had absolute neutrophil counts less than 1500/μl. Four patients with newly diagnosed ANLL were also studied. All of these patients were untreated at the time the studies were carried out.

The technique of bone marrow culture has been described in detail elsewhere (Pike and Robinson, 1970). The stimulus for colony growth was peripheral white blood cell feeder layers derived from normal humans. Peripheral blood was collected in heparin, allowed to sediment by gravity at room temperature, and the buffy coat aspirated. One ml feeder layers containing 1 million nucleated peripheral blood cells in 0.5% agar in McCoy's 5A medium were prepared in 35 mm plastic petri dishes. To these feeder layers were added various concentrations of lithium carbonate or lithium chloride ranging from 1 to 33 meq/liter. Bone marrow from the patients described above was aspirated through the posterior iliac crest into heparinized syringes, allowed to sediment by gravity at room temperature, and the buffy coat removed. No separation or adherence techniques were undertaken. Bone marrow cells in autologous plasma were added as overlays to the feeder layers in 1 ml aliquots of 0.3% agar in McCoy's 5A medium at a concentration of 250,000 nucleated cells per ml. Plates were then incubated in a fully humidified incubator with a constant flow of 7.5% CO_2 in air for 12-14 days at which time colony counts were done. Only colonies containing 50 or more cells were counted. Values have been expressed as a percent of colonies stimulated in the presence of lithium as compared to controls without lithium (always indicated as 100%).

Eight patients with Felty's syndrome were studied. The diagnosis of Felty's syndrome was based upon a classical history of rheumatoid arthritis, clinical splenomegaly, and spontaneous sustained neutropenia. After written informed consent, as approved by the Human Subject Committee, University of Colorado Medical Center, all patients were given lithium carbonate orally in a dose of 300 mg three times daily for six weeks. Weekly blood counts with differentials were performed and serum and urine samples obtained for measurement of lithium levels and CSA. The method for measuring serum and urinary CSA has been described elsewhere (Robinson and Pike, 1970). One-tenth ml of untreated serum or 0.15 ml of dialyzed, sedimented, filter sterilized urine was placed in triplicate 35 mm plastic petri dishes to which was added a mixture of 0.3% agar and McCoy's 5A medium containing 75,000 nucleated bone marrow cells from the femurs of C57 black mice. After mixing of the serum and/or urine and culture medium, the plates were allowed to gel at room temperature and incubated as described above for 7 days at which time colony counts were performed. As described above, only colonies containing 50 or more cells were counted.

RESULTS

Table I shows the effect of the addition of lithium chloride in a concentration of 1 meq/liter on colony formation by bone marrow cells from patients with a wide variety of neutropenic disorders. As indicated previously, these studies were done using as a source of CSA normal human peripheral white blood cell feeder layers. Results are expressed as the change in colony numbers compared to control plates without lithium. The data show only a single concentration of lithium chloride (1 meq/liter) but the results were similar with other concentrations, although at high concentrations, i.e. 10-30 meq/liter, inhibition of colony formation was observed. The patients studied included one patient with cyclic neutropenia, 4 patients with idiopathic neutropenia and 2 patients with preleukemia characterized by refractory, hypercellular megaloblastic bone marrows. In no instance did the addition of lithium increase colony formation.

The effect of lithium chloride on bone marrow colony formation in four patients with ANLL is shown in Table II. As above, only one concentration of lithium carbonate is shown (1 meq/liter), but the results were similar regardless of the level of lithium present in plates. Previous studies have shown that cells from patients with ANLL rarely undergo colony formation *in vitro*. In the studies shown here, no significant increase in colony formation was noted when lithium was added to culture plates. The data would appear to show great changes when given in percent of control. The number of colonies present in plates without lithium was, however, very low (1 to 10) and the changes noted are not significant.

TABLE I

THE EFFECT OF LITHIUM CARBONATE ON GRANULOCYTE COLONY FORMATION BY BONE MARROW CELLS FROM PATIENTS WITH NEUTROPENIA

Patient	Nature of Neutropenia	Colony Formation	
		Control*	LiCl (1 meq/L)
1	Cyclic neutropenia	100%	72%
2	Idiopathic	100%	71%
3	Idiopathic	100%	84%
4	Idiopathic	100%	90%
5	Idiopathic	100%	97%
6	Preleukemia	100%	104%
7	Preleukemia	100%	112%

* Control values are number of colonies stimulated by human peripheral WBC feeder layers in the absence of lithium.

TABLE II

THE EFFECT OF LITHIUM CARBONATE ON COLONY FORMATION BY BONE MARROW CELLS FROM HUMANS WITH ACUTE NONLYMPHOCYTIC LEUKEMIA

Patient	Type of Leukemia	Colony Formation	
		Control*	LiCl (1 meq/L)
1	Acute myelomonocytic	100%	94%
2	Acute meylomonocytic	100%	150%
3	Acute undifferentiated	100%	154%
4	Acute undifferentiated	100%	181%

* Control values are the number of colonies stimulated by human peripheral WBC feeder layers in the absence of lithium.

Simultaneous studies (not shown) were undertaken to determine the serum and urinary CSA levels in the above patients with neutropenia and ANLL. All the patients studied had CSA values which were elevated or within the normal range for our laboratory. These results have been presented elsewhere (Robinson et al., 1972; Gupta et al., 1975).

Table III shows the effect of administration of lithium carbonate on peripheral blood neutrophil levels in patients with Felty's syndrome. Shown are the mean pre-lithium values and the highest neutrophil level after lithium administration. All eight patients responded to lithium with a rise in neutrophil counts. Neutrophil levels rose from 38 to 517% with a median of 126%.

Table IV shows changes in urinary and serum CSA values in patients with Felty's syndrome before and after the administration of lithium carbonate. The mean urinary CSA in the prelithium period was 5.2 with a rise to a mean of 22.6 after the administration of lithium carbonate. This increase was highly significant ($p < 0.01$). The mean serum CSA activity during the prelithium period was 6.1 and during lithium therapy was 36.5, again highly significant ($p < 0.01$). It should be noted that both the urinary and serum CSA values are low compared to other neutropenic disorders (urinary CSA 27 and serum CSA mean 10) as measured in our laboratory (Robinson and Pike, 1970; Robinson et al., 1972, Gupta et al., 1975).

DISCUSSION

It has been clearly shown that the administration of lithium salts to humans increases peripheral blood neutrophil levels due to an increase in total neutrophil mass (O'Connell, 1970; Shopsin et al., 1971; Tisman et al., 1973; Rothstein et al., 1978). The mechanism of action of lithium appears to result from an effect on CSF producing cells. Addition of lithium to culture plates containing CSF producing cells increases colony formation (Joyce and Chervenick, 1975; Harker et al., 1977; Morley and Galbraith, 1978; Spitzer et al., in press). Removal of adherent cells, which are the

TABLE III

THE EFFECT OF ADMINISTRATION OF LITHIUM CARBONATE ON PERIPHERAL BLOOD NEUTROPHIL COUNTS IN EIGHT PATIENTS WITH FELTY'S SYNDROME

	Absolute neutrophil counts/mm^3		Per cent increase	
	Range	Mean	Range	Mean
Pre-lithium	746-2692	1355	----	----
On-lithium	940-4491	2476	38-517%	126%

TABLE IV

CHANGES IN URINE AND SERUM COLONY STIMULATING ACTIVITY (CSA) IN EIGHT PATIENTS WITH FELTY'S SYNDROME BEFORE AND AFTER LITHIUM CARBONATE

	Urine CSA			Serum CSA		
	Range	Mean	Per cent Increase	Range	Mean	Per cent Increase
Pre-lithium	1-15	5.2	----	1-17	6.1	----
On-lithium	8-48	22.6	435%	4-85	36.5	598%

sources of CSF, results in no effect of lithium. Likewise, addition of lithium to cultures containing no adherent cells and a preformed source of CSA (human placenta conditioned medium) does not enhance colony formation. The clinical usefulness of lithium carbonate would then seem to be most beneficial in neutropenic disorders when CSA production is reduced. The present studies have corroborated this suggestion.

The present, and previous studies, have shown that serum and urinary CSA levels are reduced in patients with Felty's syndrome (Gupta et al., 1975). The nature of this defect in Felty's syndrome is unknown but it is presumed to be due to a defect in the monocyte-macrophage system in this disorder and the ability of these cells to produce CSA. Administration of lithium carbonate to patients with Felty's syndrome increases peripheral neutrophil numbers concomitant with a rise in serum and urinary CSA levels. The presumed mechanism of action of lithium is, therefore, through increased production of CSA in this syndrome.

In the majority of other neutropenic disorders, serum and urinary CSA levels and production do not appear to be the result of altered production of CSA, but the result of intrinsic cellular abnormalities with poor responsiveness to granulopoietic factors. Previous studies in this laboratory have shown that in the majority of idiopathic neutropenias, serum and urinary CSA levels are high (Robinson et al., 1972; Gupta et al., 1975). The present studies were carried out to determine whether the administration of lithium carbonate might be beneficial even in the face of these findings. It has not been shown, however, that lithium enhances granulocyte colony formation when added to cultures of bone marrow cells from patients with a wide variety of neutropenias or ANLL when an adequate source of CSA is present.

It would appear from the present studies that lithium may be most beneficial in neutropenic disorders in which it can be demonstrated that CSA levels are reduced and/or CSA production altered. Administration to patients with normal or increased serum CSA levels would not appear to be beneficial in the majority of instances. It is of interest, however, that recent studies by Van Zant et al. (1979) have suggested there is a competition between CSA and erythropoietin for multipotential stem cells. Dependent upon the levels of each of these factors present, multipotential stem cells can be "forced" into committed cell lines. It is conceivable that administration of lithium, by enhancing CSA levels even in the presence of already normal or elevated CSA, may increase neutrophil production at the expense of other cell lines by increasing the inflow into the committed granulocyte cell line. From the theoretical standpoint, this might be beneficial since decreased red blood cell production can be compensated for easily by blood transfusions. The total spectrum of neutropenic disorders in which lithium will be beneficial remains, however, to be determined.

SUMMARY

Studies have been carried out to determine the *in vivo* and *in vitro* effects of lithium carbonate in various neutropenic disorders. Addition of lithium to cultures of bone marrow from patients with a variety of neutropenic disorders and ANLL in which normal or elevated serum and/or urinary CSA levels were present did not enhance granulocyte colony formation. Administration of lithium carbonate to patients with Felty's syndrome, in which serum and urinary CSA levels are reduced, enhanced peripheral blood neutrophil levels and serum and urinary CSA values. Lithium administration appears to be most beneficial in neutropenic patients in whom it can be demonstrated that CSA production is reduced.

ACKNOWLEDGEMENTS

This work was supported by grants from the National Institutes of Health, National Cancer Institute (1R01CA23552-02), American Cancer Society #CH-81, and by grant (RR-51) from the General Clinical Research Centers Program of the Division of Research Resources, National Institutes of Health.

REFERENCES

Barrett, A.J., Hugh-Jones, K., Newton, K., and Watson, J.G., 1977, Lithium therapy in aplastic anemia, The Lancet 1:202.

Catane, R., Kaufman, J., Mittelman, A., and Murphy, G.P., 1977, Attenuation of myelosuppression with lithium, N. Engl. J. Med. 297:452.

Charron, D., Barrett, A.J., Faille, A., Alby, N., Schmidt, T., and Degos, L., 1977, Lithium in acute myeloid leukemia, The Lancet 1:1307.

Cohen, M.S., Zakhireh, B., Metcalf, J.A., and Root, R.K., 1979, Granulocyte function during lithium therapy, Blood 53:913.

Gupta, R., Robinson, W.A., and Albrecht, D., 1975, Granulpoietic activity in Felty's syndrome, Ann. Rheum. Dis. 34:156.

Gupta, R.C., Robinson, W.A., and Smyth, C.J., 1975, Efficacy of lithium in rheumatoid arthritis with granulocytopenia (Felty's syndrome), Arth. Rheum. 18:179.

Gupta, R.C., Robinson, W.A., and Kurnick, J.E., 1976, Felty's syndrome, Am. J. Med. 61:29.

Harker, W.G., Rothstein, G., Clarkson, D.W., Athens, J.W., and Macfarlane, J.L., 1977, Enhancement of colony-stimulating activity production by lithium, Blood 49:263.

Joyce, R.A. and Chervenick, P.A., 1975, Effect of lithium on the release of colony stimulating activity (CSA) from blood leukocytes, Proc. Am. Soc. Haematol. 18:126.

Metcalf, D., 1977, "Hemopoietic Colonies," Springer-Verlag, Berlin, Heidelberg, New York.

Morley, Jr., D.C. and Galbraith, P.R., 1978, Effect of lithium on granulopoiesis in culture, Can. Med. Assoc. J. 118:288.

O'Connell, R.A., 1970, Leukocytosis during lithium carbonate treatment, Int. J. Pharmacopsychiatry 4:30.

Pike, B.L. and Robinson, W.A., 1970, Human bone marrow colony growth in agar-gel, J. Cell. Physiol. 76:77.

Robinson, W.A. and Pike, B.L., 1970, Leukopoietic activity in human urine. The granulocytic leukemias, N. Engl. J. Med. 282:1291.

Robinson, W.A., Entringer, M.A., and Otsuka, A.L., 1972, In vitro studies in acute granulocytic leukaemia in humans, in "The Nature of Leukaemia" (P.C. Vincent, ed.), pp. 151-161, V.C.N. Blight, Sydney, N.S.W., Australia.

Robinson, W.A. and Mangalik, A., 1975, The kinetics and regulation of granulopoiesis, Semin. Hematol. 12:7.

Rossof, A.H. and Coltman, Jr., C.A., 1976, The effect of lithium carbonate on the granulocyte phagocytic index, Experientia 32:238.

Rothstein, G., Clarkson, D.R., Larsen, W., Grosser, B.I., and Athens, J.W., 1978, Effect of lithium on neutrophil mass and production, N. Engl. J. Med. 298:178.

Shopsin, S., Friedman, R., and Gershon, S., 1971, Lithium and leukocytosis, Clin. Pharmacol. Ther. 12:923.

Spitzer, G., Verma, D.S., Barlogie, B., McCredie, K.G., and Dicke, K., 1979, Possible mechanisms of action involved in the augmentatioin of in vitro spontaneous myeloid colony formation by lithium, Cancer Res., in press.

Stein, R.S., Beaman, C., Ali, M.Y., Hansen, R., Jenkins, D.D., and Jume'an, H.G., 1977, Lithium carbonate attenuation of chemotherapy-induced neutropenia, N. Engl. J. Med. 297:430.

Tisman, G., Herbert, V., and Rosenblatt, S., 1973, Evidence that lithium induces human granulocyte proliferation: Elevated serum vitamin B12 binding capacity in vivo and granulocyte colony proliferation in vitro, Br. J. Haematol. 24:767.

Tisman, G., 1974, Lithium carbonate protection against drug-induced leukopenia in lymphosarcoma patients, IRCS 2:1509.

Van Zant, G and Goldwasser, E., 1979, Competition between erythropoietin and colony-stimulating factor for target cells in mouse marrow, Blood 53:946.

STIMULATION OF GRANULOPOIESIS *IN VITRO* AND *IN VIVO* USING LITHIUM IN CHILDREN WITH CHRONIC NEUTROPENIA

Helen S.L. Chan, Melvin H. Freedman, and
E. Fred Saunders

Division of Hematology
Hospital for Sick Children and the
Department of Pediatrics
University of Toronto
Toronto, Ontario M5G 1X8
Canada

Psychiatric patients have been observed to have a dramatic increase in their neutrophil counts while on lithium (Li) therapy (Mayfield and Brown, 1966). There are reports of the ability of lithium to improve chemotherapy-induced neutropenia in cancer patients (Greco *et al.*, 1976; Stein *et al.*, 1977) and in Felty's syndrome (Gupta *et al.*, 1975). Lithium appears to act through a direct stimulation of committed granulocytic progenitors (CFU-c) (Tisman *et al.*, 1973; Morley and Galbraith, 1978) as well as an increase of colony-stimulating activity (CSA), the humoral stimulator of granulopoiesis (Harker *et al.*, 1977; Gupta *et al.*, 1976). Our purpose was to study and correlate the *in vitro* and *in vivo* effect of lithium on granulopoiesis in children with chronic neutropenia.

TABLE I

PATIENT DATA AT TIME OF STUDY

Patient No.	Diagnosis	Sex	Age Yrs	Neutrophil $/mm^3$	Marrow Cellularity	Marrow Remarks
Aplastic Anemia						
1	Fanconi	F	6	700	D	
2	Fanconi	F	16	900	D	
3	Fanconi	F	8	700	D	
4	Fanconi	F	5	1200	D	
5	Fanconi	F	7	1100	D	
6	Severe Acquired	M	7	700	D	
7	Severe Acquired	M	10	0	D	
8	Severe Acquired	F	7	600	D	
9	Mild Acquired	F	13	1000	N	
10	Mild Acquired	F	4	1000	N	
11	Mild Acquired	M	2	1800	N	

Neutropenia						
12	Kostmann	F	1	0	N	Maturation arrest at myelocyte
13	Shwachman	M	11	400	D	Decreased granulocyte series
14	Idiopathic	F	2	200	N	Normal granulocyte series
15	Idiopathic	M	8	700	N	Decreased granulocyte series
16	Idiopathic	M	1	300	I	Decreased neutrophils
17	Idiopathic	F	1	300	I	Decreased neutrophils

F: female; M: male; D: decreased; N: normal; I: increased

MATERIALS AND METHODS

Subjects

Studies were done in seventeen children with chronic neutropenia and their clinical data are summarized in Table I. At the time of study, the patients were free of infection and taking no medication except patient 14 who was receiving antibiotics for pneumonia.

Patients 1 to 5 had classical Fanconi's aplastic anemia with congenital anomalies, increased chromosomal breaks, and progressive pancytopenia. Patients 6 to 8 had severe idiopathic acquired aplastic anemia with marked marrow hypoplasia, requiring red cell and platelet transfusions. Patients 9 to 11 had mild idiopathic acquired aplastic anemia with mild pancytopenia and with minimal or no reduction in marrow cellularity. They did not require blood products for support. Patient 12 had autosomal recessive neutropenia of the Kostmann type with a characteristic maturation arrest in the marrow at the early myelocyte stage. At no time were mature neutrophils present in the marrow or in the peripheral blood. Patient 13 had exocrine pancreatic insufficiency associated with chronic neutropenia (Shwachman syndrome). The marrow showed a reduced granulocytic series. Patients 14 to 17 had idiopathic neutropenia which did not fit a recognized syndrome. Their marrows showed depletion of mature neutrophils or a symmetrical reduction in the granulocytic series with normal cellularity.

Control bone marrow was obtained from 5 children ranging from 1 to 13 years of age without hematological disease or infection who had aspirates performed as part of their medical investigation.

Consent

These studies were approved by the Human Experimentation Committee of the Hospital for Sick Children and informed consent was obtained from parents of children who received a trial of lithium therapy.

CFU-c Assay

Nucleated marrow and peripheral blood cells were concentrated by layering over Ficoll-Paque (Pharmacia Fine Chemicals) and centrifuged (200 g, 10°C) for 20 minutes. The cells were incubated twice in plastic culture plates at 37°C for 30 minutes to remove adherent cells (Messner et al., 1973). One-hundred-thousand nucleated marrow cells or 5×10^5 nucleated peripheral blood cells were cultured in 0.8% methylcellulose (Iscove et al., 1971), 30% fetal calf serum and alpha medium conditioned with a standard CSA made from the peripheral blood leukocytes of a normal adult volunteer (Amato et al., 1976). Cultures were incubated at 37°C for 14 days in air with 5% CO_2 and high humidity. Colonies were counted directly in the culture plates using an inverted microscope. A CFU-c colony was defined as a cluster of 20 or more granulocytes (Iscove et al., 1971). The results were expressed as mean colony number of duplicate plates per 10^5 cells cultured.

CSA Assay

To test the patients' ability to produce colony-stimulating activity, CSA from their peripheral blood leukocytes was tested in the CFU-c assay system using 3 control marrows and compared with the standard CSA which was defined as 100% activity (Amato et al., 1976).

Lithium Stimulation of Granulopoiesis In Vitro

To establish the optimal dose of Li for in vitro stimulation of CFU-c, dose-response studies were performed on marrows from five controls and patient 12. Lithium chloride (Fisher Scientific) was freshly dissolved in alpha medium and added to the plates in concentrations from 5×10^{-2} to 5×10^{-5}M.

Protocol for Lithium Therapy

Five patients (1, 2, 8, 12, and 14) received a clinical trial of lithium therapy. Complete blood counts, marrow morphology, CSA from peripheral blood leukocytes, and marrow and blood CFU-c numbers were determined before and during therapy. The dose of lithium carbonate required to maintain serum levels between 0.5 to 1 meq/liter ranged from 20-100 mg/kg/day. Serum electrolytes, BUN, creatinine, thyroid function tests, and urine specific gravity were monitored.

RESULTS

Lithium Stimulation of Granulopoiesis In Vitro

CFU-c grew only in the presence of added CSA. Lithium dose-response studies (Table II) showed that the concentration of Li that produced a maximum increase in CFU-c numbers over the controls with CSA alone was 5×10^{-3}M. Bone marrows from the 17 patients were then tested with this dose of Li and the results are shown in Table III. Patients 1 to 8, with severe acquired and Fanconi's aplastic anemia, had very low CFU-c numbers which did not increase when Li was added to the cultures. Patients 9 to 11 with mild aplastic anemia and patients 12 to 17 with miscellaneous neutropenias had low to low normal CFU-c numbers which increased significantly with Li.

TABLE II

LITHIUM DOSE-RESPONSE STUDY ON GROWTH OF CFU-C FROM BONE MARROWS OF 5 CONTROLS AND PATIENT 12

	CFU-c	
Concentration	Controls	Patient 12
0	64 ± 26	58 ± 4
5×10^{-5} M	59 ± 16	68 ± 2
5×10^{-4}M	65 ± 12	86 ± 12
5×10^{-3}M	97 ± 31	100 ± 2
5×10^{-2}M	0	0

Results are expressed as mean ± standard deviation/10^5 cells cultured.

TABLE III

EFFECT OF LITHIUM (5×10^{-3}M) ON MARROW CFU-C IN VITRO

	Without Li	With Li
Patients 1 to 8	5 ± 6	4 ± 6
Patients 9 to 11	23 ± 8	35 ± 9
Patients 12 to 17	30 ± 21	57 ± 35

Results are expressed as mean ± SD/10^5 cells.

Lithium Therapy in Neutropenic Patients

When serum Li levels are maintained between 0.5-1 meq/liter, the patients did not manifest any toxic side effects and their hemoglobin levels and platelet counts did not change significantly from pre-treatment levels. In patient 1, with Fanconi's aplastic anemia, marrow cellularity did not improve. Bone marrow CFU-c numbers remained low (5/10^5 cells before Li -vs- 3/10^5 cells after one month of Li). As shown in Figure 1, CSA increased by 66% but peripheral blood CFU-c remained low and the neutropenia persisted. Patient 2, with Fanconi's aplastic anemia, and patient 8, with severe acquired aplastic anemia, had identical patterns of response. In patient 12, with Kostmann neutropenia, four weeks of Li did not change the bone marrow morphology; however, there was a striking increase in bone marrow CFU-c from 57 to 93/10^5 cells. CSA increased by 91% (Figure 2) and peripheral blood CFU-c increased from 6 to 75/5 x 10^5cells. Nevertheless, the agranulocytosis persisted. In patient 14, with idiopathic neutropenia, marrow morphology remained unchanged on lithium. After 4 weeks of therapy, bone marrow CFU-c increased from 8 to 64/10^5 cells. As shown in Figure 3, CSA increased from 37% to 162% and peripheral blood CFU-c from 18 to 82/5 x 10^5 cells. Neutrophils increased from 180 to a maximum of 14,000/mm^3. During a 3-month period when Li was stopped, CSA and CFU-c promptly decreased to pre-treatment levels and the neutrophil count fell to less than 500/mm^3. Subsequently, on Li maintenance for 6 months, neutrophils remained over 3,500/mm^3.

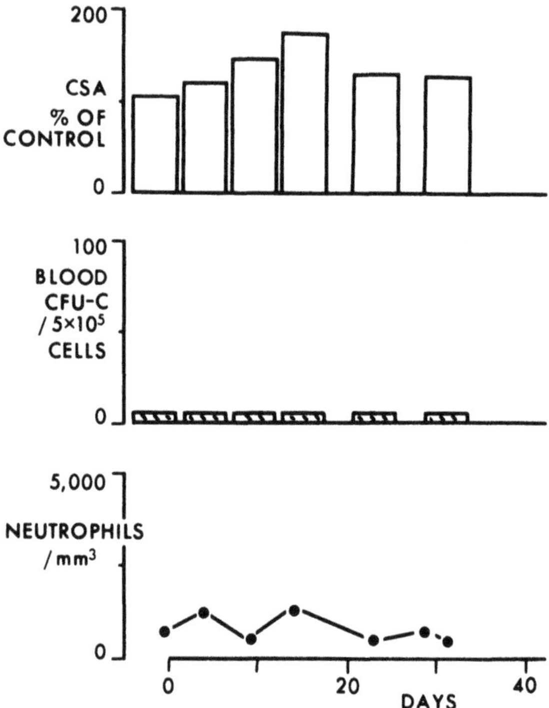

Figure 1. Peripheral blood CSA, CFU-c and neutrophil counts of patient 1 during 30 days of lithium therapy.

DISCUSSION

From the experience using lithium in psychiatric patients, it appears that the drug stimulates granulopoiesis in vivo and therefore may be useful in the treatment of neutropenia. Preliminary data have indicated success in management of chemotherapy-induced neutropenia. However, the effect of lithium on abnormal granulopoiesis has not been determined, and no criteria have been developed for selection of neutropenic patients suitable for a trial of lithium therapy.

We studied the in vitro effect of lithium on 17 patients with various types of neutropenias. Patients with Fanconi's and severe acquired aplastic

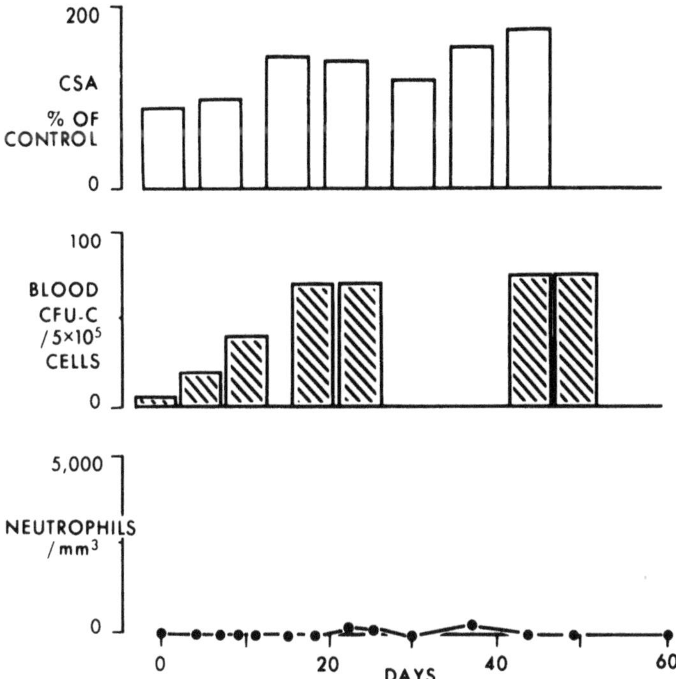

Figure 2. Peripheral blood CSA, CFU-c and neutrophil counts of patient 12 during 50 days of lithium therapy.

anemia have markedly reduced or undetectable granulopoietic stem cells (Saunders and Freedman, 1978; Freedman et al., 1979) and, from our data, failed to respond to added lithium in vitro. In contrast, patients with mild aplastic anemia who had mildly reduced CFU-c did show a significant increase in the presence of lithium. A similar increase in CFU-c was seen in the patients with congenital or acquired neutropenia. An obvious conclusion is that if patients have very few or no granulopoietic precursors, lithium is ineffective.

We gave lithium to 5 patients with different forms of neutropenia as a therapeutic trial, and 3 patterns of response were seen. In the 3 patients with Fanconi's and severe acquired neutropenia, there was a prompt and significant increase in CSA levels; however, blood and marrow CFU-c remained low and the neutrophil counts were unchanged. In contrast, in the patient with Kostmann neutropenia, although there was an increase in both CSA and blood and marrow CFU-c, the patient did not produce mature neutrophils *in vivo*. A third form of response was seen in the patient with idiopathic neutropenia in whom CSA and CFU-c increased, and neutrophil counts responded dramatically. The effect was reversible on stopping lithium, and was reproducible when lithium was restarted.

The *in vitro* testing of lithium on marrow cultures prior to therapy was predictive in all the patients except the one with Kostmann neutropenia. It was expected that the patients with aplastic anemia would not

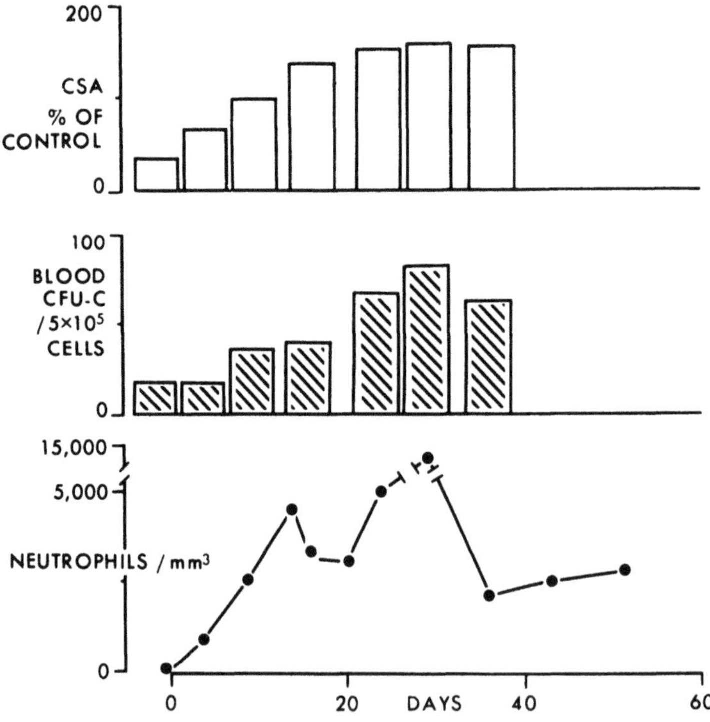

Figure 3. Peripheral blood CSA, CFU-c and neutrophil counts in patient 14 during 50 days of lithium therapy.

improve because there was no stem cell compartment for the lithium or the increased CSA level to stimulate. Granulopoiesis in Kostmann neutropenia is unique in that granulopoietic progenitors are plentiful and are capable of maturation to the neutrophil stage in vitro (Barak et al., 1971; Amato et al., 1976), but not in vivo. The defect in this condition would not appear to be intrinsic to the stem cell, but more likely, in the hematopoietic microenvironment. The discrepancy between in vivo and in vitro granulopoiesis led to misleading predictive testing.

In the patient with a beneficial clinical result with lithium treatment, the in vitro testing predicted the response. This patient had a low CSA level which increased to normal with lithium, and as there was an adequate stem cell compartment able to respond to the CSA, production of normal neutrophil numbers resulted.

We conclude that a trial of lithium is safe for children with chronic neutropenia. Long term effects remain unknown, however. We recommend the following preliminary criteria for a trial of lithium therapy in neutropenic patients: a sufficient granulocytic stem cell compartment, low CSA, and an in vitro response to Li.

REFERENCES

Amato, D., Freedman, M.H., and Saunders, E.F., 1976, Granulopoiesis in severe congenital neutropenia, Blood 47:531.

Barak, Y., Paran, M., Levin, S., and Sachs, L., 1971, In vitro induction of myeloid proliferation and maturation in infantile genetic agranulocytosis, Blood 38:74.

Freedman, M.H., Gelfand, E.W., and Saunders, E.F., 1979, Acquired aplastic anemia: antibody-mediated hematopoietic failure, Am. J. Hemat., in press.

Greco, F.A., Brereton, H.D., and Pomeroy, T., 1976, Lithium carbonate attenuation of neutropenia from cancer chemotherapy, Proc. Amer. Assoc. Canc. Res. 17:250.

Gupta, R.C., Robinson, W.A., and Smyth, C.J., 1975, Efficacy of lithium in rheumatoid arthritis with granulocytopenia (Felty's syndrome), Arthritis Rheum. 18:179.

Gupta, R.C., Robinson, W.A., and Kurnick, J.E., 1976, Felty's syndrome: effect of lithium on granulopoiesis, Am. J. Med. 61:29.

Harker, W.G., Rothstein, G., Clarkson, D., Athens, J.W., and MacFarlane, J.L., 1977, Enhancement of colony-stimulating activity production by lithium, Blood 49:263.

Iscove, N.N., Senn, J.S., Till, J.E., and McCulloch, E.A., 1971, Colony formation by normal and leukemic human marrow cells in culture: effect of conditioned medium from human leukocytes, Blood 37:1

Mayfield, D. and Brown, R.G., 1966, The clinical laboratory and electroencephalographic effects of lithium, J. Psychiat. Res. 4:207.

Messner, H.A., Till, J.E., and McCulloch, E.A., 1973, Interacting cell populations affecting granulopoietic colony formation by normal and leukemic human marrow cells, Blood 42:701

Morley, D.C., Jr. and Galbraith, P.R., 1978, Effect of lithium on granulopoiesis in culture, Canad. Med. Assoc. J. 118:288.

Saunders, E.F. and Freedman, M.H., 1978, Constitutional aplastic anemia: defective hematopoietic stem cell growth in vitro, Br. J. Haematol. 40:277.

Stein, R.S., Beaman, C., Ali, M.Y. Hansen, R., Jenkins, D.D., and Jume'an, H.G., 1977, Lithium carbonate attenuation of chemotherapy-induced neutropenia, New Engl. J. Med. 297:430.

Tisman, G., Herbert, V., and Rosenblatt, S., 1973, Evidence that lithium induces human granulocyte proliferation: elevated serum vitamin B12 binding capacity in vivo and granulocyte colony proliferation in vitro, Br. J. Haematol. 24:767.

CLINICAL EXPERIENCE WITH LITHIUM IN APLASTIC ANEMIA AND CONGENITAL NEUTROPENIA

Austin John Barrett

Department of Hematology
Westminster Medical School
London S.W.1

The ability of lithium salts to stimulate granulopoiesis in hematologically normal subjects with psychiatric disorders (Shopsin *et al.*, 1971) encourages attempts to use lithium to stimulate granulopoiesis in patients with neutropenia. We have studied the *in vivo* and *in vitro* effects of lithium salts in aplastic anemia and congenital neutropenia in order to establish the mode of action of lithium and to evaluate its therapeutic role in neutropenic disorders. This paper summarizes clinical experience with lithium in two European centers. The hematological effects of treatment are defined. In addition, in several patients bone marrow culture studies were carried out in order to develop *in vitro* tests that could predict clinical response to lithium. Ten patients with hypoplastic anemia were seen and treated at the Westminster Hospital and Westminster Children's Hospital in London and two patients with congenital neutropenia are reported from the Hopital Necker des Enfants Malades, Paris. In addition, seven hematologically normal patients taking lithium for psychiatric disorders were studied at the Westminster Hospital.

Hematological changes were monitored by blood counts and bone marrow examinations. *In vitro* studies of bone marrow culture followed the technique of Pike and Robinson (1970) using peripheral blood feeder layers as a source of colony stimulating factor. Bone marrow cultures were plated in triplicate at a cell concentration of 2×10^5 cells per plate and counted after 10 days of incubation. Tests for hemolysis, haptoglobin levels and red cell osmotic fragility were carried out using techniques described by Dacie and Lewis (1975).

LITHIUM TREATMENT

Before starting treatment, electrolytes and thyroid status were checked. Lithium carbonate was given at a dose of 750 mg per m^2 per day in divided doses. Serum lithium levels were checked weekly and the dose adjusted to obtain serum levels of 0.8 mmole/liter. Treatment was stopped if serious side effects occurred.

In general, lithium treatment was well tolerated but most patients developed thirst, polyuria and lassitude especially during the first week of treatment. These side effects were considered acceptable and no dose reductions were made. Two patients developed dyskinesia which abated after reducing the dose. One infant with congenital neutropenia developed a nephrotic syndrome which necessitated stopping treatment.

CASE HISTORIES AND RESULTS OF TREATMENT IN APLASTIC ANEMIA

Case 1

A 27 year old male developed severe aplastic anemia following hepatitis. He failed to respond to androgen treatment or a course of horse antilymphocyte globulin. Lithium carbonate was given over an eight week trial period. At the time of treatment, he required regular blood transfusions and had recurrent infective episodes. He was on a regular dose of 7.5 mg prednisolone daily. There was a modest rise in neutrophils and a gradual improvement occurred. Transfusion requirements decreased 18 months later, in association with a partial autologous recovery. He remains well and has not required any further specific treatment. His latest blood count showed: hemoglobin 12.4 g/dl, white cell count 3.8×10^9/liter with 60% neutrophils, platelets 60×10^9/liter.

Case 2

A 39 year old man with severe idiopathic aplastic anemia of one year's duration had shown no response to oxymethalone treatment, and had received a course of horse antilymphocyte globulin with no hematological improvement. At the time of treatment, his main problem was recurrent bleeding and dependence on monthly transfusions. A six week trial of lithium carbonate was associated with a temporary cessation of gum bleeding with a modest increase in the platelet count. Platelet transfusions were unnecessary during a four week period. One year later he remains severely aplastic with persisting bleeding requiring frequent transfusions.

Case 3

A 16 year old Pakistani girl presented with a severe aplastic anemia suspected to have followed the use of antihistamines. She was admitted for consideration for bone marrow transplantation. During the period of assessment which covered six weeks, she received oxymethalone 50 mg twice daily and lithium carbonate. Her neutrophil count fell further during this time but her platelet count rose transiently to 40×10^9/liter. This was not associated with any clinical improvement. She died later after two attempted bone marrow grafts from her histocompatible brother failed to produce hematological reconstitution.

Case 4

An 11 year old boy developed severe aplastic anemia. He was referred for a bone marrow transplant from his histocompatible brother. Three attempts at transplantation failed to produce hematological reconstitution and he was given lithium carbonate six weeks after the second graft attempt, at which time he was severely pancytopenic and was nursed in a Vickers-Trexler plastic isolator. Two weeks after starting lithium treatment, reticulocytes rose on a single occasion to 20×10^9/liter. There was a slight increase in the bone marrow cellularity but no clinical improvement occurred. He was later removed from isolation and sent home where he died without achieving bone marrow reconstitution.

Case 5

A three year old girl with severe aplastic anemia received a bone marrow transplant from her histocompatible brother. In view of her age, the immunosuppressive agent cyclosporin A was used to prepare her for transplantation instead of cyclophosphamide. No hematological reconstitution followed. Four weeks after transplantation, she was given lithium carbonate for a one month period without any change in blood counts or any clinical improvement. She died two weeks after stopping treatment, from hemorrhagic complications.

Case 6

A 13 year old boy presented with Fanconi type aplastic anemia at the age of six and was controlled on androgens until he became refractory at the age of 11. On referral he had mouth ulcers and recurrent nose bleeds. Treatment with lithium carbonate and prednisolone, 15 mg daily, was started. There was a rapid rise of neutrophil, platelet and reticulocyte counts. The increase in neutrophils was sustained after prednisolone had been stopped. During the following 13 months, he developed increasing problems from bleeding and anemia, but did not develop any further infections. He died 14 months after starting lithium treatment, with hemorrhagic complications.

Case 7

A ten year old girl presented with a long history of recurrent pneumonia and unexplained fevers. She was found to be anemic with reticulocytopenia, neutropenia, and a normal platelet count. The bone marrow was hypoplastic. Her physical features suggested Fanconi type aplastic anemia: she was below the 10th centile for height, she had a sallow complexion with "cafe au lait" spots and a pointed face with prominent epicanthic folds. However, blood and bone marrow chromosomal analyses did not show the presence of breaks. Her pneumonia responded to antibiotic treatment but she remained neutropenic. Lithium carbonate was started and within ten days there was a rise of neutrophils, platelets and reticulocytes. Platelet and reticulocyte counts reached a peak within 15 days after starting treatment, and subsequently began to fall. The neutrophil count rose steadily, reaching a maximum of 2.5×10^9/liter 47 days after starting treatment. Lithium treatment was continued for four months and in the last month all treatment had been stopped and the neutrophil count still remains elevated. She has had no further infections.

Case 8

A 12 year old girl with established Fanconi type aplastic anemia was referred for consideration for bone marrow transplantation. She was refractory to androgen treatment and had major problems from hemorrhage - nose bleeds and gum bleeds. Two weeks after starting lithium treatment, her neutrophil count rose but there was no change in platelet and reticulocyte counts.

Case 9

A 42 year old woman developed chronic granulocytic leukemia and received busulphan in an approximate dose of 2 mg daily for six months. She became pancytopenic in the last two months of treatment and did not respond to prednisolone treatment. At the time of referral, she was severely pancytopenic and had two episodes of infection - a septicemia, and an infected finger. Bone marrow examination showed severe hypoplasia with presence of a Philadelphia chromosome. Prednisolone treatment was stopped and she was given lithium carbonate over a two month period. The neutrophil count rose modestly and transiently but she developed no further infections. She was discharged from hospital requiring intermittent blood and platelet transfusions support. She remains pancytopenic. Bone marrow examinations showed no change in cellularity before and after starting lithium. In both samples, the Philadelphia chromosome was detected.

Case 10

A 30 year old man presented with Stage III Hodgkin's Disease and was given three courses of nitrogen mustard, vincristine, procarbazine and prednisone with clinical improvement and regression of mediastinal lymph nodes. After the last course of treatment, he became severely pancytopenic. Repeated marrow aspirates and trephines showed profound bone marrow hypoplasia without evidence of involvement with Hodgkin's Disease. It was concluded that his aplasia was an idiosyncrasy to one of the chemotherapeutic agents and he was admitted into reverse barrier isolation for treatment. During a three months hospitalization when he was given successively oxymethalone, etiocholanolone, and high doses of methyl prednisolone in an attempt to stimulate the bone marrow, he developed recurrent pyrexias and a Klebsiella pneumonia which cavitated. He also required heavy support with blood, platelets and leucocyte transfusions. Lithium carbonate was started during methyl prednisolone treatment and has been continued to date after other treatments were stopped. There has been no hematological improvement but he has been discharged from hospital without further infectious episodes. He has now become refractory to platelet transfusions and remains severely pancytopenic.

The hematological and clinical changes occuring with lithium treatment are summarized in Tables I, II and III.

LITHIUM TREATMENT IN CONGENITAL NEUTROPENIA

The data have been reported elsewhere (Barrett et al., 1977). The results are summarized in Table IV. Bone marrow culture studies were carried out in two patients to determine whether the addition of lithium to their mononuclear cell feeder layers increased normal or autologous bone marrow colony growth. We have previously shown that feeder layers from normal subjects only show enhancement of colony stimulating activity at sub-optimal cell concentrations in the feeder layer. The two patients with congenital neutropenia differed quantitatively from normal in the CSA activity of their mononuclear cells, and the feeder cells of Case 11 (who had a clinical response to lithium) showed a large increase in the colony growth of normal and autologous bone marrow cells when lithium was

TABLE I

HEMATOLOGICAL CHANGES AFTER LITHIUM TREATMENT

No.	Patient Age	Patient Sex	Diagnosis	Neutrophils x $10^9/l$ Pre	Neutrophils x $10^9/l$ Post	Platelets x $10^9/l$ Pre	Platelets x $10^9/l$ Post	Reticulocytes x $10^9/l$ Pre	Reticulocytes x $10^9/l$ Post
1	27	M	H	0.25	0.8	10-80	125	17	85
2	31	M	I	0.3-0.7	1.1	10-30	40	2	74
3	16	F	I	0.0-0.4	0.3	7-15	40	0-0.5%	0.5%
4	11	M	I	0.0-0.6	0.65	10-25	20(100)	10	20
5	4	F	I	0.0-0.05	0.02	26-(70)	25(75)	10	10
6	13	M	F	0.1-0.3	4.2	10-20	80	5-17	85
7	8	F	F	0.1-0.6	3.2	140-250	525	10	5.8
8	12	F	F	0.5-0.7	1.0	7-(45)	12	10	10
9	42	F	D	0.0-0.1	0.3	3-25	(90)	10	10
10	30	M	D	0.1-0.6	0.6	15-(102)	(75)	10	10

"Pre" figures are the range of counts in 6 weeks pre-treatment. "Post" figures are the maximum values reached. Brackets indicate transfused values. Underlined figures indicate rise in blood counts.

H: hepatitis; I: idiopathic; F: Fanconi; D: drug-induced causes of neutropenia.

TABLE II

BONE MARROW CHANGES AFTER LITHIUM TREATMENT

Patient	Diagnosis	Bone Marrow Cellularity	
		Pre	Post
1	H	↓↓	↓↓
2	I	↓↓↓	↓↓↓
3	I	↓↓↓	↓↓↓
4	I	↓↓↓	↓↓
5	I	↓↓	↓↓
6	F	↓↓	↓↓
7	F	↓	↓
8	F	↓	Not tested
9	D	↓↓	↓↓
10	D	↓↓↓	↓↓↓

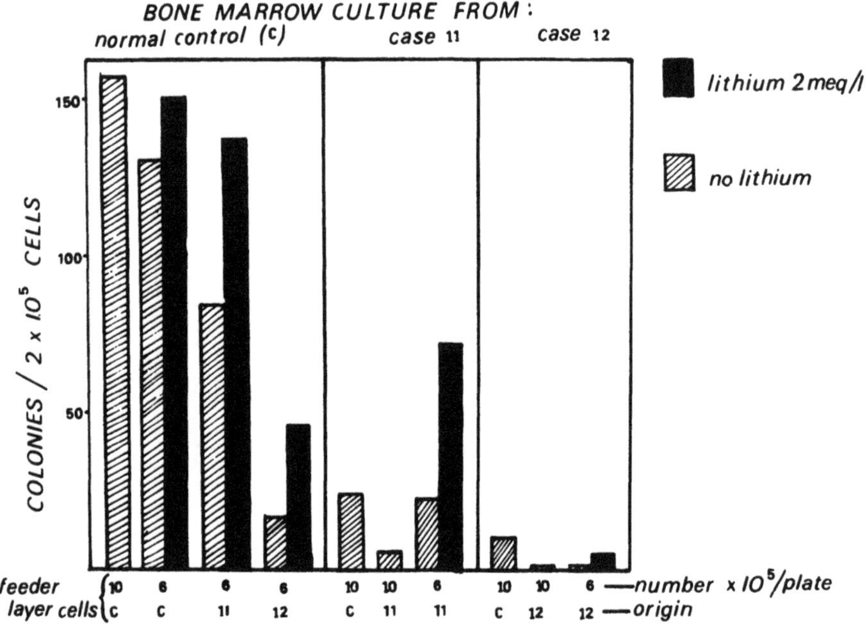

Figure 1. In vitro effect of lithium on CFU-C growth in congenital neutropenia.

TABLE III

CLINICAL CHANGES WITH LITHIUM TREATMENT

	Age	Sex	Dx	DOT	RTR		Reduced		Outcome	Surv.
				(Months)	BLD	PLTS	Bld	Inf		(Months)
1	27	M	H	2	NO	NO	NO	---	Autologous recovery	49+
2	31	M	I	1½	NO	YES(T)	YES(T)	---	Remains severely aplastic	11+
3	16	F	I	1½	NO	NO	NO	NO	Rejected marrow graft	2 (dead)
4	11	M	I	5	NO	NO	NO	NO	Rejected marrow graft	5 (dead)
5	3	F	I	1	NO	NO	NO	NO	Rejected marrow graft	1½(dead)
6	13	M	F	13	NO	YES(T)	YES(T)	YES	Thrombytocopenia recurred	14 (dead)
7	8	F	F	4	YES	---	---	YES	Well	5+
8	12	F	F	1+	NO	NO	---	---	Bleeding persists	1+
9	42	F	D	2	NO	NO	---	YES	Remains aplastic	5+
10	30	M	D	2½+	NO	NO	NO	---	Remains aplastic	2½+

T = transient: 2-3 weeks duration; --- = Unassessable or not relevant; Dx = diagnosis; DOT = duration of treatment; RTR = reduced transfusion requirement; BLD = blood; PLTS = platelets; Bld = bleeding; Inf = infection; Surv. = survival from starting treatment.

TABLE IV

LITHIUM IN CONGENITAL NEUTROPENIA

Patient 11	Pre-Lithium	1 Week After Stopping	3 Weeks After Stopping
F 2 yrs	Neutrophils $0.0 \times 10^9/1$	$2.0 \times 10^9/1$	$0.2 \times 10^9/1$
Marrow arrest at promyelocyte; 3 weeks lithium treatment	Recurrent pneumonia and Skin abscesses	Infections cleared	Recurrence of infection
Patient 12			
F 1½ yrs	Neutrophils $0.0 \times 10^9/1$	$0.0 \times 10^9/1$	
Marrow arrest at promyelocyte; 4 weeks lithium treatment	Recurrent pneumonia and Skin abscessess	No response	

added to the feeder layer. Both patients had sub-normal numbers of CFU-C on normal and autologous feeder layers but in Case 11, lithium was shown to enhance colony forming ability in vitro (Figure 1).

HEMATOLOGICAL EFFECTS OF LITHIUM IN PATIENTS WITH PSYCHIATRIC DISORDERS

Seven patients receiving lithium for manic-depressive disorders were studied. Table V shows their hematological characteristics. Not all patients showed a neutrophil leucocytosis. Some had modest rises in the reticulocyte and platelet count. Blood CFU-C levels were within the normal limits. Red cell osmotic fragility, haptoglobin levels, and hemopexin levels were normal and the direct Coomb's test was negative in five patients tested.

TABLE V

BLOOD CHANGES IN SEVEN HEMATOLOGICALLY NORMAL PATIENTS TAKING LITHIUM

	Mean ± SD	Range	Normal Upper Limit (95% Confidence Limits)
Neutrophils x $10^9/l$	8.2 ± 1.6	5.8 - 10.4	7.5
Reticulocytes x $10^9/l$	96 ± 42	36 - 140	100
Platelets x $10^9/l$	272 ± 77	202 - 414	400
CFU-C per ml	27 ± 21	6 - 49	88 ± 69 (Men) 44 ± 43 (Women)
Lithium level	0.75 ± 0.1	0.6 - 0.9	--

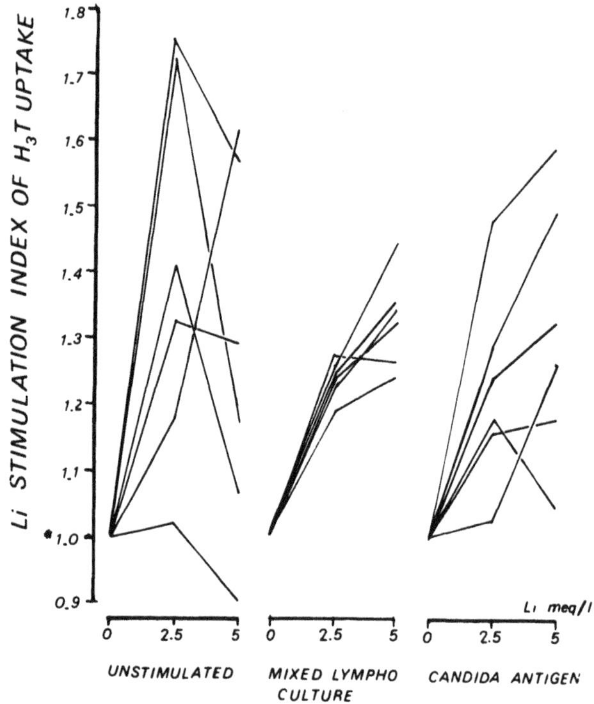

Figure 2. Lithium dependent increase in tritiated thymidine uptake by lymphocytes from six normal subjects in mixed lymphocyte and candida antigen responses. *: "No lithium" counts normalized to 1.0.

DISCUSSION

Mode of Action of Lithium

The mode of action of lithium on granulopoiesis was first investigated by Tisman et al. (1973) who showed that lithium stimulated bone marrow CFU-C growth in vitro. Harker et al. (1977) showed that lithium enhanced colony stimulating activity (CSA) of mononuclear cells. We have shown similar effects of lithium on CFU-C, and by incorporating lithium in blood mononuclear cell feeder layers in normal subjects and in patients with congenital neutropenia, examined the ability of lithium to stimulate colony growth in this disorder. The neutrophil response to lithium in Case 11 was associated with a larger than normal enhancement by lithium of normal and patient CFU-C growth suggesting that the therapeutic effect observed was due to lithium-enhanced CSA activity.

In normal subjects, the neutrophil response to lithium may be due to enhanced CSA production. This probably accounts for the neutrophil increment with lithium in aplastic anemia where CSA levels are normal (Kern et al., 1977).

A second possible mode of action of lithium is via inhibition of suppressor T lymphocytes (Gelfand et al., 1979). We have shown that lithium can increase lymphocyte tritiated thymidine uptake in a dose-dependent fashion in one-way mixed lymphocyte reactions and in vitro lymphocyte response to candida antigen (Figure 2). The in vitro inhibition of suppressor cells may explain these phenomena. There is also indirect evidence of suppressor cell inhibition in the known association of autoimmune thyroid disorders with long-term lithium treatment, and, recently, patients taking lithium have been found to have a high frequency of tissue specific autoantibodies (Franks, personal communication). Thymus derived cells are thought to be important in the regulation of hematopoiesis in mice (Sharkis et al., 1978) and suppressor lymphocytes have been implicated in the etiopathogenesis of aplastic anemia (Ascensao et al., 1976; Hoffman et al., 1977) and Diamond-Blackfan pure red cell aplasia (Hoffman et al., 1976). However, the evidence for a suppressor lymphocyte role in the causation of aplastic anemia has been challenged (Singer et al., 1978; Barrett et al., in press). It is possible that the reticulocytosis, thrombocytosis, and, perhaps, neutrophil leucocytosis seen in some hematologically normal and abnormal patients on lithium may be due to inhibition of a hemopoietic suppressor cell of the T lymphocyte category. This hypothesis raises the interesting possibility of using lithium in disorders due to abnormal suppressor cell activity such as pure red cell aplasia and some types of hypogammaglobulinemia.

Impaired immunity has been reported in Fanconi aplastic anemia (Pederson et al., 1977). It is possible that lithium inhibition of a suppressor lymphocyte may have produced the hematological effects seen in the patients we treated. However, it is also possible that the neutrophil leucocyte increase was caused by enhancement of CSA since feeder layer activity is low in this condition (Gupta, personal communication).

Clinical Results

Lithium has produced increases in the neutrophil count in Felty's syndrome (Gupta et al., 1975), and neutropenia following chemotherapy (Greco and Brereton, 1977; Charron et al., 1977). In this series of patients, the results of lithium therapy were disappointing. In patients with acquired severe marrow hypoplasia, neutrophil response was modest and increments in platelets and reticulocytes were small and transient. In no patient was an autologous recovery obtained that could be ascribed to lithium, and clinical benefit was minimal. In contrast, neutrophil increments were greater in patients with Fanconi aplasia. However, despite reticulocytosis, no lengthening of the transfusion interval occurred and clinical benefit was largely restricted to the reduction in the occurrence of bacterial infection. It should be pointed out that the patients studied had severe marrow aplasia and had failed to respond to other therapeutic maneuvers. A possible therapeutic role of lithium in less severe aplasia is not, therefore, ruled out by our results. The neutrophil rise seen in Case 11 with congenital neutropenia encourages further use of lithium in other neutropenias of uncertain etiology.

In conclusion, the hematological use of lithium may be restricted to conditions where colony stimulating activity is low or where there is myelosuppression due to over-activity of suppressor lymphocytes. Colony forming assays can be adapted to examine both these mechanisms in vitro, and used to predict a therapeutic response to lithium. Further clinical trials of lithium in other hematological disorders in association with in vitro tests are indicated.

ACKNOWLEDGEMENTS

I wish to thank Dr. C. Griscelli, Dr. K. Hugh-Jones, Dr. K. Newton, Dr. R. Powles, and Dr. S. Retsas for permission to report their patients and I wish to acknowledge the cooperation of Dr. A. Faille, D. Buriot, and Dr. M.Y. Gordon in these studies. This work was supported by grants from the Andrew Bostic Fund and the Leukemia Research Fund of Great Britain.

REFERENCES

Ascensao, J., Pahwa, R.N., Kagan, W.A., Hansen, J.A., Moore, M.A.S., and Good, R., 1976, Aplastic anemia: Evidence of an immunological mechanism, Lancet 1:669.

Barrett, A.J., Griscelli, C., Buriot, D., and Faille, A., 1977, Lithium therapy in congenital neutropenia, Lancet 2:1357.

Barrett, A.J., Faille, A., Balitrand, N., Ketels, F., and Najean, Y., 1979, Bone marrow culture in aplastic anemia, J. Clin. Path., in press.

Charron, D., Barrett, A.J., Faille, A., Alby, A., Schmidt, T., and Degos, L., 1977, Lithium in acute myeloid leukemia, Lancet 1:1387.

Dacie, J.V. and Lewis, S.M., 1975, Practical Hematology, 5th Edition, p. 12, Churchill Livingstone, Edinburgh.

Gelfand, E.W., Dosch, H-M., Hastings, D., and Shore, A., 1979, Lithium: A modulator of cyclic AMP-dependent events in lymphocytes, Science 203:367.

Greco, F.A. and Brereton, H., 1977, Lithium carbonate, attentuation of neutropenia from cancer therapy, Oncology 34:153.

Gupta, R.C., Robinson, W.A., and Albrecht, D., 1975, Efficacy of lithium in rheumatoid arthritis with granulocytopenia (Felty's Syndrome), Ann. Rheum. Dis. 34:156.

Harker, W.G., Rothstein, G., Clarkson, J., Athens, J.W., and MacFarlane, J.L., 1977, Ehancement of colony stimulating activity production by lithium, Blood 49:263.

Hoffman, R., Zanjani, E.D., Vila, J., Zalusky, R., Lutton, J.D., and Wasserman, L.R., 1976, Diamond-Blackfan syndrome: Lymphocyte mediated suppression of erythropoiesis, Science 193:899.

Hoffman, R., Zanjani, E.D., Lutton, J.D., Zalusky, R., and Wasserman, L.R., 1977, Suppression of erythroid colony formation by lymphocytes from patients with aplastic anemia, New Eng. J. Med. 296:10.

Kern, P., Heimpel, H., Heit, W., and Kubanek, B., 1977, Granulocyte progenitor cells in aplastic anemia, Brit. J. Hematol. 35:613.

Pederson, F.K., Hertz, H., Lundsteen, C., Platz, P., and Thomsen, M., 1977, Indication of primary immunodeficiency in Fanconi's anemia, Acta Ped. Scand. 66:745.

Pike, B.L. and Robinson, W.A., 1970, Human bone marrow colony growth in agar-gel, J. Cell. Physiol. 76:77.

Sharkis, S.J., Ahmed, A., Sensenbrenner, L.L., Jedrezejczak, W.W., Goldstein, A.L., and Sell, K.W., 1978, The regulation of hemopoiesis: Effect of thymosin or thymocytes in a diffusion chamber, in "Experimental Hematology Today, 1978," p.17-22, (S.J. Baum and G.D. Ledney, eds.) Springer-Verlag, New York.

Shopsin, B., Friedmann, R., and Gershon, S., 1971, Lithium and leucocytosis, Clin. Pharmacol. Therap. 12:923.

Singer, J.W., Brown, J.E., James, M.C., Doney, K., Warren, R.P., Storb, R., and Thomas, E.D., 1978, Effect of peripheral blood lymphocytes from patients with aplastic anemia on granulocyte colony growth from HLA-matched and mismatched marrows: Effect of transfusion sensitization, Blood 52:37.

Tisman, G., Herbert, V., and Rosenblatt, S., 1973, Evidence that lithium increases human granulocyte proliferation: Elevated serum vitamin B12 binding capacity in vivo, and granulocyte colony proliferation in vitro, Brit. J. Hematol. 24:767.

LITHIUM THERAPY OF CHRONIC NEUTROPENIA

Richard S. Stein and Carol A. Howard

Department of Medicine
Vanderbilt University School of Medicine
Nashville, Tennessee 37232

Lithium carbonate can increase granulocyte production in psychiatric patients (Rothstein *et al.*, 1978) and normal subjects (Stein *et al.*, 1978b). Administration of lithium has improved neutropenia in cases of Felty's syndrome (Gupta *et al.*, 1975), aplastic anemia (Barrett *et al.*, 1977; Blum, 1979), and congenital neutropenia (Barrett *et al.*, 1977). On this basis, we instituted a pilot study to determine the efficacy of lithium in the treatment of neutropenia or diverse etiologies. This report presents the results of that trial.

METHODS

Patients

Twenty-seven subjects were studied. Patients were eligible if they had been neutropenic, granulocytes < $1500/mm^3$, for at least one month, and if no history of drug induced neutropenia was obtained. All patients gave informed consent. On the basis of history and bone marrow examination, patients were classified as to etiology of neutropenia. The categories which were used are as follows: 1) acute myelogenous leukemia - hypercellular marrow with > 50% blasts; 2) aplastic anemia - severely hypoplastic marrow; 3) pre-leukemia/smoldering leukemia - a bone marrow which had > 50% blasts but was hypocellular or which showed only 5-50%

blasts; 4) hairy cell leukemia, post-splenectomy; 5) massive splenomegaly - patients not included in categories 1 to 4 having a spleen palpable 6 cm below the costal margin; and 6) idiopathic neutropenia - patients without a specific diagnosis.

Procedures

All patients underwent a baseline bone marrow examination. The circulating granulocyte count was determined as the mean of two measurements. A baseline hydrocortisone challenge test for marrow reserve and an epinephrine challenge test for marginated granulocytes were performed. The procedure for the hydrocortisone test is as follows: hydrocortisone, 100 mg, was injected intravenously. Leukocyte counts and differentials were obtained at 0, 60, 120, and 180 minutes. The marrow reserve was defined as the maximum increase in total granulocytes (Dale et al., 1975). In our experience the normal response to this challenge is 3950 cells/mm^3. The epinephrine test is performed by administering aqueous epinephrine 1:1000, 0.4 ml/m^2, subcutaneously. Leukocyte counts and differentials were obtained at 0, 15, 30, 45, and 60 minutes. The marginated granulocytes were defined as the maximum increase in total granulocytes (Samuels, 1951). In our experience, the normal response to this challenge is 1880 cell/mm^3. In patients over age 60, epinephrine challenge tests were not performed.

Lithium carbonate, 300 mg t.i.d., was administered by mouth for 21 days. Lithium levels were monitored at least weekly. After 21 days circulating granulocytes were measured; hydrocortisone and epinephrine challenge tests were repeated. Lithium was then discontinued and a follow-up circulating granulocyte count was obtained 21 days after lithium had been discontinued. No patients received chemotherapy for leukemia or other disorders during the trial. No patients were receiving androgens. One patients was receiving maintenance prednisone, 10 mg/day.

Definition of Response

A favorable response of circulating granulocytes or to the hydrocortisone or epinephrine challenge tests was arbitrarily defined as an increase on day 21 of $\geq$ 30% and $\geq$ 300 cells/mm^3 over baseline values. An unfavorable response required decreases of a similar magnitude. All other responses were considered no change.

RESULTS

The response of the circulating granulocytes to lithium for the entire group of patients, and for responders and non-responders, is presented in Table I. For the entire series of patients, the average granulocyte increase after three weeks of lithium adminstration was 84%; however, among responders the increase was 389%. Granulocyte counts on day 42 were not significantly different than baseline granulocyte counts, although this approached statistical significance among responders.

TABLE I

CIRCULATING GRANULOCYTE RESPONSE TO LITHIUM

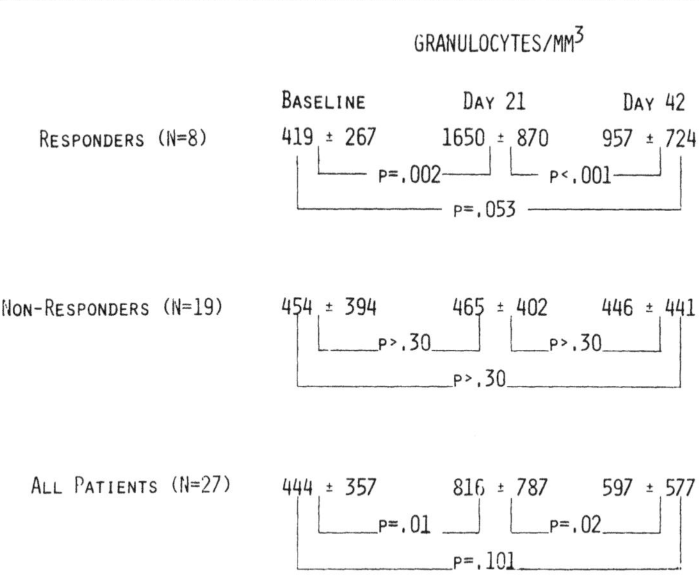

	Granulocytes/mm^3					
	Baseline	Day 21	Day 42	Baseline vs Day 21	Day 21 vs Day 42	Baseline vs Day 42
Responders (N=8)	419 ± 267	1650 ± 870	957 ± 724	p=.002	p<.001	p=.053
Non-Responders (N=19)	454 ± 394	465 ± 402	446 ± 441	p>.30	p>.30	p>.30
All Patients (N=27)	444 ± 357	816 ± 787	597 ± 577	p=.01	p=.02	p=.101

TABLE II

GRANULOCYTE RESPONSE TO LITHIUM: INDIVIDUAL PATIENTS

Etiology and Patient	Circulating Granulocytes/mm^3			Response to Lithium*		
	Baseline	On Lithium x 21 days	Lithium Stopped x 21 days	Circulating Granulocytes	Marrow Reserve	Marginated Granulocytes
Acute Myelogenous Leukemia						
1	98	108	169	0	0	0
2	81	108	170	0	ND	ND
3	0	0	0	0	ND	ND
4	98	0	0	0	ND	ND
5	731	663	600	0	ND	ND
Aplastic Anemia						
6	150	704	260	+	ND	ND
7	225	1400	703	+	ND	ND
8	792	1066	476	0	0	0
9	20	196	20	0	0	0
Pre-Leukemia, Smoldering Leukemia						
10	440	806	765	+	0	ND
11	1021	1326	1330	0	-	0
12	819	846	344	0	+	ND
13	213	2460	1748	+	ND	ND
14	1053	780	1376	0	-	ND
15	450	1045	198	+	0	ND
16	792	779	434	0	+	ND
17	495	660	263	0	ND	ND
Hairy Cell Leukemia: Post Splenectomy						
18	864	2309	1008	+	+	+
19	246	1377	680	+	+	ND
20	765	3100	2300	+	0	+
Massive Splenomegaly						
21	62	135	100	0	0	ND
22	817	464	861	-	+	+
23	552	342	350	0	-	+
24	40	25	32	0	0	0
Idiopathic Neutropenia						
25	176	114	594	0	0	0
26	78	343	200	0	ND	ND
27	918	884	1161	0	-	0

+ Favorable, - Unfavorable, 0: No change, ND: Not Done, see methods section for response criterion.

Granulocyte responses of individual patients to the administration of lithium are presented in Table II. The median values of circulating granulocytes for each diagnostic group are presented in Table III. For the entire series of 27 patients, 8 favorable responses were seen. Favorable responses to lithium were not seen in patients with acute myelogenous leukemia (0/5), massive splenomegaly (0/4), or idiopathic neutropenia (0/3). Favorable responses were limited to patients with aplastic anemia (2/4), pre-leukemia/smoldering leukemia (3/8), and hairy cell leukemia - post splenectomy (3/3). This association of response and diagnostic category was statistically highly significant, p = 0.003 (Fisher Exact Test).

TABLE III

CIRCULATING GRANULOCYTES DURING LITHIUM STUDY: DIAGNOSTIC CATEGORIES

	Baseline	On Lithium x 21 days	Lithium Stopped x 21 days	Favorable Responses Number of Patients
Acute Myelogenous Leukemia	202	176	188	0/5
Aplastic Anemia	272	841	365	2/4
Pre-Leukemia/Smoldering Leukemia	660	1087	806	3/8
Hairy Cell Leukemia, Post-Splenectomy	625	2262	1329	3/3
Massive Splenomegaly	368	242	285	0/4
Idiopathic Neutropenia	391	447	652	0/3
All Patients				8/27

As shown in Table IV, favorable responses were not seen in patients with baseline granulocyte counts less than 100 cell/mm^3, but this tendency only approached statistical significance, p = 0.06. As shown in Tables V and VI, neither baseline marrow reserve nor baseline marginated granulocytes, as measured by hydrocortisone and epinephrine challenges, predicted response to lithium.

Responders and non-responders to lithium were compared with respect to a number of variables. Age, sex, baseline monocyte count, baseline granulocyte count, and baseline response to hydrocortisone and epinephrine were not significantly different for responders or non-responders (Table VII).

The data were also subjected to linear regression analysis. The magnitude of the change in circulating granulocytes in response to lithium therapy was independent of baseline granulocyte count, ($r = 0.003$, $p = 0.99$), and showed only weak statistically insignificant correlations with baseline marrow reserve ($r = 0.355$, $p = 0.105$), and baseline marginated granulocytes ($r = 0.498$, $p = 0.059$).

TABLE IV

RESPONSE TO LITHIUM AS RELATED TO BASELINE GRANULOCYTE COUNT

Baseline Circulating Granulocytes	Favorable Responses/ Patients Studied
<100/mm^3	0/8
100-499/mm^3	6/8
500-999/mm^3	2/9
1000-1500/mm^3	0/2

TABLE V

RESPONSE TO LITHIUM AS RELATED TO BASELINE MARROW RESERVE

Baseline Marrow Reserve Granulocytes*	Favorable Responses/ Patients Studied
0-500/mm^3	4/13
500-1000/mm^3	2/3
1000-1500/mm^3	0/1
>1500/mm^3	2/6
Not done	0/4

*Hydrocortisone Challenge Test Response

TABLE VI

RESPONSE TO LITHIUM AS RELATED TO BASELINE MARGINATED GRANULOCYTES

Baseline Marginated Granulocytes*	Favorable Responses/ Patients Studied
<100/mm^3	1/2
100-500/mm^3	3/9
500-1000/mm^3	0/1
1000-2000/mm^3	0/2
>2000/mm^3	2/2
Not done	2/11

* Epinephrine Challenge Test Response

TABLE VII

CHARACTERISTICS OF RESPONDERS AND NON-RESPONDERS TO LITHIUM

	Responders	Non Responders	
Number	8	19	
Age (Range)	(23-70)	(17-73)	
Median	50	55	p>.30
Sex: Males	6	17	p>.30
Females	2	2	
Baseline Circulating Granulocytes (Mean)	419 ± 267	454 ± 394	p>.30
Baseline Hydrocortisone Response (Mean)	878 ± 936	889 ± 1049	p>.30
Baseline Epinephrine Response (Mean)	914 ± 1006	515 ± 518	p>.30
Baseline Monocytes (Mean)	506 ± 797	162 ± 183	p=.26

Lithium Levels and Toxicity

Lithium levels between 0.5 and 1.0 meq/L were obtained in 26 of 27 patients. One patient achieved a maximum serum level of only 0.4 meq/L. Tremor, which improved following transfusions of packed red blood cells, was noted in three patients with hematocrits between 18 and 25. Additional toxicity definitely attributable to lithium was not seen.

DISCUSSION

Lithium carbonate previously has been shown to increase granulocyte production in psychiatric patients and normal volunteers (Rothstein et al., 1978; Stein et al., 1978b). This phenomenon has been used to attenuate neutropenia in patients receiving myelotoxic chemotherapy for cancer (Stein et al., 1977; Greco and Brereton, 1977; Lyman et al., 1978) and for acute leukemia (Stein et al., 1978). In small studies, lithium has led to increased granulocyte counts in neutropenic patients with Felty's syndrome, aplastic anemia, and congenital neutropenia.

Since positive results are more likely to be reported than negative results, the actual efficacy of lithium in these situations is unknown. For this reason, we instituted a broad pilot study of lithium in all types of chronic neutropenia. Since neutropenia may occur in a number of clinical settings and by a number of mechanisms, our patients were stratified by clinical diagnosis as well as by degree of neutropenia. To aid in our interpretation of this clinical trial, hydrocortisone and epinephrine challenge tests were used to measure marrow reserve and marginated granulocytes before and after the administration of lithium.

Although our study is preliminary, with only a few patients in each diagnostic category, certain preliminary observations can be made. For the entire series of patients, the mean granulocyte count after 3 weeks of lithium therapy was higher than the baseline granulocyte count (816 granulocytes/mm^3 vs 444 granulocytes/mm^3, $p < 0.01$). However, only 8 of 27 patients had a favorable response to lithium, defined as an increase in circulating granulocytes of $\geq$ 30% and $\geq$ 300 cells/mm^3, over baseline values. Among responders, the mean increase in granulocytes was 389% (1650 granulocytes/mm^3 vs 419 granulocytes/mm^3).

As with the administration of lithium to normal subjects, in all 8 responders the circulating granulocyte count decreased following discontinuation of lithium. This suggests that we are seeing a real response to lithium and not just spontaneous granulocyte recovery. However, since the day 42 granulocyte counts among responders had not completely returned to baseline values (957 granulocytes/mm^3 vs 419 granulocytes/mm^3, p = 0.053), we cannot yet determine if lithium alters granulocyte production in a manner which is self-sustaining following discontinuation of the drug. Although the lithium effect is not self-sustaining in normal subjects, in patients with abnormal granulocyte production, it is conceivable that stem cells might be affected in such a way that the benefit of lithium would be sustained. At this time, the data are not adequate to fully evaluate this possibility.

Responses were seen only in patients with pre-leukemia/smoldering leukemia, aplastic anemia, and hairy cell leukemia post splenectomy. Responses were not seen in patients with acute myelogenous leukemia (AML), patients with massive splenomegaly, or patients with idiopathic neutropenia. This association of response with diagnostic category was statistically highly significant, p = 0.003. This finding is compatible with the hypothesis that lithium acts by augmenting the production of colony stimulating activity by monocytes (Joyce and Chervenick, 1975; Harker et al., 1977) although alternative or additional mechanisms of action are not excluded. In patients whose marrows are packed with AML there is likely no room for increased granulocyte production; in cases of massive splenomegaly, increased production may be masked by splenic pooling of granulocytes. The variable responses which we observed in the other diagnostic categories may reflect variations in the numerous factors which regulate granulocyte production, such as availability of stem cells, levels of colony stimulating activity, adequate "soil" for granulopoiesis and presence of inhibitors to granulopoiesis. Thus far, however, we have been unable to identify factors other than diagnostic category to aid in the selection of patients likely to respond to lithium. Age, sex, baseline granulocyte counts, baseline monocyte counts, and baseline responses to hydrocortisone and epinephrine were similar among responders and non-responders. However, since only a small number of patients have been evaluated, it is possible that further studies will demonstrate statistically significant relationships between baseline granulocyte pools and the response to lithium.

While assessment of marrow reserve and marginated granulocytes did not help predict the response to lithium, in no case did a patient showing a favorable response of circulating granulocytes show a decreased response to hydrocortisone or epinephrine challenge. This supports the hypothesis that, as in normal subjects, lithium induced granulocytosis reflects increased production of granulocytes and not merely redistribution of granulocytes.

The lithium dose, duration of lithium administration, and serum lithium levels needed to produce optimal hematologic effects are unknown and alternate schedules of drug administration might produce different results. For purposes of safety we used a lithium dose of 300 mg t.i.d., a dose which has been associated with favorable results in other clinical trials (Gupta et al., 1975; Stein et al., 1977). Using this dose, lithium levels between 0.5 and 1.0 meq/L were acheived in 26 of 27 patients. Other than tremor, which occurred in three anemic patients (hematocrits 18 - 25%) and which was reversed with transfusion of packed red cells, significant toxicity attributable to lithium was not observed.

Since lithium therapy has minimal toxicity, and since our sample size is limited, we cannot conclude that lithium therapy should not be attempted in patients with packed marrows, massive splenomegaly, or idiopathic neutropenia. However, we suspect that responses in such patients are unlikely to occur, and we feel that when alternative measures such as splenectomy are contemplated, the decision to try lithium must carefully consider the risks in delaying effective therapy.

In the diagnostic categories in which we observed responses, lithium would appear to be a useful clinical option. In patients with hairy cell leukemia, chemotherapy has been associated with considerable toxicity. The favorable responses we have seen in patients remaining neutropenic following splenectomy may represent a useful therapeutic advance for these patients. In aplastic anemia, androgens have not been shown to affect survival and, other than marrow transplantation, no effective therapy is available. Trials of lithium in this disease would appear indicated. At the present time, there is no effective therapy for patients with pre-leukemia. Since neutropenia may be a major source of morbidity in these patients, further evaluation of lithium in pre-leukemia and smoldering leukemia seems appropriate. It is also possible that the response to lithium in this group of patients may have prognostic value, but at this time, adequate data are not available to evaluate this hypothesis.

In this preliminary report, we have been concerned only with the short term response to lithium. Obviously, if lithium is to be of clinical value, its long term effects on granulopoiesis and upon the incidence of infection are of interest. The degree of granulocytosis produced by lithium suggests, but does not prove, that lithium induced granulocytosis will be of clinical value, but only clinical trials can evaluate this issue. Such long term trials are in progress. Hopefully, these studies, and further studies of the mechanism of action of lithium, will further clarify the circumstances in which the administration of lithium is likely to be of clinical value.

ACKNOWLEDGEMENTS

This work was supported by research grant 1RO1CA 23971-01 from the National Cancer Institute, the National Institutes of Health and Public Health Service Grant No. 5MO1 RR-95 from the General Clinical Research Center Branch of the Division of Research Resources, National Institutes of Health.

REFERENCES

Barrett, A.J., Hugh-Jones, K., Newton, K., and Watson, J.G., 1977, Lithium therapy in aplastic anemia, Lancet 1:202.

Barrett, A.J., Griscelli, C., Buriot, D., and Faille, A., 1977, Lithium therapy in congenital neutropenia, Lancet 2:1357.

Blum, S.F., 1979, Lithium therapy of aplastic anemia, N. Eng. J. Med. 300:677.

Dale, D.C., Fauci, A.S., Guerry, D., and Wolfe, S.M., 1975, Comparison of agents producing a neutrophilic leukocytosis in man. Hydrocortisone, prednisone, endotoxin, and etiocholanolone, J. Clin. Invest. 56:808.

Greco, F.A. and Brereton, H.D., 1977, Effect of lithium carbonate on the neutropenia caused by chemotherapy: a preliminary clinical trial, Oncology 34:154.

Gupta, R.C., Robinson, W.A., and Smyth, C.J., 1975, Efficacy of lithium in rheumatoid arthritis with granulocytopenia, Arthritis Rheum. 18:179.

Harker, W.G., Rothstein, G., Clarkson, D., Athens, J.W., and Macfarlane, J.L., 1977, Enhancement of colony stimulating activity production by lithium, Blood 49:263.

Joyce, R.A. and Chervenick, P.A., 1975, Effect of lithium on the release of colony stimulating activity (CSA) from blood leukocytes, Proc. Am. Soc. Hematol. 18:126.

Lyman, G.H., Williams, C.C., and Preston, D., 1978, A prospective randomized study of the effect of lithium carbonate on the granulocytopenia and incidence of infection associated with intensive chemotherapy and radiation therapy for undifferentiated small cell bronchogenic carcinoma, Blood 52:277 (Supplement 1).

Rothstein, G., Clarkson, D., Larsen, W., Grosser, B.I., and Athens, J.W., 1978, Effect of lithium on neutrophil mass and production, N. Eng. J. Med. 298:178.

Samuels, A.J., 1951, Primary and secondary leukocyte changes following the intramuscular injection of epinephrine hydrochloride, J. Clin. Invest. 30:941.

Stein, R.S., Beaman, C., Ali, M.Y., Hansen, R., Jenkins, D.D., and Jume'an, H.G., 1977, Lithium carbonate attenuation of chemotherapy induced neutropenia, N. Eng. J. Med. 297:430.

Stein, R.S., Flexner, J.M., and Graber, S.E., 1978a, Lithium and granulocytopenia during induction therapy of acute myelogenous leukemia, Blood 52:277 (Supplement 1).

Stein, R.S., Hanson, G., Koethe, S., and Hansen, R., 1978b, Lithium induced granulocytosis, Ann. Int. Med. 88:809.

LITHIUM CARBONATE THERAPY OF APLASTIC ANEMIA

S.F. Blum

Section of Hematology
Department of Medicine
Cooper Medical Center
Camden, NJ. 08103

A fifty-eight year old female with known aplastic anemia of four years duration was treated with lithium carbonate, 900 mgs. daily. Within fifteen days the hemoglobin stabilized and transfusions were not longer required. The white blood count rose from $2100/mm^3$ to $5400/mm^3$ and the neutrophil percentage rose from 27% to 73%. The platelet count which had been below $4000/mm^3$ for several months rose to $87{,}000/mm^3$. The lithium level ranged from 0.45 to 1.3 meq/L. Thirty days after the initiation of lithium carbonate the hemoglobin was 11.6 gms/dl, white blood count $5100/mm^3$ and platelet count $134{,}000/mm^3$. Over the succeeding four months the hemoglobin and white count remained stable and no transfusions were required. The platelet count gradually fell to $31{,}000/mm^3$ and the development of hypothyroidism was noted. The lithium level during this period was below 1.0 meq/L. An increased dose of lithium carbonate raised the lithium level to 1.07 meq/L and Synthroid was given. The platelet count subsequently rose to $64{,}000/mm^3$. Aside from the hypothyroidism the patient has suffered no significant side effects from the lithium carbonate therapy and is asymptomatic.

(Abstract only)

GRANULOCYTE FUNCTION IN PATIENTS RECEIVING LITHIUM CARBONATE

Myron S. Cohen, M.D., Behnam Zahkireh, M.D.,
Julia A. Metcalf, B.A., and Richard K. Root, M.D.

Department of Internal Medicine
Yale University School of Medicine
New Haven, Connecticut

Phagocytic cells provide protection against a wide variety of microbial pathogens. A depletion of polymorphonuclear leukocytes (PMNs) below a critical number (Bodey et al., 1966) and/or abnormality in their cellular function (Quie, 1975) is associated with serious infection. Therefore, agents capable of enhancing phagocyte number and function are of importance. The lithium ion (Li^+) induces leukocytosis (Shopsin et al., 1971) and may diminish the neutropenia associated with cancer chemotherapy (Greco and Brereton, 1977; Charron et al., 1977; Stein et al., 1977). While such effects appear desirable, it is equally important that the functions of these phagocytic cells are preserved in their contribution to the host defense system. In this paper we shall report our investigation into the microbicidal ability of neutrophils obtained from patients receiving lithium carbonate (Li_2CO_3), and the in vitro effects of lithium chloride (LiCl) on several PMN functions.

MATERIALS AND METHODS

Four men and one woman who were receiving Li_2CO_3 (Lithane, Roerig Corp., New York, N.Y.) in the therapy of affective disorders were studied (Table I). Their ages ranged from 20 to 51 years. The Li_2CO_3

TABLE I

AGE, SEX, LITHIUM DOSAGE AND CONCENTRATION AND LEUKOCYTE COUNT OF THE PATIENT POPULATION*

Patient	Age	Sex	Li_2CO_3 Dosage (Gm/Day)	Serum Li^+** (meq/L)	Leukocyte Count ($x\ 10^3$)	
					Before Li_2CO_3	During Li_2CO_3
J.L.	22	M	0.9	0.68	8.0 (55)	14.5(79)***
M.S.	37	F	1.5	0.88	9.9 (64)	13.2(72)
C.D.	42	F	1.5	1.14	unknown	8.7 (72)
R.D.	51	F	1.5 - 2.1	1.7	unknown	8.3 (78)
K.S.	20	F	1.8	1.7	6.6 (55)	12.8(74)

* All patients had been receiving Li_2CO_3 for at least eight weeks prior to this study.

** Serum Li^+ concentration was determined at the time of neutrophil function studies.

*** Segmented and band polymorphonuclear leukocytes as a percent of the total leukocyte count.

dosage ranged from 0.9 to 1.8 grams per day with a mean of 1.5 ± 0.15 grams per day. On the day of the study, serum Li^+ concentration ranged from 0.68 to 1.7 meq/liter with a mean of 1.2 ± 0.21 meq/liter. All patients had been receiving Li_2CO_3 for at least eight weeks. Four patients were using other psychoactive agents which included benztropine, tranylcypromine, perphenazine, and tryptophan.

Preparation of Leukocytes

Two-hundred ml of heparinized whole blood were obtained by venipuncture and PMNs were separated by dextran sedimentation and hypotonic lysis of contaminating erythrocytes (Root et al., 1972). Cell populations from normal volunteers not using medication were prepared in an identical fashion for use as a control. Differential counts were determined by examination of a Wright's stained smear.

Locomotion

Random migration and chemotaxis were evaluated by the modified Boyden chamber-micropore technique of Zigmond and Hirsch (1973). Chambers were prepared by placing cells (3×10^6/ml) in the upper compartments separated from the lower compartments by 1.2 μm pore filters (Millipore Corp., Bedford, Mass.). In the lower compartment either Gey's medium (random migration) or 5% E. coli endotoxin activated sera (activated chemotaxis) were added. Endotoxin activated sera were prepared as previously described (Clark and Kimball, 1971). After a 50 minute incubation at 37°C cell migration into the filters was measured by the leading front technique (Zigmond and Hirsch, 1973). All experiments were run in duplicate.

Phagocytosis

The phagocytic activity of PMNs was determined by measuring the cellular uptake of S. aureus 502A radiolabelled with a ^{14}C-amino acid mixture (Root et al., 1972). Heat killed bacteria (1.25×10^9) were tumbled at 37° in 12 x 75 mm glass tubes that contained 2.5×10^6 PMN in

Hanks Balanced Salt Solution (HBSS, Flow Labs., Rockville, Maryland) with 10% patient or control sera (see Experimental Design); the final volume was 1 ml and the bacteria to cell ratio was 500/1. Tubes were preincubated for 10 minutes before the addition of bacteria, and ingestion was halted at 10 and 20 minutes by the addition of cold sodium fluoride (Fisher Scientific Co., Fair Lawn, New Jersey). Percent association of bacteria was calculated as previously described (Root *et al.*, 1972). All tests were run in duplicate.

Measurement of Bactericidal Ability

The ability of PMNs to kill *S. aureus* 502A was assessed by a method previously described (Hymans *et al.*, 1978). Killing was determined by measuring the survival of bacteria after 20, 30 and 60 minute incubations with PMNs and calculated as: % bacteria killed = 100% - % bacteria surviving. The bacteria to cell ratio was 10/1; all experiments were run in duplicate.

Experimental Design

Patient cells were compared to normal cells in preparations containing either patient or normal sera. By comparing the function of normal cells suspended in either homologous or autologous (patient) sera, and patient cells in homologous and autologous (normal) sera, the effect of patient sera itself on PMN function was determined.

Effect of In Vitro Lithium

To ascertain the effect of the *in vitro* addition of Li^+, LiCl (Fischer Chemical Co., Fair Lawn, New Jersey) in final concentrations of either 0.5 or 2.0 mmolar was incubated for 30 minutes with normal PMNs. Identical preparations free of LiCl served as controls, and all tests were run in duplicate.

Presentation of Results

To eliminate the impact of day to day variation on absolute results, all observations are reported as percent of the defined control. When we compared patient cells to normal cells they were both suspended in normal sera (normal cells in normal sera = 100% control) and patient sera (normal cells in patient sera = 100% control). When we compared the effects of the different sera on cell function, normal cells were suspended in the two serum sources (normal cells in normal sera = 100% control) as were patient cells (patient cells in normal sera = 100% control). See Tables II and III.

Statistics

The paired t test was used to compare patient and control preparations, and $p < 0.05$ was considered statistically significant.

RESULTS

Leukocyte counts among the patients ranged from 8,300 to 14,500/mm^3 with absolute granulocyte counts (segmented and band forms) 6,300 to 11,400/mm^3. Three of the five patients had leukocytosis (leukocyte count greater than 10,000/mm^3) which developed as a consequence of lithium therapy (Table I). The results of assays comparing the functions of patient and normal cells, and the effect of patient sera on these functions are summarized in Tables II and III.

Locomotion

Random migration of patient PMNs was 112.2 ± 5.8% (mean ± 1 SEM) of normal cells. Activated chemotaxis of patient PMNs was 111.0 ± 8.5% and 113.0 ± 5.9% of control in normal and patient activated sera, respectively (Table II); these differences were not statistically significant. Patient sera produced no direct change in patient or normal cells when compared to normal sera (Table III).

Phagocytosis

Normal and patient cells had equivalent phagocytic activity at 10 and 20 minutes when suspended in patient or normal sera (Table II). Cells obtained from the five patients and four of five volunteers demonstrated

TABLE II

EFFECT OF Li_2CO_3 THERAPY ON THE FUNCTION OF PATIENT NEUTROPHILS*

Serum Source	Phagocytic Activity of Patient Cells+		Bactericidal Ability of Patient Cells+			Chemotaxis of Patient Cells+
	10'	20'	20'	30'	60'	
Normal Sera (100% = normal cells and normal sera)	102.6 ± 0.4	101 ± 8.5	116.2 ± 23.6	98.6 ± 15	100 ± 0.44	111.0 ± 8.5
Patient Sera (100% = normal cells and patient sera)	119.4 ± 0.89	109.6 ± 12.3	119.4 ± 21.9	87.8 ± 1.24	99.6 ± 0.4	113.0 ± 5.9

*Values given are mean ± SEM of percent of control. The control for patient cells in normal sera was normal cells in normal sera. The control for patient cells in patient sera was normal cells in patient sera. Neutrophils from five patients and five normal volunteers were compared.

+No parameters compared were statistically different using the paired t test.

TABLE III

EFFECT OF SERUM FROM LITHIUM TREATED PATIENTS ON THE FUNCTION OF NORMAL AND PATIENT NEUTROPHILS*

	Phagocytosis in Patient Sera+		Bactericidal Ability in Patient Sera+			Chemotaxis in Patient Sera+
Cell Source	10'	20'	20'	30'	60'	
Normal Cells (100% = normal cells in normal sera)	111.6 ± 5.8	96 ± 5.8	97 ± 3.0	99.4 ± 6.8	100.2 ± 0.37	98.6 ± 2.1
Patient Cells (100% = patient cells in normal sera)	132.4 ± 17.8	104 ± 9.3	102.4 ± 4.7	101.1 ± 3.1	101 ± 2.37	101.2 ± 4.6

*Values given are mean ± SEM of percent of control. The control for normal cells in patient sera was normal cells in normal sera. The control for patient cells in patients sera was patient cells in normal sera. Neutrophils from five patients and five normal volunteers were compared.

+No parameters compared were statistically significant using the paired t test.

Reprinted with the permission of Blood, 53:913, 1979.

increased phagocytosis at 10 minutes when suspended in patient sera (Table III, Fig. 1). The mean differences between cells suspended in patient sera compared to those suspended in normal sera are not significant, and increased phagocytosis in individual patients was not related to leukocyte count.

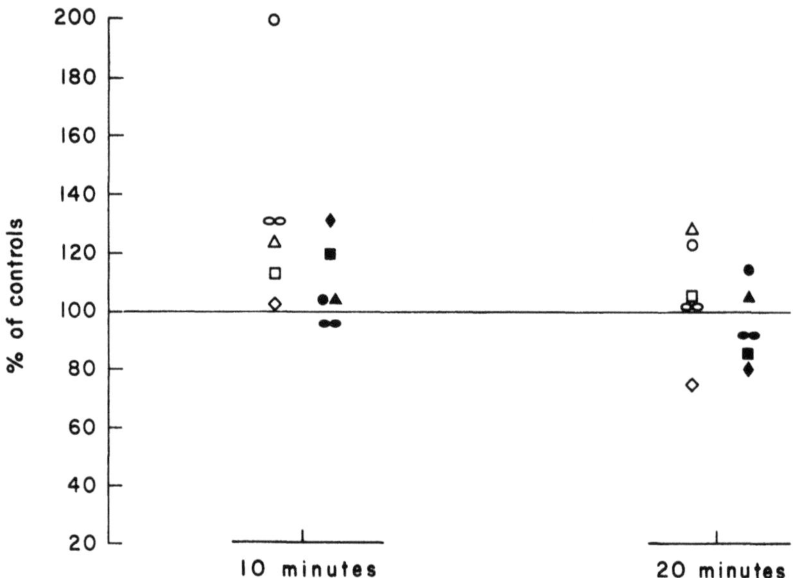

Figure 1. Phagocytosis by cells suspended in patient and normal sera (100% = control) were compared at 10 and 20 minutes. PMNs obtained from the five patients receiving lithium (and suspended in patient sera) are represented by open symbols whereas PMNs from five normal volunteers (and suspended in patient sera) are represented by dark symbols.

Bactericidal Activity

Although patient cells suspended in both normal and homologous sera killed S. aureus slightly better than normal cells at 20 minutes (116.2 ± 23.6% and 119.4 ± 21.9% of control, respectively), killing of bacteria over 60 minutes by both populations was equivalent (Table II). Patient sera had no effect on bactericidal ability (Table III).

Effect of LiCl

Chemotaxis, bactericidal ability, and phagocytosis of normal cells were compared after incubation of cells in 0.5 and 2.0 mmolar LiCl. No adverse or beneficial effects of LiCl on these functions were observed (Data not shown).

DICUSSION

Although Li^+ may produce leukocytosis (Shopsin *et al.*, 1971, Rothstein *et al.*, 1978) and offset the neutropenia associated with cancer chemotherapy (Charron *et al.*, 1977; Greco and Brereton, 1977; Stein *et al.*, 1977), thorough evaluation of PMN function during Li_2CO_3 therapy has not been performed. Whereas Stein and his colleagues (1978) reported normal ingestion of yeast by PMNs obtained from patients receiving Li_2CO_3, MacGregor and Dyson (1978) observed decreased adherence of PMNs to nylon fibers among psychiatric patients using Li_2CO_3. This effect was not mediated directly by Li^+, but rather by a plasma factor; adherence improved significantly after dialysis of patient plasma. Adherence of PMNs to venule walls *in vivo* appears important in the inflammatory response (Marchesi and Florey, 1960). In contrast to the findings of MacGregor and Dyson (1978), however, a study by Rothstein and coworkers (1978) revealed normal or increased migration of neutrophils into inflammatory sites during Li_2CO_3 therapy. These observations are particularly intriguing in light of the fact that altered levels of cyclic AMP or more specifically the cyclic AMP/GMP ratio may affect PMN chemotaxis (Perez *et al.*, 1979; Miller, 1975) and degranulation (Oliver, 1978). Li^+ is known to decrease cyclic AMP concentrations in several tissues (Singer and Rotenberg, 1973), including lymphocytes (Gelfand *et al.*, 1979). Lithium might then be expected to enhance the inflammatory response, as suggested by the findings of Rothstein *et al.*, 1978.

To clarify further the effects of lithium, we chose to investigate a variety of *in vitro* PMN functions during Li_2CO_3 therapy. These included random migration and activated chemotaxis, phagocytosis and bactericidal activity. Cells from five psychiatric patients studied performed as well as normal cells in all assays. Three patients had leukocytosis as a consequence of lithium therapy; these cells were functionally equivalent to those without leukocytosis and to normal cells in each parameter examined.

The experimental design allowed us to judge not only patient cell function, but the effect of sera obtained from these patients on their own and normal PMNs. We noted that both patient and normal cells had slightly increased phagocytic activity at 10 minutes when cells were suspended in patient sera compared to cells suspended in normal sera. No such changes were observed in phagocytosis at 20 minutes, or bactericidal activity. Furthermore, the mean differences in phagocytosis (for all studies as a group) between cells suspended in patient or normal sera was not statistically significant ($p > 0.05$).

To evaluate the possibility that the lithium ion itself enhanced phagocytosis or other functions, Li^+ in concentrations equivalent to those achieved _in vivo_ with therapeutic dosages of Li_2CO_3 was incubated with normal PMNs for 30 minutes. In these experiments cellular locomotion, phagocytosis and bactericidal ability at low (0.5 mmolar) or high (2.0 mmolar) concentration had no significant effect. These results are in agreement with a recent report by Perez and his colleagues (1979). They found that chemotaxis by normal PMNs exposed to lithium _in vitro_ was unchanged by such treatment, whereas a chemotactic defect in a young woman with recurrent infections resolved during lithium therapy, perhaps secondary to an alteration of PMN cyclic AMP concentration. Shenkman and his coworkers (1978) observed an increase in phagocytosis of latex particles by cultured macrophages directly related to the lithium concentration in the media which ranged from 0.6 to 10.0 meq/liter. These cells were exposed to lithium for three days, and phagocytosis was reported at 30 minutes only, making comparison of these results and our own observations impossible.

In summary, we observed no defects among PMNs harvested from patients ingesting Li_2CO_3 (regardless of leukocytosis) or exposed to Li^+ _in vitro_. Therefore, cells recruited in response to lithium therapy would be expected to contribute fully to the phagocyte host defense system. The observation that sera from patients ingesting Li_2CO_3, or that lithium itself (Shenkman et al., 1978) may enhance phagocytosis requires further evaluation.

ACKNOWLEDGEMENTS

The authors wish to thank Mr. Thomas Hitchcock and Drs. Julian Lieb and Raymond Anton for bringing the patients who volunteered for this study to our attention. We also wish to thank Ms. Lil Chapman and Ms. Patty Lincoln for their help in the preparation of the original manuscript.

REFERENCES

Bodey, G.P., Buckley, M., Sathe, Y.S., and Freireich, E.J., 1966, Quantitative relationships between circulating leukocytes and infection in patients with acute leukemia, Ann. Intern. Med. 64:328.

Charron, D., Barrett, A.J., Faille, A., Alby, N., Schmitt, T., and Degos, L., 1977, Lithium in acute myeloid leukemia, The Lancet 1:1307.

Clark, R.A. and Kimball, H.R., 1971, Defective granulocyte chemotaxis in Chediak-Higashi Syndrome, J. Clin. Invest. 50:2645.

Gelfand, E.W., Dosch, H., Hastings, D., and Shore, A., 1979, Lithium: A modulator of cyclic AMP-dependent events in lymphocytes?, Science 203:365.

Greco, F.A. and Brereton, H.D., 1977, Effect of lithium carbonate on the neutropenia caused by chemotherapy: A preliminary clinical trial, Oncology 34:153.

Hyams, J.S., Donaldson, M.H., Metcalf, J.A., and Root, R.K., 1978, Inhibition of human granulocyte function by methotrexate, Cancer Res. 38:650.

MacGregor, R.R. and Dyson, W.L., 1978, Effect of lithium on granulocyte adherence, Clin. Res. 26:352A.

Marchesi, J.T. and Florey, H.W., 1960, Electron micrographic observations on the emigration of leukocytes, Quart. Journ. Expt. Physio. 45:343.

Miller, M.E., 1975, Pathology of chemotaxis and random mobility, Seminars in Hematology 12:59.

Oliver, J.M., 1978, Cell biology of leukocyte abnormalities-membrane and cytoskeletal function in normal and defective cells, Am. J. Path. 93:221.

Perez, H.D., Kaplan, H., Shenkman, L., Borkowsky, W., and Goldstein, I.M., 1979, Reversal of an abnormality of polymorphonuclear leukocyte chemotaxis with lithium, Clin. Res. 27:353A.

Quie, P.G., 1975, Pathology of bactericidal power of neutrophils, Seminars in Hematology 12:143.

Rothstein, G., Clarkson, D.R., Larsen, W., Grosser, B.I., and Athens, J.W., 1978, Effect of lithium on neutrophil mass and production, N. Eng. J. Med. 298:178.

Root, R.K., Rosenthal, A.S., Balestran, D.J., 1972, Abnormal bactericidal, metabolic, and lysosomal functions of Chediak-Higashi syndrome leukocytes, J. Clin, Invest. 51:649.

Shenkman, L., Borkowsky, W., Holzman, R.S., and Shopsin, B., 1978, Enhancement of lymphocyte and macrophage function in vitro by lithium chloride, Clin. Immunol. Immunopath. 10:187.

Shopsin, B., Friedman, R., and Gershon, S., 1971, Lithium and leukocytosis, Clin. Pharmcol. Ther. 12:923.

Singer, I. and Rotenberg, D., 1973, Mechanism of lithium action, New Eng. J. Med. 289:254.

Stein, R.S., Beaman, C., Ali, M.Y., Hansen, R., Jenkins, D.D., and Jume'am, H.G., 1977, Lithium carbonate attenuation of chemotherapy-induced neutropenia, New. Eng. J. Med. 297:430.

Stein, R.S., Hansen, G.H., Koethe, S., and Hansen, R., 1978, Lithium induced granulocytosis, Ann. Intern. Med. 88:1978.

Zigmond, S.H. and Hirsch, J.G., 1973, Leukocyte locomotion and chemotaxis. New methods for evaluation and demonstration of a cell derived chemotactic factor, J. Exp. Med. 137:387.

INHIBITION OF GRANULOCYTE ADHERENCE BY LITHIUM: POSSIBLE RELATIONSHIP TO LITHIUM-INDUCED LEUKOCYTOSIS

Rob Roy MacGregor and William L. Dyson

Departments of Medicine, Surgery and Psychiatry
University of Pennsylvania School of Medicine
Philadelphia, Pennsylvania

Many patients receiving lithium carbonate therapy for psychiatric disorders develop increased neutrophil counts in their peripheral blood (O'Connell, 1970; Shopsin et al., 1971). The mechanism for this neutrophilia is thought to involve the stimulation of increased neutrophil production by the marrow. Addition of lithium carbonate in therapeutic concentrations to soft agar cultures of bone marrow promotes granulocyte colony growth (Tisman et al., 1973) and this promotion has been shown to result from the production of increased colony-stimulating activity (Harker et al., 1977). A recent study of granulocyte kinetics in patients treated with lithium has shown that they develop an increased total blood granulocyte pool, an increased marginal pool, and accelerated granulocyte production (Rothstein et al., 1978). Thus, the mechanism for lithium-induced neutrophilia appears to be the stimulation of increased marrow production, with a resultant increase in total intravascular neutrophil pool.

While these data were still unreported, we became interested in lithium-induced neutrophilia because of work from our laboratory showing that demargination of PMNs was often accompanied by decreased granulocyte adherence (GA) (MacGregor, 1977; Gluckman and MacGregor,

1978). Theorizing that inhibition of GA by lithium could shift PMNs from the marginal to circulating neutrophil pool, thereby causing a shift neutrophilia, we investigated the in vitro and in vivo effects of lithium on GA.

MATERIALS AND METHODS

The nylon fiber column assay for granulocyte adherence has been described in detail previously (MacGregor et al., 1974). Briefly, carefully weighed amounts of spun nylon fiber are packed into Pasteur pipettes to a column length of exactly 15 mm. One ml volumes of heparinized whole blood are applied to the top of triplicate columns and allowed to flow through by gravity at 37°C. Comparison of the pre- and post-column granulocyte counts permits calculation of the percent of granulocytes adhering to the column. Results of the triplicate columns are averaged for each blood specimen and expressed as the percent granulocyte adherence. GA is proportional to the weight of fiber in the column. Because we were anticipating an inhibition in GA, we used "high-adherence" columns, those which lead to the adherence of the majority of PMNs (76.0 ± 12% adherence for men, 70.8 ± 4.3% for women).

In the studies of in vitro lithium effect, heparinized whole blood (5 U/ml) was drawn from normal laboratory personnel (20-40 years of age), and lithium chloride was added to reach a final concentration of 0.01, 0.1, 1.0, and 10.0 millimolar lithium. The blood was then incubated for 30 minutes at 37°C, and tested for GA.

Patients were chosen from the out-patient practice of one of us, on the basis of having taken lithium carbonate for more than 6 months at a daily dose of 600-1500 mg/day without known side effects. Twenty-five patients were studied, 17 women and 8 men. Mean age was 48.5 years, with a range of 24-77. None had serious underlying disease, nor were any taking medications known to affect GA. Mean serum lithium concentration on the day of study was 0.83 meq/liter with a range of 0.14-1.54, measured by atomic absorption spectrophotometry.

To determine whether changes in adherence were due to direct effects of lithium therapy on the PMNs or were mediated through a plasma factor, cells were separated from plasma by centrifugation at 80 g for 10 minutes. The cell button was then washed x 3 with modified Hank's solution, and resuspended in autologous plasma, serum, or ABO-compatible normal plasma. (Previous reports from our laboratory have shown that washing and recombination does not affect the adherence of normal cells, Lentnek et al., 1976). To study the effect of dialysis on the plasma factor inhibiting adherence, 5 ml of heparinized plasma were dialyzed at 4°C vs 500 ml of modified Hank's solution for 24 hours, utilizing cellulose dialysis tubing (No. 3787-020, Arthur H. Thomas, Philadelphia, Pa.).

RESULTS

Addition of lithium carbonate to heparinized whole blood caused a dose-dependent inhibition of granulocyte adherence, significant ($p < 0.02$, Student t test) at the 0.1 mM concentration and above (Fig. 1).

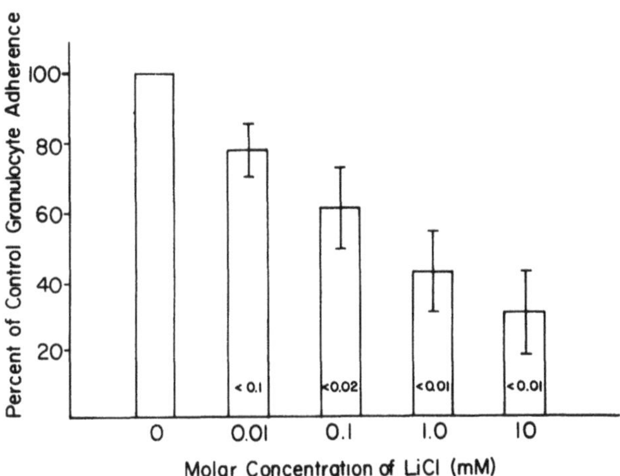

Figure 1. The incubation of heparinized whole blood with lithium chloride inibits granulocyte adherence. Isobars represent mean adherence values for 4 experiments, brackets ± the standard error of the mean. Inhibition is significant as noted on isobars at concentrations of 0.1 mM and above (Student t test).

In testing the 25 lithium-treated patients, we arbitrarily set an adherence value of < 50% on high-adherence columns as abnormally low (normal values for men are 76.0 ± 12%, for women 70.8± 4.3%). By these criteria, 13 of the 25 had inhibited GA, 11 of the 17 women and 2 of the 8 men. Mean serum lithium concentration was similar for the 2 groups: 0.85 meq/liter in the group with < 50%, and 0.80 in those with GA > 50%. Figure 2 shows the relationship between the individual's GA value and his serum lithium concentration. Mean PMN count in the patient group with GA < 50% was $5138/mm^3$, and $5442/mm^3$ in the group with GA > 50%. Only 3 patients in each group had PMN counts > $6{,}000/mm^3$.

The consistency of abnormally low GA tests was examined in 7 patients measured from 2-4 times at monthly intervals: 6 of the 7 maintained GA values below 50% on follow-up testing; one, who originally had GA of 36%, increased to 52 and 53% on subsequent determinations.

Separation and recombination studies demonstrated that GA was inhibited by a plasma factor, and that the inhibition was reversible. Figure 3 shows that cells from 5 lithium-treated patients (chosen for their low GA values when whole blood was tested) had a mean GA of 34.2 ± 2.9% when washed and resuspended in their own plasma. When ABO-compatible normal plasma was used, their GA increased to 53.3 ± 7.4%, an improvement significant at the 0.05 level (Student t test). Of interest, the same patient cells showed a mean GA of 57.3 ± 3.7% when resuspended in their own serum, indicating that the inhibiting factor was only operative in plasma. Mean GA of normal cells in their own plasma was 70.5 ± 3.5% but fell to 48.1 ± 3.4% when suspended in plasma from the lithium-treated patients ($p < 0.01$, Student t test). Thus, plasma from lithium-treated patients who have low GA contains a factor which inhibits adherence of their own and normal cells; moreover, the inhibition of GA demonstrated by their cells is reversible on washing and resuspension in normal plasma.

Three patients with previously low GA had plasma obtained for dialysis against modified Hank's solution. Mean adherence of normal ABO-compatible PMNs in their undialyzed plasma was 48.0 ± 3.2%, vs 60.3 ±

2.4% in their dialyzed plasma ($p < 0.05$, Student t test). Thus, the adherence-inhibiting plasma factor could be dialyzed significantly.

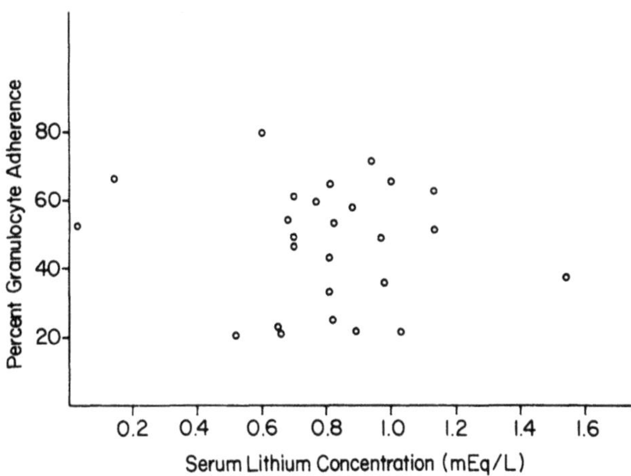

Figure 2. Relationship between patients' serum lithium concentrations and the intensity of their granulocyte adherence.

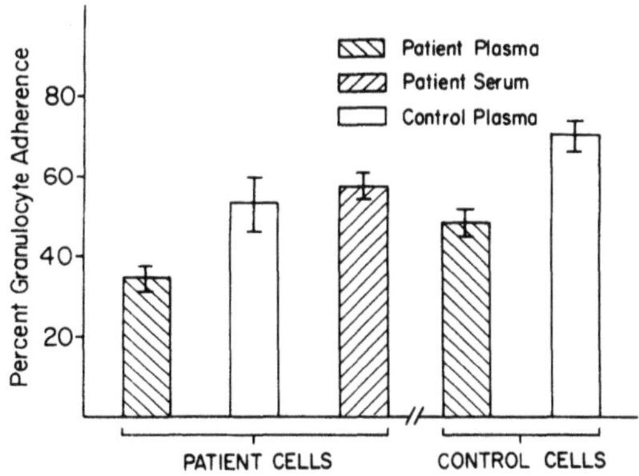

Figure 3. The relative contribution of PMNs and plasma to the impaired granulocyte adherence of lithium-treated patients. Isobars represent mean adherence for 4 experiments, brackets ± the standard error of the mean. Adherence of patients' and normal cells is inhibited by patients' plasma.

In a final series of experiments, we tried to correct the poor GA in two patients by administration of ascorbic acid 4 g/day orally for 6 weeks. In one, pre-ascorbic acid adherence was 48.1%, and after 6 weeks of treatment 45.2%. In the other, values went from 31.0% pre-treatment to 23.8% post. Thus, ascorbic acid failed to increase their GA values.

DISCUSSION

The predominant mechanism for lithium-induced neutrophilia appears to be the stimulation of bone marrow cells to produce increased numbers of circulating PMNs (Tisman et al., 1973; Rothstein et al., 1978). In describing the background for their studies, both authors discussed demargination of PMNs, resulting in a "pseudoleukocytosis" as a reasonable possibility to explain the clinically increased PMN counts. As evidence against this thesis, Tisman (1973) showed that serum B_{12} binding capacity was increased in lithium-induced leukocytosis, indirectly demonstrating a true increase in the number of circulating PMNs. Then Rothstein's work (1978) showed by direct measurement that the total blood granulocyte pool was indeed increased and that the marginal pool was also increased, in contrast to the decrease which would have been expected if demargination were the mechanism for leukocytosis.

It is not clear how to fit our finding of decreased GA into the above information. In general, we have found poor GA in situations of demargination, e.g. following epinephrine administration (MacGregor, 1977), steroid therapy (MacGregor et al., 1974; MacGregor, 1976a), and acute intoxication (Gluckman and MacGregor, 1978). In fact, this relationship between impaired GA and demargination had proven so constant that we have developed an operating hypothesis that the body regulates the distribution of PMNs between the CGP and MGP at least partially by modulating the intensity of granulocyte adherence. Although we do not have GA values on the patients studied by Rothsten et al., (1978), it is likely from our data that half had inhibited GA, and yet maintained an enlarged MGP. This indicates either that our hypothesis is wrong, or that unmeasured complicating variables are involved in determining pool size.

The mechanism for the impaired GA is unclear. The addition of lithium to normal blood *in vitro* caused a dose-dependent suppression of GA, suggesting a direct effect of lithium. Also, the improved GA of normal cells in patient plasma which had been dialyzed showed that the inhibiting factor was a small molecule, perhaps lithium itself. However, to confound this simple theory, we found that in contrast to plasma, serum from patients with poor GA did not inhibit normal cells, although both serum and plasma would be expected to have equal lithium concentrations. Also, we found no relationship between the plasma lithium concentration and the intensity of GA.

Our attempt to improve GA with ascorbic acid therapy had several origins. Earlier work in our laboratory had shown that cyclic GMP and its agonists increased GA, and antagonized adherence-inhibiting plasma factors *in vitro* (MacGregor, 1976b). Because ascorbic acid had been used recently to improve cGMP concentration and PMN function in a patient with Chediak-Higashi syndrome (Boxer, 1978) we administered 4 g of ascorbic acid orally to renal transplant patients in a successful attempt to improve their GA and granulocyte delivery (Thorner *et al.*, 1978). Therefore, we also attempted to improve GA in two of the lithium-treated patients, but were unsuccessful.

In summary, our studies showed that lithium inhibits GA *in vitro*, that lithium carbonate therapy is associated with inhibited GA in approximately half of patients taking it, but that the blood lithium concentration was not predictive of the patient's GA value. The relationship of these findings to the mechanism for lithium-induced neutrophilia remains unclear.

ACKNOWLEDGEMENTS

We wish to thank the patients who contributed their time and interest to the study. Mrs. Elvira Ventura provided expert technical assistance, and Mrs. Mary Jane Welsh typed the original manuscript.

REFERENCES

Boxer, L.A., Watanabe, A.M., Rister, M., Besch, H.R., Allen, J., and Baehner, R.L., 1978, Correction of leukocyte function in Chediak-Higashi syndrome with ascorbate, N. Eng. J. Med. 295:1041.

Gluckman, S.J., and MacGregor, R.R., 1978, The effect of acute alcohol intoxication on granulocyte mobilization and kinetics, Blood 52:551.

Harker, W.B., Rothstein, G., Clarkson, D., Athens, J.W., and Macfarlane, J.L., 1977, Enhancement of colony-stimulating activity production by lithium, Blood 49:263.

Lentnek, A.L., Schreiber, A.D., and MacGregor, R.R., 1976, The induction of augmented granulocyte adherence by inflammation. Mediation by a plasma factor, J. Clin. Invest. 57:1098.

MacGregor, R.R., 1976a, The effect of anti-inflammatory drugs and inflammation on granulocyte adherence, Amer. J. Med. 61:597.

MacGregor, R.R., 1976b, Cyclic nucleotide induction as the mechanism for modification of granulocyte adherence by plasma factors, Clin. Res. 24:348A.

MacGregor, R.R., 1977, Granulocyte adherence changes induced by hemodialysis, endotoxin, epinephrine, and glucocorticoids, Ann. Intern. Med. 86:35.

MacGregor, R.R., Spagnuolo, P.J., and Lentnek, A.L., 1974, Inhibition of granulocyte adherence by ethanol, prednisone, and aspirin, measured with a new assay system, N. Eng. J. Med. 291:642.

O'Connell, R.A., 1970, Leukocytosis during lithium carbonate treatment, Int. Pharmacopsychiat. 4:30.

Rothstein, G., Clarkson, D.R., Larson, W., Grosser, B.I., and Athens, J.W., 1978, Effect of lithium on neutrophil mass and production, N. Eng. J. Med. 298:178.

Shopsin, B., Friedmann, R., and Gershon, S., 1971, Lithium and leukocytosis, Clin. Pharm. Therapeut. 12:923.

Thorner, R.E., Barker, C.F., and MacGregor, R.R., 1978, Improvement in steroid-induced granulocyte dysfunction with ascorbic acid, Interscience Conference on Antimicrobial Agents and Chemotherapy, Atlanta, Ga., October, 1978.

Tisman, G., Herbert, V., and Rosenblatt, S., 1973, Evidence that lithium induces human granulocyte proliferation: elevated serum vitamin B12 binding capacity _in vivo_ and granulocyte colony proliferation _in vitro_, _Brit. J. Haematol._ 24:767.

EFFECTS OF LITHIUM ON POLYMORPHONUCLEAR LEUKOCYTE CHEMOTAXIS

H. Daniel Perez, Howard B. Kaplan, Ira M. Goldstein,
Louis Shenkman, and William Borkowsky

Department of Medicine
New York University Medical Center
New York, New York 10016

Lithium, known best for its efficacy in the treatment of neuropsychiatric disorders, also is capable of influencing the function of a variety of non-neural cells. Shenkman et al. (1978), for example, demonstrated that lithium was capable of enhancing several functions of human peripheral blood mononuclear cells. Lithium chloride, in vitro, augmented thymidine incorporation by phytohemagglutinin-stimulated human lymphocytes and increased the ability of these cells to form rosettes with sheep erythrocytes. Lithium also stimulated phagocytosis of polystyrene latex particles by cultured human macrophages. Finally, lithium was found capable of reversing the inhibitory effects of prostaglandin E_1 and theophylline on the response of human lymphocytes to phytohemagglutinin. Since these inhibitory effects were very likely mediated by increased cellular levels of cyclic 3',5'-adenosine monophosphate (cAMP), the authors concluded that lithium acted by interfering in some fashion with adenylate cyclase activity. A similar conclusion was reached more recently by Gelfand et al. (1979). These authors found that theophylline, salbutamol, isoproterenol, and dibutyryl cAMP inhibited sheep erythrocyte rosette formation by human T lymphocytes as well as secretion of immunoglobulin M from plaque-forming B cells. Consistent with an ability to inhibit adenylate cyclase, lithium prevented the effects of all the drugs except dibutyryl cAMP.

Several functions of human peripheral blood polymorphonuclear leukocytes (PMN) are inhibited by elevated cellular levels of cAMP. For example, it has now been demonstrated that exogenous cAMP, as well as agents that raise levels of this cyclic nucleotide within cells, inhibit PMN adhesiveness (MacGregor et al., 1978), phagocytosis (Cox and Karnovsky, 1973), oxidative metabolism (Lehmeyer and Johnston, 1978), release of lysosomal enzymes (Zurier et al., 1974), and chemotaxis (Hill et al., 1975). In this report we describe the effects of lithium in vitro and in vivo on some of these PMN functions. We have found PMN chemotactic responsiveness to be particularly susceptible to inhibition by cAMP. We also have found that whereas lithium has no effect on chemotaxis by normal PMN in vitro or in vivo, it is capable of preventing the cAMP-dependent inhibition of chemotaxis by cells exposed to β-adrenergic agonists. Finally, administration of lithium to a patient with abnormal PMN chemotaxis and recurrent infections associated with increased cellular levels of cAMP, resulted in a diminution of cAMP levels, a return to normal of PMN chemotactic responsiveness, and a favorable clinical response.

EFFECTS OF LITHIUM ON FUNCTIONS OF NORMAL PMN

Lithium in vitro failed to influence normal PMN random motility and chemotaxis (Table I). As a chemoattractant in these experiments, we employed fresh autologous serum in which the alternative complement pathway had been activated by treatment with zymosan (Goldstein et al., 1973; Perez et al., 1978). Chemotaxis was assayed by the "leading front" method of Zigmond and Hirsch (1973). Results are expressed as the distance (μm/45 min) that the leading front of cells migrated into micropore filters separating the upper, or cell compartments, from the lower, or stimulus compartments of modified Boyden chambers. As can be seen in Table 1, incubation of normal PMN with lithium (10^{-3} M) did not influence either the random motility of these cells or their chemotactic response to zymosan-treated serum.

TABLE I

FAILURE OF LITHIUM TO INFLUENCE PMN RANDOM MOTILITY AND CHEMOTAXIS

Additions to: Upper Compartment	Lower Compartment	PMN Migration μm/45 min ± SEM
Normal PMN	Buffer (random motility)	84.7 ± 2.5
Normal PMN + $Li^+(10^{-3}M)$	Buffer (random motility)	84.3 ± 2.7
Normal PMN	Zymosan-treated serum (2.0%, v/v)	116.1 ± 4.0[a]
Normal PMN + $Li^+(10^{-3}M)$	Zymosan-treated serum (2.0%, v/v)	115.9 ± 4.9[a]

[a] p -vs- buffer < 0.01 (Student's t test)

When human PMN are exposed to serum-treated (or opsonized) zymosan particles, the cells generate superoxide anion radicals and degranulate, that is, selectively release lysozomal enzymes, such as β-glucuronidase (Goldstein et al., 1975). In conjunction with phagocytosis, these PMN functions are necessary for optimal microbicidal activity (Oliver, 1978). Shown in Table II are the results of experiments in which we examined the effects in vitro of lithium on superoxide anion production and degranulation by normal human PMN. As was the case with chemotaxis, lithium (10^{-3} M) had no effect on these normal PMN functions.

TABLE II

EFFECT OF LITHIUM, EPINEPHRINE, AND cAMP ON PMN SUPEROXIDE ANION GENERATION AND DEGRANULATION

Additions to PMN[a]:	Superoxide Anion Generation[b]	Degranulation[c]
None (Control)	15.4 ± 0.6	9.3 ± 0.7
Li^+ (10^{-3}M)	15.5 ± 0.5	9.9 ± 0.5
Epinephrine (10^{-5}M)	15.7 ± 0.9	8.3 ± 0.8
cAMP (10^{-5}M)	15.0 ± 0.1	10.0 ± 0.7

[a]PMN were preincubated with cytochalasin B (5.0 μg/ml) for 10 min and with other additions for 5 min at 37°C before exposure to serum-treated zymosan for 15 min. Superoxide anion generation and degranulation were measured as described previously (Goldstein et al., 1975).

[b]Nanomoles cytochrome c reduced/10^6 PMN, Mean ± SEM, n = 5.

[c]Percent of total β-glucuronidase released, Mean ± SEM, n = 5.

Not shown are experiments in which we examined the effects of lithium in vivo on PMN functions. Lithium carbonate was administered to normal volunteers in doses adjusted to yield levels in serum of approximately 10^{-3} M. Isolated PMN from these subjects were studied in vitro and were found to be comparable to PMN obtained from control subjects with respect to their ability to respond to chemoattractants, to generate superoxide anion radicals, and to degranulate. These results are in accordance with those described previously by Cohen et al. (1979).

EFFECTS OF LITHIUM ON FUNCTIONS OF PMN EXPOSED TO EPINEPHRINE AND cAMP

To examine the possibility that lithium might interfere with PMN adenylate cyclase activity, we studied the effects of lithium on the inhibition of chemotaxis mediated by epinephrine and cAMP. Results of these experiments (Figure 1) are expressed as net PMN migration beyond that accounted for by random motility (Zigmond and Hirsch, 1973). Both epinephrine (10^{-5} M) and cAMP (10^{-5} M) significantly inhibited chemotaxis. However, the inhibition of chemotaxis observed when PMN were exposed to epinephrine was prevented completely by lithium (10^{-3} M). Epinephrine and other β-adrenergic agonists have been demonstrated previously to activate adenylate cyclase in human PMN and thereby increase cellular levels of cAMP (Zurier et al., 1974; Hill et al., 1975). The possibility that

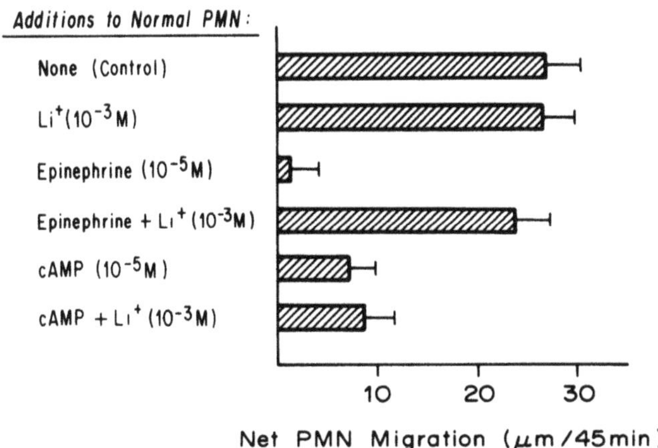

Figure 1. Effects of lithium on the inhibition of PMN chemotaxis mediated by epinephrine and cAMP. Normal PMN were preincubated with additions for five minutes at 37°C before being placed into the cell compartments of modified Boyden chambers. Chemotaxis was measured as described previously (Zigmond and Hirsch, 1973; Perez et al., 1978).

lithium interferes with this action of epinephrine is supported by the results obtained when PMN were exposed directly to exogenous cAMP. As shown in Figure 1, lithium was incapable of preventing the inhibition of chemotaxis induced by this cyclic nucleotide.

Epinephrine and exogenous cAMP, at concentrations that inhibited chemotaxis, failed to influence superoxide anion generation and degranulation by normal PMN (Table II). Degranulation could be inhibited, albeit modestly, only when PMN were exposed to very high concentrations of exogenous cAMP (10^{-3} M) in the presence of the phosphodiesterase inhibitor, theophylline (5×10^{-4} M) (Zurier et al., 1974). Thus, superoxide anion generation and degranulation by PMN appeared to be less susceptible than chemotaxis to inhibition by minimally elevated cellular levels of cAMP.

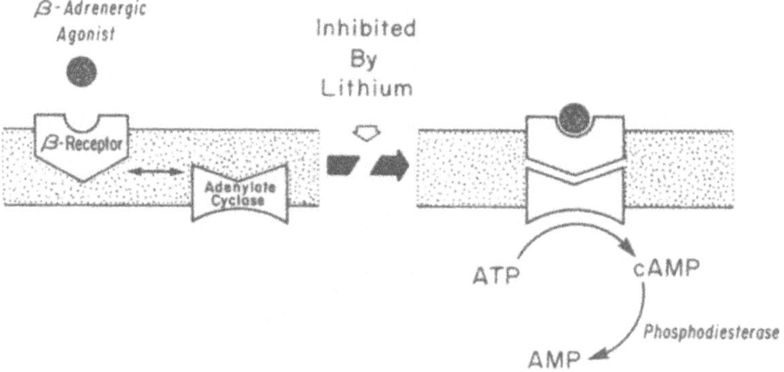

Figure 2. One proposed site of action of lithium .

These data support the conclusion that stimulation of adenylate cyclase activity in normal human PMN by β-adrenergic agonists results in small increments in cellular levels of cAMP and inhibition of chemotactic responsiveness. As in other cell types, lithium appears capable of interfering with this phenomenon in human PMN (Figure 2). These data also suggested that some, as yet unexplained, abnormalities of chemotaxis in patients might be due to altered cyclic nucleotide metabolism which would be influenced similarly by lithium. Indeed, we recently have had the opportunity of studying such a patient.

A PATIENT WITH ABNORMAL CHEMOTAXIS

A 29-year-old white woman was admitted to New York University Medical Center in November, 1977, complaining of recurrent streptococcal and staphyloccocal skin infections of seven years duration, requiring almost continuous administration of antibiotics. No other members of her family had been affected by a similar condition. Physical examination at the time of admission was remarkable for the presence of scaling and crusting lesions over her scalp and external nares. Numerous pustular lesions were present over her back, breasts, pubic area, and extremities. Abscesses were present in both axillae and tender lymphadenopathy was detected in areas draining infected lesions.

An extensive evaluation revealed normal serum levels of immunoglobulins (IgM, IgG, IgA, and IgE) and complement (C3, C4, and CH_{50}). In addition, PMN obtained from this patient were comparable to normal cells with respect to their ability to generate superoxide anion radicals and to degranulate (Table III). Furthermore, isolated PMN from this patient were perfectly capable of killing *Staphylococcus aureus in vitro* (Figure 3) and of ingesting opsonized zymosan particles (not shown). The cells had normal morphology as determined by light and by transmission electron microscopy. The patient's PMN, however, exhibited abnormal chemotactic responsiveness (Table IV). Although the cells exhibited normal random motility, directed migration toward zymosan-treated serum was sig-

TABLE III

SUPEROXIDE ANION GENERATION AND DEGRANULATION BY NORMAL AND PATIENT PMN

	Superoxide anion generation [a]	Degranulation [b]
Normal PMN	15.5 ± 3.4	10.3 ± 2.3
Patient PMN	16.1 ± 2.1	11.6 ± 1.1

[a]nmol cytochrome C reduced/10^6 PMN/15 min

[b]percent total β-glucuronidase released/15 min

nificantly less than that observed with normal PMN. Similar results were observed when the patient's cells were exposed either to the bacterial chemotactic factor from *Escherichia coli* (Ward *et al.*, 1968) or the synthetic chemotactic peptide, N-formyl-methionyl-leucyl-phenylalanine (Schiffman *et al.*, 1975). This defect in chemotaxis could not be attributed to the presence in the patient's serum of an irreversible inhibitor of PMN motility.

Effect of Lithium on Abnormal PMN Chemotaxis

The abnormality of chemotaxis exhibited by the patient's PMN could be corrected *in vitro* almost completely with the addition of lithium (10^{-3} M) (Table IV). Consequently, we began administering lithium carbonate to this patient in doses sufficient to achieve serum levels of approximately 10^{-3} M. After five weeks of therapy with lithium, PMN from the patient were as capable as normal cells of migrating in a directed

TABLE IV

AN ABNORMALITY OF PMN CHEMOTAXIS: CORRECTION IN VITRO AND IN VIVO WITH LITHIUM

Additions to:		PMN Migration
Upper Compartment	Lower Compartment	μm/45 min ± SEM
Normal PMN	Buffer (random motility)	93.3 ± 1.5
Patient PMN	Buffer (random motility)	95.8 ± 1.4
Normal PMN	Zymosan-treated serum (2.0%, v/v)	117.4 ± 2.7
Patient PMN	Zymosan-treated serum (2.0%, v/v)	102.2 ± 1.4[a]
Patient PMN + Li^+ (10^{-3}M)	Zymosan-treated serum (2.0%, v/v)	117.8 ± 0.3
Patient PMN (after therapy with lithium)[b]	Zymosan-treated serum (2.0%, v/v)	115.3 ± 2.6

[a] p -vs- normal PMN < 0.01 (Student's t test)

[b] Serum lithium concentration = 0.8 x 10^{-3}M

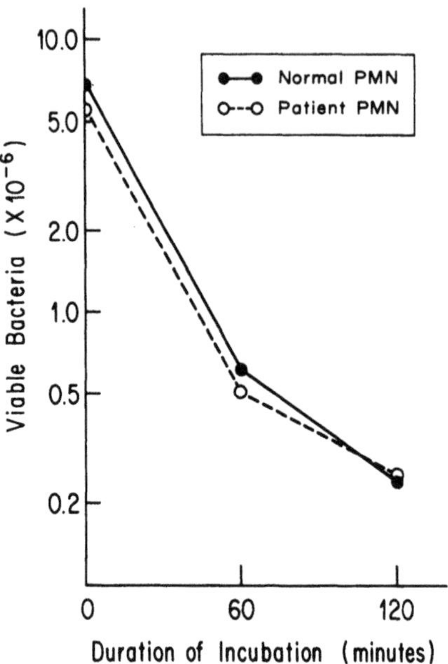

Figure 3. Bactericidal activity of normal and patient's PMN. Cells were incubated for 120 minutes at 37°C with an equal number of opsonized Staphylococcus aureus, 502A. Bactericidal activity was measured as described previously (Root et al., 1972).

TABLE V

LEVELS OF cAMP IN NORMAL AND PATIENT PMN: EFFECT OF THERAPY WITH LITHIUM

	cAMP (pmol/10^7 cells)	Serum Li^+ (mol/L)
Normal PMN	6.1 ± 0.9[a]	-----
Patient PMN (before therapy)	10.3 ± 0.1	0
Patient PMN (after therapy)	7.1 ± 0.4	0.8×10^{-3}

[a] Mean ± SEM, n = 15

fashion toward zymosan-treated serum (Table IV). Coincidentally, she became free of infections. Subsequent withdrawal of lithium therapy resulted in a relapse clinically (within two weeks) and a return of the PMN chemotactic abnormality. Addition of lithium to her PMN _in vitro_ again restored their ability to respond to chemoattractants.

During the past eight months, the patient has received lithium carbonate continuously (maintaining serum levels of approximately 0.8×10^{-3} M). While on therapy, she has been able to discontinue antibiotics for the first time since the onset of her disease and she has remained free of infections.

Effect of Lithium on PMN cAMP Levels

Before therapy with lithium, measurements of cAMP in the patient's PMN revealed levels of 10.3 picomoles per 10^7 cells, almost twice that observed in normal cells (Table V). After five weeks of therapy, at a time when her serum lithium concentration was 0.8×10^{-3} M, levels of cAMP in the patient's PMN were 7.1 picomoles, a level closer to that observed in normal cells.

SUMMARY AND CONCLUSIONS

The studies described in the report indicate that normal human PMN chemotactic responsiveness is particularly susceptible to inhibiton by minimally elevated cellular levels of cAMP. Furthermore, the data indicate that whereas lithium _in vitro_ does not affect chemotaxis _per se_, it does interfere with the cAMP-dependent inhibition of chemotaxis observed when PMN are exposed to epinephrine. In contrast, lithium does not prevent the inhibition of chemotaxis observed when cells are exposed directly to exogenous cAMP. These data support the hypothesis that lithium acts on PMN, as it does on other cell types (Shenkman _et al._, 1978; Gelfand _et al._, 1979; Dousa and Hetcher, 1970), by interfering in some fashion with the activity of adenylate cyclase.

The finding of a patient with abnormal PMN chemotaxis associated with modestly elevated cellular levels of cAMP confirmed our suspicion that some chemotactic defects observed in patients with recurrent infections may be due primarily to altered PMN cyclic nucleotide metabolism. Moreover, as in our in vitro studies, PMN from this patient were perfectly capable of generating superoxide anion radicals and of degranulating in response to contact with opsonized zymosan particles. Very high levels of cAMP appear to be required for inhibition of these PMN functions. Lithium in vitro was capable of correcting the abnormality of chemotaxis exhibited by this patient's PMN. Furthermore, administration of lithium to the patient resulted in diminution of PMN cAMP levels, a return to normal of PMN chemotactic responsiveness, and a favorable clinical response.

Several abnormalities of PMN chemotaxis have been associated with increased susceptibility to bacterial infections (Hogan and Hill, 1978; Wright et al., 1977; Stanley et al., 1978). Although several drugs have been reported to be capable of correcting abnormal PMN functions in vitro and in vivo (Goetzl et al., 1974; Wright et al., 1977; Hogan and HIll, 1978), administration of these agents leads to considerable side effects. The patient reported here responded quite dramatically to the administration of lithium carbonate in doses sufficient to achieve serum levels of approximately 0.8×10^{-3} M. This is a concentration that is easily achieved in vivo and one that does not ordinarily produce toxic side effects. Consequently, we suggest that lithium may prove to be useful for the treatment of other patients with similar abnormalities.

ACKNOWLEDGEMENTS

This research was supported by grants from the United States Public Health Service, National Institutes of Health (AM-18531, AM-25374, AM-11949, and HL-19721).

Dr. Perez is the recipient of a Clinical Investigator Award (AM-00463) from the National Institutes of Health (NIAMDD).

Dr. Goldstein and Dr. Shenkman are recipients of Career Scientist Awards from the Irma T. Hirschl Trust.

REFERENCES

Cohen, M.S., Zakhireh, B., Metcalf, J.A., and Root, R.K., 1979, Granulocyte function during lithium therapy, Blood 53:913.

Cox, J.P. and Karnovsky, M.L., 1973, The depression of phagocytosis by exogenous cyclic nucleotides, prostaglandins and theophylline, J. Cell Biol. 59:480.

Dousa, T. and Hetcher, O., 1970, The effect of NaCl and LiCl on vasopressin-sensitive adenyl cyclase, Life Sci. 9:765.

Gelfand, E.W., Dosch, H-M., Hastings, D., and Shore, A., 1979, Lithium: A modulator of cyclic AMP-dependent events in lymphocytes?, Science 203:365.

Goetzl, E.J., Wasserman, S.I., Gigli, I., and Austen, K.F., 1974, Enhancement of random migration and chemotactic response of human leukocytes by ascorbic acid, J. Clin. Invest. 53:813.

Goldstein, I.M., Hoffstein, S., Gallin, J., and Weissmann, G., 1973, Mechanisms of lysosomal enzyme release from human leukocyte: microtubule assembly and membrane fusion induced by a component of complement, Proc. Natl. Acad. Sci. USA 70:2916.

Goldstein, I.M., Roos, D., Kaplan, H.B., and Weissmann, G., 1975, Complement and immunoglobulins stimulate superoxide production by human leukocytes independently of phagocytosis, J. Clin. Invest. 56:1155.

Hill, H., Estensen, R.D., Quie, P.G., Hogan, N.A., and Goldberg, N.D., 1975, Modulation of human neutrophil chemotactic response by cyclic 3', 5'-guanosine monophosphate and cyclic 3', 5'-adenosine monophosphate, Metabolism 24:447.

Hogan, N.A. and Hill, H., 1978, Enhancement of neutrophil chemotaxis and alteration of levels of cellular cyclic nucleotides by levamisole, J. Infect. Dis. 138:437.

Lehmeyer, J.E. and Johnston, R.B., 1978, Effect of anti-inflammatory drugs and agents that elevate intracellular levels of cyclic AMP on the release of toxic oxygen metabolites by phagocytes: Studies in a model of tissue-bound IgG, Clin. Immunol. Immunopathol. 9:482.

MacGregor, R.R., Macarak, E.J., and Kefalides, N.A., 1978, Comparative adherence of granulocytes to endothelial monolayers and nylon fibers. J. Clin. Invest. 61:697.

Oliver, J.M., 1978, Cell Biology of leukocyte abnormalities-membrane and cytoskeletal function in normal and defective cells, Am. J. Pathol. 93:221.

Perez, H.D., Lipton, M., and Goldstein, I.M., 1978, A specific inhibitor of complement (C5)-derived chemotactic activity in serum from patients with systemic lupus erythematosus, J. Clin. Invest. 62:29.

Root, R.K., Rosenthal, A.S., and Balestra, D.J., 1972, Abnormal bactericidal, metabolic, and lysosomal functions of Chediak-Higashi Syndrome leukocytes, J. Clin. Invest. 51:649.

Schiffmann, E., Corcoran, B.A., and Wahl, S.M., 1975, N-formyl methionyl peptides as chemoattractants for leukocytes, Proc. Natl. Acad. Sci. U.S.A. 79:1059.

Shenkman, L., Borkowsky, W., Holzman, R.S., and Shopsin, B., 1978, Enhancement of lymphocyte and macrophage function in vitro by lithium chloride, Clin. Immunol. Immunopathol. 10:187.

Stanley, J., Perez, H.D., Gigli, I., Goldstein, I.M., and Baer, R.L., 1978, Hyperimmunoglobulin E Syndrome, Arch. Dermatol. 114:765.

Ward, P.A., Lepow, I.H., and Newman, L.J., 1968, Bacterial factor chemotactic for polymorphonuclear leukocytes, Am. J. Pathol. 52:725.

Wright, D.G., Kirkpatrick, C.H., and Gallin, J.I., 1977, Effects of levamisole on normal and abnormal leukocyte locomotion, J. Clin. Invest. 59:941.

Zigmond, S. and Hirsch, J.G., 1973, Leukocyte locomotion and chemotaxis: new methods for evaluation and demonstration of a cell-derived chemotactic factor, J. Exp. Med. 137:387.

Zurier, R.B., Weissmann, G., Hoffstein, S., Kammerman, S., and Tai, H.H., 1974, Mechanisms of lysosomal enzyme release from human leukocytes. II. Effects of cAMP and cGMP, autonomic agonists, and agents which affect microtubule function, J. Clin. Invest. 53:297.

EFFECTS OF LITHIUM ON NEUTROPHIL METABOLISM IN VITRO AND ON NEUTROPHIL FUNCTION DURING THERAPY

J.N. Siegel, R.B. Johnston Jr., R.S. Lowe,
P.S. Epstein, and A.H. Rossof

Rush-Presbyterian-St. Luke's Medical Center
Chicago,Illinois,
National Jewish Hospital and Research Center
Denver, Colorado, and
Wilford Hall USAF Medical Center
San Antonio, Texas

Lithium carbonate (LC), an effective therapeutic agent for manic depressive psychosis, induces neutrophilia associated with an increased blood neutrophil pool and survival *in vivo* (Rothstein *et al.*, 1978) and with enhanced growth of granulocyte committed stem cells *in vitro* (Rossof and Fehir, 1979). Despite these well documented effects on the granulocyte population, few studies have investigated the interactions of lithium and granulocyte function. Reports of lithium effects on the metabolic function of a variety of relatively homogeneous cell populations have shown that lithium increases the adhesion of nervous system cells and interferes with the effects of colcemid *in vitro* (Reiser *et al.*, 1975), increases the intensity of platelet aggregation and prolongs the duration of disaggregation *in vitro* (Imandt *et al.*, 1977), inhibits mitogen-induced lymphocyte proliferation and suppressor T-cell activity *in vitro* (Gelfand *et al.*, 1979) and enhances neutrophil skin window migration *in vivo* (Rothstein *et al.*, 1978).

Biologic interactions of lithium in intermediary metabolism may occur via substitution for cations serving such functions as enzyme activators, charge carriers and membrane stabilizers. One mechanism of lithium action is an interaction with the adenyl cyclase-cAMP system. Lithium has been reported to inhibit hormone-induced adenyl cyclase activation in brain, kidney and thyroid tissue enzyme systems (Singer and Rotenberg, 1973), to inhibit PGE_1 stimulated adenyl cyclase in platelets (Wang et al., 1974), to reverse theophylline, salbutamol and isoproterenol inhibition of E-rosette formation (Gelfand et al., 1979) and to reduce internal cAMP levels correlated with an abnormality of PMN chemotaxis (Perez et al., 1979).

A number of preliminary clinical trials have suggested a role for LC in the adjuvant treatment of patients receiving myelosuppressive chemotherapy (Tisman, 1974; Charron et al., 1977; Stein et al., 1977; Greco and Brereton, 1977; Stein et al., 1978; Lyman et al., 1978; Turner et al., 1979; Visca et al., 1979) and in the management of certain neutropenic disorders (Gupta et al., 1976; Rampon et al., 1976; Schapira et al., 1977; Barrett et al., 1977; Blum, 1979). Before this treatment can be advocated on a large scale, it is imperative to determine that the functional integrity of the PMN population is maintained in the presence of Li^+. We undertook an investigation of the effects of Li^+ on oxidative metabolism and membrane-dependent functions of normal PMN *in vitro* and on the metabolic activity *in vitro* and membrane responsiveness *in vivo* of PMN obtained before and during LC therapy. It is the purpose of this paper to present the results of these investigations which indicate the preservation of PMN function in the presence of Li^+ in the customary therapeutic range.

MATERIALS AND METHODS

Blood from healthy donors or patients on lithium therapy was obtained by venipuncture in preservative-free heparin (100 u/10 ml). Granulocytes were isolated by Ficoll-Hypaque and dextran sedimentation (Boyum, 1968) followed by hypotonic lysis (Zurier et al., 1973) or by dextran sedimentation alone. The final cell suspension of 10^7 PMN/ml in the assay buffer showed > 97% viability by Trypan blue dye exclusion.

Superoxide Generation

The generation of the superoxide anion radical, $\cdot O_2^-$, was assayed as the superoxide dismutase-inhibitable reduction of ferricytochrome C according to Babior et al. (1973). The single phagocytic stimulus was boiled washed zymosan (Henson, 1971) opsonized with autologous serum (10^9 particles/ml serum) at 37°C for 30 min, washed thoroughly and resuspended to 10^9 particles/ml assay buffer. PMN (2×10^6), opsonized zymosan (Z*) at a 30:1 particle:cell ratio and 0.5-5.0 meq/l LC in PBS adjusted to pH 7.4 were incubated in a total volume of 1.0 ml for 15 min at 37° C. Reduced cytochrome c in supernatants was measured at 550 nm.

Hexose Monophosphate Shunt (HMP)

Glucose-1-^{14}C oxidation was assayed according to Stjernholm and Manak (1970). PMN (5×10^6), Z* at a 30:1 particle:cell ratio and 0.5-5.0 meq/l LC were incubated for 30 min at 37°C while shaking in 2.0 ml PBS. $^{14}CO_2$ produced is reported as $^{14}CO_2$ cpm/5×10^6 PMN/30 minutes.

Chemiluminescence

Chemiluminescence produced by the decay of high energy oxidative intermediates was measured with a liquid scintillation system in the out-of-coincidence mode as described by Johnston et al. (1975). PMN (5×10^6) were preincubated with LC (0.5-5.0 meq/l) for one hour prior to the addition of the phagocytic (Z*) or nonphagocytic (phorbol myristate acetate (PMA)) stimulus. Counts were recorded at 3.5 minute intervals after the addition of the stimulus.

Candidacidal Activity

Oxygen dependent killing capacity of PMN were monitored by the method of Lehrer and Cline (1969). Buffy coat PMN were obtained by dextran sedimentation and adjusted to the standard concentration in AB serum.

These PMN, from normal donors, were incubated with 0.5-5.0 meq/l LC for one hour prior to the addition of viable Candida at 1:1 Candida:PMN ratio with continued incubation for an additional hour. Nonviable yeast in a deoxycholate lysate were counted using methylene blue.

Aggregation

PMN aggregation was studied with platelet aggregometry techniques using a Payton 300 dual channel aggregometer-recorder system (Craddock et al., 1978). Highly purified PMN are suspended at 10^7 PMN/ml in Hanks-Hepes (20 mM) buffer without calcium or magnesium, containing 1% human serum albumin and treated with cytochalasin B at 5 &g/ml for 15 min at 37°C. Cytochalasin B treated PMN (PMN-CB) in the presence or absence of LC and/or Ca were placed in a siliconized cuvette and stirred at 600 RPM at 37°C for 3 min prior to the addition of the aggregating stimulus. To provide necessary amplification for recording, the experimental system is calibrated against a 70% cell suspension. Aggregating agents used include zymosan activated autologous serum (ZTS), the chemotactic peptide formyl-methionyl-phenylalanine (FMP) and PMA.

Phagocytic Index

Ingestion was assayed with a modification of the procedure of Berg and Brandt (1973). Buffy coat cells were suspended to 10^4 PMN/µl in autologous plasma and incubated with 0.5-5.0 meq/l LC in PBS for 1,2, or 4 hours prior to the addition of heat killed Torulopsis glabrata at an 8:1 yeast:cell ratio. The phagocytic index was recorded as mean number of yeast per cell as visualized in a stained preparation under oil immersion.

Degranulation

In vitro degranulation studies utilized purified PMN (5 x 10^6) in PBS incubated while shaking at 37°C in the presence or absence of LC for 30 min prior to the addition of Z* at a 30:1 particle:cell ratio. When theophylline was included, it was added to the PMN/LC suspension 15 minutes before the addition of the Z*. After an additional 30 min of incubation with Z* at $37^{o}C$, supernatants were assayed for cytoplasmic LDH (Wroblewski and LaDue, 1953) and the granular enzymes β-glucuronidase (Brittinger et al., 1978) and lysozyme (Smolelis and Hartsell, 1949). Activities are expressed as the percent of total activity obtained from 5 x 10^6 PMN lysed with Triton X-100.

Skin Chamber Migration

Leukocyte mobilization of normal and patients' PMN was studied by a modification of the skin chamber technique of Holland et al. (1971). Two sites on the flexor surface of the forearm were abraded by scraping with a #11 scalpel blade. Chambers, with a capacity of 1.0 ml, were made from the distal ends of syringes filled with saline, and secured with colostomy glue. Chamber fluid collections for cell counts were made at 4 hours.

RESULTS

PMN Oxidative Metabolism

$\cdot O_2^-$ generation is a primary event in the respiratory burst of the stimulated PMN. Results obtained by activating cells with or without a preincubation in LC are shown in Table I. The normal value range of 4.9-11.1 nmoles cytochrome c reduced/10^6PMN/hr represents at least 10 assays on 10 individual normal volunteers. Li^+ between 0.5 and 5.0 meq/l had no effect on the activity of unstimulated PMN or Z* activated PMN in these serum free assay systems. Results of a single representative experiment are shown in Table I.

Li^+ has no effect on glucose-1-^{14}C oxidation of resting PMN but does enhance $^{14}CO_2$ production by Z* activated cells up to 50% (Table I). While this effect is reproducible within an experiment, the HMP activity still falls within the range of the normal population tested concurrently.

Results of a representative experiment measuring the effects of Li^+ on the chemiluminescence of stimulated PMN are shown in Figure 1. No reproducible, significant variations from control values are seen with either Z* or PMA stimulated cells.

TABLE I

LITHIUM AND OXIDATIVE METABOLISM OF NORMAL PMN

		$\cdot O_2^-$ Generation	HMP
PMN	+ 0 meq/l Li^+	0.6	0.1×10^3
	+ 0.5 meq/l Li^+	0.3	0.1×10^3
	+ 1.0 meq/l Li^+	0.5	0.2×10^3
	+ 2.0 meq/l Li^+	0.6	0.2×10^3
	+ 5.0 meq/l Li^+	0.6	0.2×10^3
PMN + Z*	+ 0 meq/l Li^+	6.7	6.2×10^3
	+ 0.5 meq/l Li^+	6.5	7.5×10^3
	+ 1.0 meq/l Li^+	6.9	8.6×10^3
	+ 2.0 meq/l Li^+	6.7	9.8×10^3
	+ 5.0 meq/l Li^+	6.9	9.0×10^3

$\cdot O_2^-$ generation reported as nmoles cytochrome c reduced per 10^6 PMN over 1 hour; range in 10 normal volunteers: 4 - 11 with mean = 5.6. Hexose monophosphate shunt activity (HMP) reported as cpm of $^{14}CO_2$ generated per 5×10^6 PMN over 30 minutes; range in 10 normal volunteers: 4.6 - 14.6 with mean = 8.0×10^3.

Oxygen-dependent candidacidal capacity was similarly unaffected by preincubation of cells with LC at concentrations as high as 5 meq/l for one hour prior to the addition of Candida (Table II).

Membrane-Dependent PMN Activity

Cell-cell adhesion, i.e. aggregation, of cytochalasin B treated PMN reflects a surface membrane response to an external stimulus. The aggregation response induced by the chemotactic peptide FMP reaches a maximum within 30 seconds and is dependent upon externally supplied divalent cations (Figure 2A). Aggregation induced by PMA however is

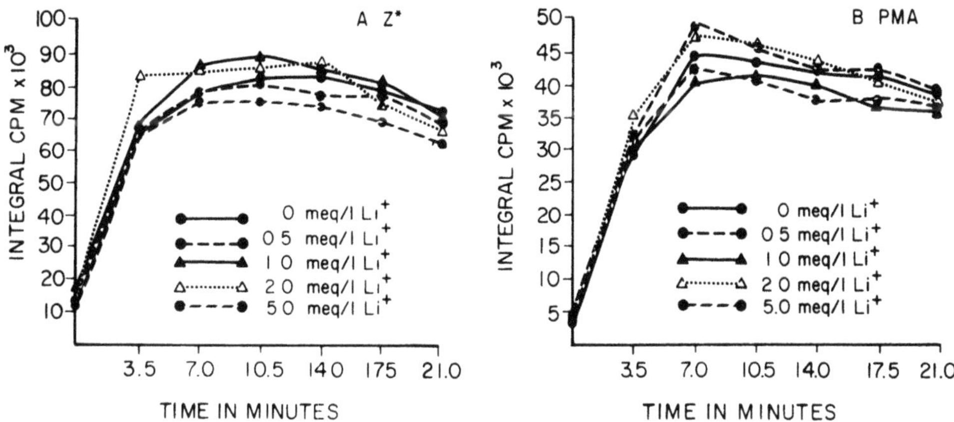

Figure 1. Representative experiment demonstrating chemiluminescence of stimulated PMNs after incubation in varying concentrations of lithium. See text for details.

TABLE II

LITHIUM AND CANDIDA KILLING BY PMN

Li^+ meq/l	% Candida Killed PBS	Puck's
0	18.7 ± 5.4	15.6 ± 2.1
0.5	20.9 ± 9.5	19.0 ± 8.5
1.0	15.7 ± 3.2	13.1 ± 3.6
2.0	16.0 ± 9.0	13.2 ± 6.2
5.0	14.5 ± 9.3	12.4 ± 5.1
Control Mean	18.9 ± 5.4	17.3 ± 3.0

Eleven separate experiments were done in PBS and nine in Puck's solution. Values reported are mean ± 1 standard deviation.

kinetically distinct, developing slowly over time and appears unaffected by the absence of an external supply of calcium and magnesium (Figure 2A). Preincubation of PMN with LC over the same concentration range for 3 min or one hour in buffer containing 0.6 mM Ca and 1.0 mM Mg results in insignificant changes in the aggregation response to FMP (data not shown). However, the inclusion of lithium in a reaction system lacking added divalent cations resulted in enhanced kinetics and magnitude of the limited response initiated by FMP (Figure 2B). Lithium has no effect on PMA-induced aggregation even under conditions of limited divalent cations (Figure 2C).

The effects of LC on ingestion, measured as the granulocyte phagocytic index (PI) are shown in Table III. Li^+ had no effect in this system.

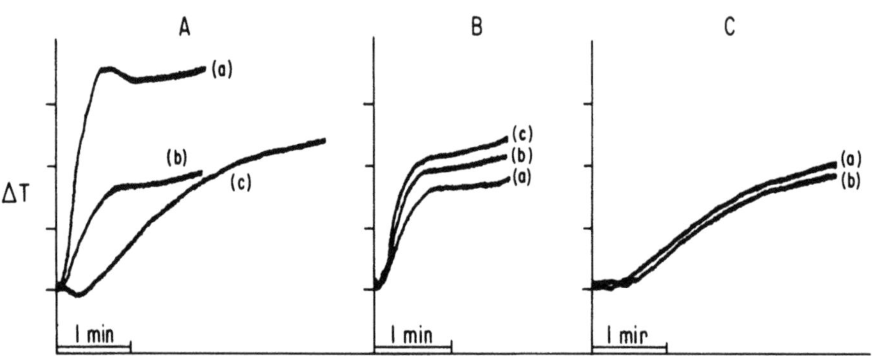

Figure 2. Panel A - Effects of calcium on FMP- and PMA-induced aggregation: (a) FMP with calcium and magnesium; (b) FMP without calcium and magnesium; (c) PMA with or without calcium and magnesium. Panel B - Effects of lithium on FMP aggregation in absence of calcium and magnesium: (a) 0.0 and 5.0 meq/L Li^+; (b) 1.0 and 2.0 meq/L Li^+; (c) 0.5 meq/L Li^+. Panel C - Effects of lithium on PMA aggregation in absence of calcium and magnesium: (a) 1.0, 2.0, and 5.0 meq/L Li^+; (b) 0.0 and 0.5 meq/L Li^+.

The effects of LC on lysosomal enzyme release of unstimulated and phagocytically stimulated normal PMN are shown in Table IV. Concentrations of 0.5 - 5.0 meq/l Li^+ had no effect on the energy-dependent release of granular ¢-glucuronidase or lysozyme from resting or phagocytically stimulated PMN. Li^+ between 0.5 and 5.0 meq/l had no effect on the viability of resting or stimulated PMN as indicated by release of lactate dehydrogenase (LDH). A concentration of 10 meq/l is lethal to the intact human PMN and results in 50 - 80% LDH release from resting and Z* stimulated cells.

TABLE III

LITHIUM AND GRANULOCYTE PHAGOCYTIC INDEX

Li^+ meq/l	Incubation period 1 h	2 h	4 h	Overall mean
0	4.13 ± 1.77	4.04 ± 1.53	4.45 ± 1.49	4.21
0.5	4.32 ± 1.69	4.11 ± 1.58	4.34 ± 1.50	4.26
1.0	3.94 ± 1.56	4.22 ± 1.42	4.15 ± 1.70	4.10
2.0	4.10 ± 1.39	4.14 ± 1.41	4.14 ± 1.52	4.13
5.0	4.31 ± 1.81	4.36 ± 1.58	4.16 ± 1.13	4.28
Overall mean	4.16	4.17	4.25	

Each value represents 6 experiments performed on PMNs from 4 normal healthy male volunteers. Values reported are means ± 1 standard deviation. Data from Rossof, A.H. and Coltman, C.A., Jr., 1976, *Experientia* 32:238.

In view of the known interaction of lithium with adenyl cyclase-cAMP mediated responses, we tested the effects of lithium on cAMP mediated inhibition of lysomal enzyme release (Table V). No data for LDH are included since release was unaffected in all experiments. The addition of theophylline to PMN prior to the addition of Z* resulted in the complete inhibition of ¢-glucuronidase release and a 40% inhibition of the release of lysozyme. Preincubation of PMN with LC, even at a concentration as low as 0.5 meq/l, partially restored ¢-glucuronidase release and elevated lysozyme release to control values (Table V).

TABLE IV

LITHIUM AND LYSOSOMAL DEGRANULATION OF NORMAL PMN

		Enzyme Release % Total Released by Triton X-100		
		β-glucuronidase	Lysozyme	LDH
PMN	+ 0 meq/l Li^+	0.7	1.1	3.0
	+ 0.5 meq/l Li^+	0.9	2.2	5.0
	+ 1.0 meq/l Li^+	0.6	2.2	3.0
	+ 2.0 meq/l Li^+	0.7	2.2	3.0
	+ 5.0 meq/l Li^+	0.3	1.1	5.0
PMN + Z*	+ 0 meq/l Li^+	8.0	17.4	7.0
	+ 0.5 meq/l Li^+	7.9	16.8	5.0
	+ 1.0 meq/l Li^+	8.2	17.9	0.0
	+ 2.0 meq/l Li^+	7.6	14.6	0.0
	+ 5.0 meq/l Li^+	7.9	22.4	0.0

These representative data are from one of three experiments using PMNs from normal volunteers.

Lithium Therapy and PMN Function

Our patient studies have investigated *in vitro* metabolic responsiveness of PMN of patients receiving lithium showing characteristic neutrophilia and therapeutic lithium levels between 0.7-1.4 meq/l. Mean and range values from normal volunteer donors assayed simultaneously in the *in vitro* experiments are shown in Table VI. Means of the patient PMN responses of both $\cdot O_2^-$ generation and HMP assays appear elevated although they do not significantly vary from the control range values.

A study correlating peripheral blood counts and *in vivo* skin chamber migration responsiveness of patients before and after the initiation of LC therapy is shown in Figure 3. Results of the pre- and post-lithium studies show two-fold increases in WBC and two-three-fold increases in chamber migration. The pre- and post-lithium values for two normal volunteers also show two-fold WBC changes and greater than three-fold increases in chamber migration.

DISCUSSION

The results reviewed above are consistent with all other evidence that lithium is tolerated in a concentration range similar to that of Mg^{++} and Ca^{++} suggesting possible interactions in systems regulated by those cations (Mellerup and Jorgensen, 1975). In the therapeutic concentration range and above (0.5-5.0 meq/l), lithium was neither toxic nor stimulatory to resting normal PMN in any oxidative or membrane function measured. In addition, lithium had no significant effect on $\cdot O_2^-$ generation, chemiluminescence and candidacidal activity of optimally stimulated PMN. The consistent enhancement of HMP activity is interpreted as a high normal response. The absence of a similar effect on $\cdot O_2^-$ generation could be related to the duration of the experiments which, even with a preincubation, were one hour shorter than the HMP experiments. Energy and membane-dependent activities such as aggregation and degranulation also were unaffected by lithium in optimally stimulated systems.

TABLE V

LITHIUM AND THEOPHYLLINE-INDUCED INHIBITION OF DEGRANULATION

Incubation System	% Enzyme Released	
	¢-Glucuronidase	Lysozyme
Test Experiments		
PMN → Z*	8.0	20.5
PMN → THEO → Z*	0.2	12.5
PMN + Li^+ → THEO → Z*	4.1	19.3
Control Experiments		
PMN	0.0	2.6
PMN → THEO	0.0	2.6
PMN + Li^+	0.0	0.0
PMN + Li^+ → THEO	0.0	0.0

THEO signifies theophylline studied at 10^{-3}M. Li^+ final concentration was 0.5 meq/l. The arrows signify the sequences of adding the various components to the incubation systems; see text for details.

Lithium has been shown to have a Ca^{++} like effect in some systems. For example, lithium stimulates acetylcholine secretion by cortical slices in the absence of Ca^{++} (Carmody and Gage, 1973) and both Li^+ and Ca^{++} inhibit some enzymes similarly, specifically adenyl cyclase activation in platelets (Wang et al., 1974) and in thyroid tissue (Singer and Rotenberg, 1973). In the aggregation system described, in the presence of externally limiting Ca^{++} and Mg^{++}, and an optimal stimulus (FMP), the addition of Li^+ or Ca^{++} enhanced the response. In this same system, theophylline and exogenous cAMP have the same effect (Siegel, J., unpublished data) suggesting an effect of lithium beyond the formation of cAMP. However,

TABLE VI

EFFECTS OF LITHIUM THERAPY ON PMN FUNCTION IN VITRO

Patient	$\cdot O_2^-$ Generation	HMP Activity	WBC (10^3)	Serum Li^+ (meq/l)	Drug Therapy
A.	11.8	6.6×10^3	8.3	0.87	Amitriptyline, Desipramine, Dextroamphetamine
B.	9.1	5.6×10^3	9.1	1.15	
C.	10.1	12.9×10^3	7.9	1.35	
D.	12.6	6.5×10^3	10.5	1.3	Benztropine mesylate, Norgestrel, Ethinyl estradiol
E.	5.2	9.8×10^3	9.1	1.07	Propoxyphene, Tranylcypramine
Patient:					
Mean	9.8	8.3×10^3			
Range	5.2-12.6	$5.6-12.9 \times 10^3$			
Normal:					
Mean	7.6	7.3×10^3			
Range	4.6-11.1	$4.6-14.6 \times 10^3$			

*Five normals were studied concurrently.

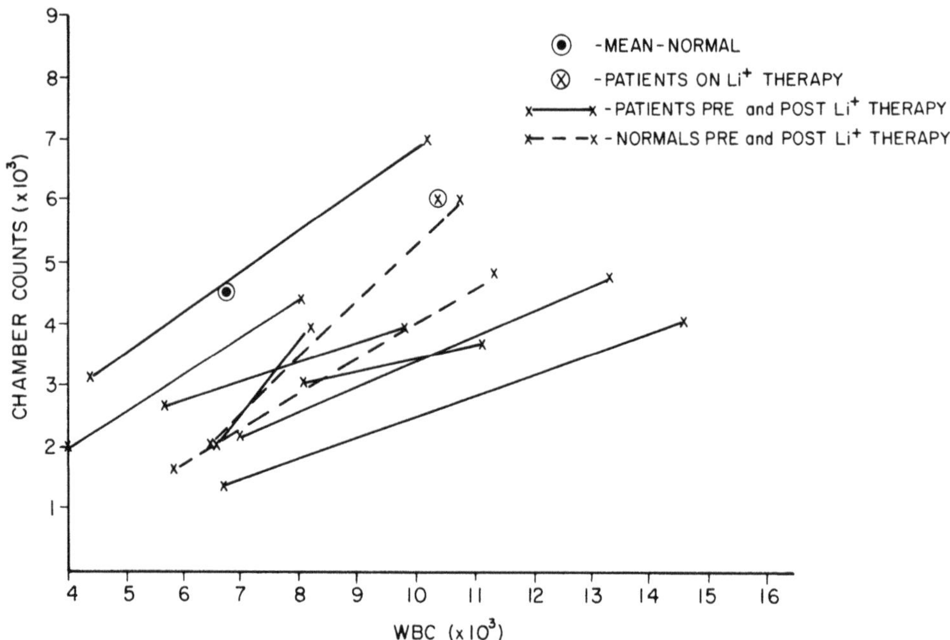

Figure 3. WBC migration into skin windows plotted against peripheral blood WBC concentrations in patients and normal volunteers before and after receiving lithium carbonate.

in agreement with the reviewed data, lithium did reverse cAMP mediated inhibition of lysosomal enzyme release induced by theophylline. This was a partial effect, most notable at relatively low levels of cell stimulation. Experiments testing the effects of lithium in the presence of limiting external divalent cations have not been done.

Studies on the in vitro metabolic responsiveness of PMN from patients receiving lithium correlated nicely with normal PMN data showing high normal $\cdot O_2^-$ generation and HMP activity. Unfortunately, we have performed studies on only two patients before and after lithium therapy. One patient with low normal $\cdot O_2^-$ generation activity before lithium showed high normal activity two weeks later; a second patient with high normal activity before therapy was unchanged after. Our studies correlating granulocyte count and in vivo chamber migration show increases in migration (2-3 fold) consistent with high normal metabolic responsiveness of the increased cell population. These values are not as great as those previously reported (Rothstein et al., 1978) of 4-55 fold increases in migration responses of patient on chronic lithium therapy.

These data demonstrate that the Li^+, in the concentration range commonly achieved in clinical practice, does not impair any aspect of PMN function so far tested. The quantitative benefit of LC in some clinical conditions is not offset by any qualitative defect, suggesting that further clinical trials can be done with safety.

REFERENCES

Babior, B.M., Kipnes, R.S., and Curnette, J.T., 1973, The production by leukocytes of superoxide, a potential agent, J. Clin. Invest. 52:741.

Barrett, A.J., Griscelli, C., Buriot, D., and Faille, A., 1977, Lithium therapy in congenital neutropenia. The Lancet 2:1357.

Berg, B. and Brandt, L., 1973, Syndrome of anemia, thrombocytopenia and subnormal granulocyte function in elderly patients, Scand. J. Haematol. 10:161.

Bille, P.E., Jensen, J.P.K., and Paulsen, J.C., 1975, Studies on the hematologic and cytogenic effect of lithium, Acta Med. Scand. 198:281.

Blum, S.F., 1979, Lithium therapy of aplastic anemia, New Eng. J. Med. 300:677.

Boyum, A, 1968, Isolation of mononuclear cells and granulocytes from human blood IV. Isolation of mononuclear cells by one centrifugation, Scand. J. Clin. Lab. Invest. 21:77 (Supplement).

Brittinger, G., Hirschorn, R., Douglas, S.D., and Weissman, G., 1968, Studies on lysosomes XI. Characterization of a hydrolase-rich fraction from human leukocytes, J. Cell Biol. 37:394.

Carmody, J.J. and Gage, P.W., 1973, Lithium stimulates secretion of acetylcholine in the absence of extracellular calcium, Brain Res. 50:476.

Charron, D., Barrett, A.J., Faille, A., Alby, N., Schmitt, T., and Degos, L., 1977, Lithium in acute myeloid leukemia, The Lancet 1:1307.

Craddock, P.R., White, J.G., and Jacob, H.S., 1978, Potentiation of complement (C5a)-induced granulocyte aggregation by cytochalasin B, J. Lab. Clin. Med. 91:490.

Gelfand, E.W., Dosche, H-M., and Hastings, D., 1979, Lithium: A modulator of cyclic AMP-dependent events in lymphocytes, Science 203:365.

Greco, F.A. and Brereton, H.D., 1977, Effect of lithium carbonate on the neutropenia caused by chemotherapy: A preliminary clinical trial, Oncology 34:153.

Gupta, R.C., Robinson, W.A., and Kurnick, J.E., 1976, Felty's syndrome - effect of lithium on granulopoiesis, Amer. J. Med. 61:29.

Henson, P.M., 1971, The immunologic release of constituents from neutrophil leukocytes I. The role of antibody and complement on non-phagocytosable surfaces or phagocytosable particles, J. Immunol. 107:1535.

Holland, J.F., Senn, H., and Banerjee, T., 1971, Quantitative studies of localized leukocyte mobilization in acute leukemia, Blood 37:499.

Imandt, L., Genders, T., Wessels, H., and Haanen, C., 1977, The effect of lithium on platelet aggregation and platelet release reaction, Thromb. Res. 11:297.

Johnston, R.B., Jr., Keele, B.B., Jr., Misra, H.P., Lehmeyer, J.E., Webb, L.S., Baehner, R.L., and Rajagopalan, K.V., 1975, The role of superoxide anion generation in phagocytic bactericidal activity. Studies with normal and chronic granulomatous disease leukocytes, J. Clin. Invest. 55:1357.

Lehrer, R.I. and Cline, M.J., 1969, Interaction of Candida albicans with human leukocytes and serum, J. Bacteriol. 98:996.

Lyman, G.H., Williams, C.C., and Preston, D., 1978, A prospective randomized study of the effect of lithium carbonate on the granulocytopenia and incidence of infection associated with intensive chemotherapy and radiation therapy for undifferentiated small cell bronchogenic carcinoma, Blood 52:228 (Supplement 1).

Mayfield, D. and Brown, R.G., 1966, The clinical laboratory and electroenephalographic effects of lithium, J. Psychiat. Res. 4:207.

Mellerup, E.T. and Jorgensen, O.S., 1975, Basic chemistry and biological effects of lithium, in: "Lithium Research and Therapy," (F.N. Johnson, ed.) p. 353, Academic Press Inc.

Perez, H.D., Kaplan, H., Shenkman, L., Borkowsky, W., and Goldstein, I.M., 1979, Reversal of an abnormality of polymorphonuclear leukocyte chemotaxis with lithium, Clin. Res. 27:353A.

Rampon, S., Bussiere, J-L., Sauvezie, B., Missioux, D., Lopitaux, R., and Prive, L., 1976, Traitement du syndrome de Felty par le lithium, La Nouvelle Presse Medicale 5:1756.

Reiser, G., Lautenschlager, E., and Hamprecht, B., 1975, Effects of colemid and lithium ions on processes of cultured cells derived from the nervous system, in: "Microtubules and Microtubule Inhibitors," (M. Borgers and M. de Brabander, eds.) North-Holland Publishing Company, Amsterdam.

Rossof, A.H. and Fehir, K.M., 1979, Lithium carbonate increases marrow granulocyte-committed colony-forming units and peripheral blood granulocytes in a canine model, Exp. Hematol. 7:255.

Rothstein, G., Clarkson, D.R., Larsen, W., Grosser, B.I., and Athens, J.W., 1978, Effect of lithium on neutrophil mass and production, New Eng. J. Med. 298:178.

Schapira, D.V., Gordon, P.A., and Herbert, F.A., 1977, Reduction of infections is Felty's sydrome through use of lithium, Arth. Rheum. 28:1556.

Shopsin, B., Friedmann, R., and Gershon, S., 1971, Lithium and leukocytosis, Clin. Pharmacol. Ther. 12:923.

Singer, I. and Rotenberg, D., 1973, Mechanisms of lithium action, New Eng. J. Med. 189:254.

Smolelis, A.N. and Hartsell, S.E., 1949, The determination of lysozyme, J. Bacteriol. 58:731.

Stein, R.S., Beaman, C., Ali, M.Y., Hansen, R., Jenkins, D.D., and Jume'an, H.G., 1977, Lithium carbonate attenuation of chemotherapy-induced neutropenia, New Eng. J. Med. 297:430.

Stein, R.S., Flexner, J.M., and Graber, S., 1978, Lithium and granulocytopenia during induction therapy of acute myelogenous leukemia, Blood 52:277 (Supplement 1).

Stjernholm, R.L. and Manak, R.C., 1970, Carbohydrate metabolism in leukocytes XIV. Regulation of pentose cycle activity and glycogen metabolism during phagocytosis, J. Reticuloendothel. Soc. 8:550.

Tisman, G., Herbert, V., and Rosenblatt, S., 1973, Evidence that lithium induces vitamin B12-binding capacity in vivo and granulocyte colony proliferation in vitro, Br. J. Haematol. 24:767.

Tisman, G., 1974, Lithium carbonate protection against drug-induced leukopenia in lymphosarcoma patients, IRCS 2:1509.

Turner, A.R., MacDonald, R.N., and McPherson, T.A., 1979, Reduction of chemotherapy-induced neutropenic complications with a short course of lithium carbonate, Clin. Invest. Med. in press.

Visca, U., Mensi, F., Spina, M.P., Bombara, R., Giraldi, B., Massari, A., Rossi, F., and Santi, G., 1979, Prevention of antiblastic neutropenia with lithium carbonate, The Lancet 1:779.

Wang, Y.C., Pandey, G.N., Mendels, J., and Frazer, A., 1974, Effect of lithium on prostaglandin E1-stimulated adenylate cyclase activity of human platelets, Biochem. Pharmacol. 23:845.

Wroblewski, F. and LaDue, J.S., 1953, Lactic dehydrogenase activity in blood, Proc. Soc. Exp. Biol. Med. 90:210.

Zurier, R.B., Hoffstein, S., and Weissman, G., 1973, Lysosomal enzyme release from human leukocytes I. Effect of cyclic nucleotides and colchicine, J. Cell Biol. 58:27.

THE BACTERICIDAL DEFECT OF NEUTROPHIL FUNCTION WITH LITHIUM THERAPY

William R. Friedenberg and James J. Marx

Marshfield Medical Foundation
510 N. St. Joseph Avenue
Marshfield, Wisconsin 54449

Lithium has been promoted for the treatment of granulocytopenia and as an adjuvant for cancer chemotherapy (Jacob and Herbert, 1974; Gupta *et al.*, 1975; Greco, 1976; Greco and Brereton, 1977; Charron *et al.*, 1977; Tisman and Wu, 1977; Catane *et al.*, 1977; Stein *et al.*, 1977). In preliminary studies of 8 normal volunteers we found a significant bactericidal defect of the granulocytes when studied after 1 week of lithium therapy. We also assessed lymphocyte subpopulations, function, and cell mediated immunity both *in vivo* and *in vitro* and could find no defect of lymphocyte function except for a reduction in the response of the lymphocytes to PPD antigen. The rational for the use of lithium is to decrease the incidence of infection in patients who have granulocytopenia. With such defects demonstrated in normals after short term doses, granulocyte and lymphocyte functions were studied in patients on long term lithium therapy.

MATERIALS AND METHODS

Study Subjects

Informed consent was obtained from either patients or their guardians, and a sample of venous blood was drawn for a battery of granulocyte and lymphocyte functional assays. Recent lithium levels had been performed on these individulas and were in the therapeutic range. Many of these individuals were taking other psychotrophic drugs as well as other medications as indicated clinically. All individuals had been taking lithium for a period of months to years. The blood for in vitro testing was obtained from normal laboratory personnel taking no medications.

Lymphocyte Function Tests

The lymphocyte system was assessed by the methods previously outlined from this laboratory (Hansen et al., 1978). Briefly, lymphocyte subpopulations were identified by surface markers after separation using a density gradient Ficoll-Hypaque column centrifuged at 400 g. Sheep red blood cell rosetting (E-RFC) was used to identify T cells, while complement receptors (EAC-RFC) and surface immunoglobulins were used to identify B cells. Percentages (mean ± S.D.) from a normal population were as follows: E-RFC = 50-75 percent; EAC-RFC = 10-34 percent; IgG = 5-20 percent; IgM = 3-15 percent; and IgA = 0-4 percent. Lymphocyte function was assessed by in vitro lymphocyte transformation to a panel of mitogens and recall antigens. Lymphocyte transformation has been previously described in detail (Hansen, 1978) and was performed as described. Each subject was tested for reactivity to phytohemagglutinin (PHA), concanavalin A (Con-A), pokeweed mitogen (PWM), streptokinase-streptodornase (SK-SD), mumps, candidin, histoplasmin, and tuberculin PPD. The results are expressed as the stimulation index (SI) or ratio of counts in the cultures with mitogen to the counts in control cultures. Greater than twofold stimulation by antigen was considered a positive test.

Granulocyte Function Tests

The functional integrity of the granulocyte system was assessed by a battery of tests including: nitroblue tetrazolium (NBT) reduction; chemotaxis in response to bacteria derived factor(s) and zymosan induced C5a; and phagocytic and bactericidal capabilities. These granulocytes were separated by sedimentation at 1 x g for 45 minutes at 37°C. The cell rich plasma was then layered on a Ficoll-Hypaque gradient and centrifuged for 10 minutes at 400 x g. The sedimented cells were 95% pure granulocytes. The cells were washed in Hank's balanced salt solution (HBSS) and resuspended to appropriate concentrations.

NBT Reduction

The model utilized for NBT reduction is that described by Park et al. (1968). Venous blood was collected with 10 units of heparin/ml. The blood was incubated with 0.2 percent NBT in normal saline at 37°C for 15 minutes. Blood smears are prepared, stained with Wright's stain, and a 200 cell differential was made noting the number of cells which have the reduced formazan deposits within the cytoplasm. These cells are easily recognized as PMNs with large irregular dark amorphous masses within the confines of the cytoplasm. A portion of whole blood was preincubated with 1 mg/ml bacterial lipopolysaccharide (LPS) (Difco, Detroit, MI) for 15 minutes at 37°C and the NBT test was repeated as above. Normal individuals routinely showed values < 20 percent in the unstimulated cultures and > 30 percent in the LPS stimulated cultures.

Chemotaxis

The chemotaxis response was determined as outlined in detail by Ward (1976). The chemotactic chambers (Bellco Glass, Vineland, NJ) are prepared using 5 micron porosity SMWP 02500 Millipore filters. The cells are cultured in RPMI 1640 buffered with bicarbonate at pH 7.3. Chemotactic factors used included a bacterial culture filtrate of E. coli, zymosan activated normal human serum, and the appropriate controls. The chambers are incubated at 37°C for 3 hours. The filters are carefully removed from the chambers, fixed in absolute propanol, stained with Wright's stain, and finally cleared in xylene. The filters are placed on conventional glass slides with mounting media and observed at 25 x magnification. A minimum of ten fields are viewed and the number of cells migrating completely through the filter are counted. The results are expressed as the ratio of the average number of cells per 25 x field and compared to controls.

Phagocytic and Bactericidal Activities

The ability of the granulocytes to ingest and kill bacteria was studied by the method outlined by Weir (1973). An 18 hour culture of Staphylococcus aureus, strain 502A, (ATCC, Bethesda, MD) was incubated with 1×10^7 granulocytes in a 1:1 ratio of bacteria to granulocytes. For phagocytic indices, aliquots of the bacteria-cell mixture were sampled at 30, 60, and 120 minutes. The cells are centrifuged at 400g and the number of bacteria remaining in the supernatant was calculated based on viable plate counts. Bactericidal abilities of these granulocytes were determined by mixing cultures of Staphylococcus aureus and granulocytes in ratio of 1:1 for 15 minutes at 37^oC. Excess bacteria were removed by washing. Aliquots were then taken at 30, 60, 90, and 120 minutes. The number of bacteria contained within the granulocytes was determined, after lysing the washed granulocytes, by viable plate counts. The results of these two assays were expressed as the phagocytic index (PI) and bactericidal index (KI). PI and KI are calculated by comparing the log number of bacteria at 0 minutes and 120 minutes. Normal linear regression lines can be plotted.

Peroxidase

Myeloperoxidase stains were performed as described by Kaplow (1965). The quantification was performed as described for the leukocyte alkaline phosphatase stain and normal values obtained in healthy laboratory personnel.

RESULTS

Granulocyte Function (Table I)

Three out of the four patients tested had a significant reduction in bactericidal capacity. There was no significant trend in the direction of either increased or reduced random mobility, chemotaxis, NBT reduction, or phagocytosis.

TABLE I

LONG TERM LITHIUM THERAPY

Granulocyte Function

	R.C.	M.H.	M.N.	G.D.
WBC	8200	8000	5700	8000
PMN	4220 (51)	5520 (69)	3480 (61)	5200 (65)
NBT (R)	9.5	1.5	4.5	6.0
NBT (S)	48.5	12.0	68.0	61.0
PI_{60}	0.44/0.57	0.63/0.61	0.36/0.47	0.35/0.37
PI_{120}	1.32/1.02	1.04/1.04	0.81/0.77	0.70/0.65
KI_{60}	0.19/0.26	0.33/0.42	0.39/0.35	0.32/0.29
KI_{120}	0.19/0.36	0.59/0.63	0.44/0.56	0.39/0.57
MI_3	0.89/0.86	2.6/2.6	0.66/0.87	0.60/0.84
MI_{24}	1.65/2.15	20.0/18.4	1.46/2.51	1.56/2.43
CI_E	2.6/2.5	2.0/14.6	5.2/7.2	6.3/6.8
CI_Z	2.4/2.0	2.3/5.2	3.5/3.2	4.7/3.6

WBC = Total white cell count/mm^3.

PMN = Total neutrophil count/mm^3. The number in parenthesis is the percent of the total white cell count.

NBT (R) and NBT (S) = The percent of neutrophils reducing NBT resting and stimulated respectively.

PI_{60} and PI_{120} = Phagocytic index at 60 and 120 minutes respectively.

KI_{60} and KI_{120} = Bactericidal index at 60 and 120 minutes respectively.

MI_3 and MI_{24} = Random migration at 3 and 24 hours respectively.

CI_E and CI_Z = Chemotactic index with endotoxin and zymosan respectively.

In each column the patient value is compared to the control value (patient/control).

Lymphocyte Function (Tables II and III)

There was no significant change in the number of T cells or B cells, or in the lymphocyte transformation to mitogens and antigens.

TABLE II

LONG TERM LITHIUM THERAPY

Lymphocyte Function I

	R.C.	M.H.	M.N.	G.D.
WBC	8280	8000	5700	8000
Lymphocytes	3230 (39)	1600 (20)	1800 (32)	1440 (18)
E-RFC	2150 (66)	1010 (63)	1120 (62)	920 (64)
EAC-RFC	160 (5)	270 (17)	280 (16)	270 (19)
Membrane Ig				
IgG	50 (1.5)	70 (4.4)	85 (4.7)	150 (10.5)
IgM	70 (2.3)	100 (6.0)	70 (3.75)	90 (6.3)
IgA	90 (2.8)	20 (1.0)	23 (1.3)	400 (28.0)
E-RFC (Active)	1100 (34)	500 (31)	420 (23.5)	400 (28.0)

WBC = Total white cell count/mm^3.

Lymphocytes = Total lymphocyte count/mm^3. The number in parenthesis is the percent of the total white cell count.

E-RFC = Total lymphocytes/mm^3 rosetting with sheep red blood cells. The number in parenthesis is the percent of the total lymphocytes.

EAC-RFC = Total lymphocytes/mm^3 rosetting with sheep cells sensitized with complement. The number in parenthesis is the percent of the total lymphocytes.

Membrane Ig = Total lymphocytes/mm^3 flourescing with the appropriate anti- serum reacting with IgG, IgM, and IgA respectively.

E-RFC (Active) = Total lymphocytes/mm^3 rosetting with sheep erythrocytes following brief incubation.

TABLE III

LONG TERM LITHIUM THERAPY

Lymphocyte Function II

	R.C.	M.H.	M.N.	G.D.
PHA	112.5	137.6	64.4	127.2
Con-A	37.0	60.4	25.2	24.2
SK-SD	11.0	20.5	1.69	8.9
Histo (yeast)	1.1	1.0	---	---
PPD	2.0	1.3	---	---
Candida	2.4	69.4	2.25	4.8
Mumps	1.2	2.6	1.12	5.6
PWM	9.5	23.8	2.51	6.9

The results are expressed as the ratio of tritiated thymidine uptake in cultures stimulated with a mitogen or antigen compared to unstimulated control cultures.

Myeloperoxidase Activity of Neutrophils (Table IV)

Isolated neutrophils were prepared and incubated with lithium carbonate at doses ranging from 1 mEq/l to 50 mEq/l. After 2 hours at 37°C, there was no difference in the scored histochemical stain for myeloperoxidase in these cells compared to controls. Leukocyte alkaline phosphatase stains were also similar in cells incubated with lithium when compared to controls.

TABLE IV

MYELOPEROXIDASE ACTIVITY WITH LITHIUM CARBONATE (IN VITRO)

Dilution of Lithium (mEq/L)	Peroxidase Score	LAP Score
50	286	115
10	292	114
5	256	109
1	257	104
0	273	127

The dilution of lithium is the final concentration in whole blood.
LAP = leukocyte alkaline phosphatase.

DISCUSSION

There have been no controlled clinical studies assessing the incidence of infection in patients with granulocytopenia after treatment with lithium. The phagocytic function of granulocytes in humans treated with lithium has been previously described (Rossof and Coltman, 1976) as normal which is also confirmed by our previous study. In previous studies we could find no impairment of chemotaxis, random mobility, or oxidative metabolism as measured by NBT reduction and chemiluminescence. These findings were essentially confirmed by the present studies. In our previous studies there was no significant change in the migration of granulocytes into skin windows (Friedenberg, 1979) and Rothstein et al. (1978) found no impairment of migration utilizing a different technique. They did suggest increased migration. Cohen et al. (1979) recently found no defect in the bactericidal capacity in 5 individuals exposed to lithium. Our assay of bactericidal capacity was significantly reduced both in the original study after short-term lithium therapy and in this study after long-term lithium. We also found a reduction in bactericidal capacity at both 1 and 2 hours. Cohen et al. (1979) reported no difference after 1 hour.

Previous studies have shown a suppression of adenyl cyclase activity and decreased intracellular cyclic AMP levels in tissues exposed to lithium (Dousa and Hechter, 1970; Forn and Valdecasas, 1971; Frazer et al., 1975; Essman, 1975; Ebstein et al., 1976). Competition with intracellular cations has been proposed as the mechanism of action of lithium (Frausto and Williams, 1976). It was possible that lithium would compete for the intracellular halide ions such as chloride and inhibit myeloperoxidase activity resulting in the reduction in bactericidal capacity. For that reason lithium was incubated with whole blood with concentrations varying between 1 mEq/liter and 50 mEq/liter for 2 hours. No reduction in myeloperoxidase activity was detected.

There is a significant reduction of bactericidal capacity in patients treated with lithium, but the mechanism and the clinical significance of this defect are unclear. It is entirely possible that there is more than sufficient reserve in the granulocytes' ability to kill with the remaining bactericidal capacity, and therefore this reduction in vitro is not significant clinically. Controlled clinical trials are indicated to assess the incidence of infection before lithium is widely used to treat either granulocytopenia or as an adjuvant to cancer chemotherapy.

REFERENCES

Catane, R., Kaufman, J., Mittelman, A., and Murphy, G.P., 1977, Attenuation of myelosuppression with lithium, N. Eng. J. Med. 297:452.

Charron, D., Barrett, A.J., Faille, A., Alby, N., Schmitt, T., and Degos, L., 1977, Lithium in acute myeloid leukemia, Lancet 1:1307.

Cohen, M.S., Zakhireh, B., Metcalf, J.A., and Root, R.K., 1979, Granulocyte function during lithium therapy, Blood 53:913.

Dousa, T., and Hechter, O., 1970, Lithium and brain adenyl cyclase, Lancet 1:834.

Ebstein, R., Belmaker, R., Grunhaus, L., and Rimon, R., 1976, Lithium inhibition of adrenalin-stimulated adenylate cyclase in humans, Nature 259:411.

Essman, W.B., 1975, Lithium, Lancet 2:547.

Forn, J., and Valdecasas, F.G., 1971, Effects of lithium on brain adenyl cyclase activity, Biochem. Pharmacol. 20:2773.

Frausto da Silva, J.J.R., and Williams, R.J.P., 1976, Possible mechanism for the biological action of lithium, Nature 263:237.

Frazer, A., Haugaard, E.S., Mendels, J., and Haugaard, N., 1975, Effects of intracellular lithium on epinephrine-induced accumulation of cyclic AMP in skeletal muscle, Biochem. Pharmacol. 24:2273.

Friedenberg, W.R., and Marx, Jr., J.J., 1979, The effect of lithium carbonate on lymphocyte, granulocyte, and platelet function, Cancer (in press).

Greco, F.A., 1976, Lithium and leukocytosis, Ann. Int. Med. 84:102.

Greco, F.A., and Brereton, H.D., 1977, Effect of lithium carbonate on the neutropenia caused by chemotherapy: A preliminary clinical trial, Oncology 34:15.

Gupta, R.C., Robinson, W.A., and Smyth, C.J., 1975, Efficacy of lithium in rheumatoid arthritis with granulocytopenia (Felty's syndrome), Arthritis Rheum. 18:179.

Hansen, R.L., Marx, Jr., J.J., Ptacek, L.J., and Roberts, R.C., 1977, Immunologic studies on an aberrant form of ataxia telangiectasia, Am. J. Dis. Child. 131:518.

Jacob, E., and Herbert, V., 1974, Lithium therapy for neutropenias, J. Clin. Invest. 53:35.

Kaplow, L.S., 1965, Simplified myeloperoxidase stains using benzidine dihydrochloride, Blood 26:215.

Park, B.H., Fikrig, S.M., and Smithwick, E.M., 1968, Infection and nitroblue-tetrazolium reduction by neutrophils. A diagnositic aid, Lancet 2:532.

Rothstein, G., Clarkson, D.R., Larsen, W., Grosser, B.I., and Athens, J.W., 1978, Effect of lithium on neutrophil mass and production, N. Engl. J. Med. 298:178.

Rossof, A.H., and Coltman, Jr., C.A., 1976, The effect of lithium carbonate on the granulocyte phagocytic index, Experientia 32:238.

Stein, R.S., Beaman, C., Ali, M.Y., Hansen, R., Jenkins, D.D., and Jume'an, H.G., 1977, Lithium carbonate attenuation of chemotherapy-induced neutropenia, N. Eng. J. Med. 297:430.

Tisman, G., and Wu, S.J.G., 1977, Lithium-induced granulocytosis, Lancet 2:251.

Ward, P.A., 1976, Chemotaxis, in: "Manual of Clinical Immunology," (N.R. Rose, and H. Friedman, eds.), p. 1109, American Society of Microbiology, Washington, DC.

Weir, D.M., 1973, "Handbook of Experimental Immunology," Blackwell Scientific Publication, Oxford.

EFFECT OF LITHIUM ON ACUTE MYELOCYTIC LEUKEMIA CELLS IN TISSUE CULTURE - A PRELIMINARY STUDY

J. Rosenstock, J. Archer and E. Pequignot

Hahnemann Medical College and Hospital
230 North Broad Street
Philadelphia, Pennsylvania 19102

Lithium was observed to increase the number of peripheral neutrophils in hematologically normal individuals (Shopsin *et al.*, 1971; Bille *et al.*, 1975) and in several primary neutropenic conditions (Tisman and Show-Jen, 1977; Barrett, *et al.*, 1977). When this effect is analysed in people receiving lithium for psychiatric reasons, it appeared to involve predominantly the myeloid cell line, though platelet counts were also increased (Bille *et al.*, 1975). Lithium apparently causes increased neutrophil production by increasing colony stimulating activity (Turner *et al.*, 1978).

Iatrogenic and myelophistic neutropenias are common in patients with cancer and are a major cause of morbidity and mortality. An agent with low toxicity which could specifically decrease the degree or duration of neutropenia would potentially have great therapeutic value.

The present studies were begun in an attempt to determine whether the growth stimulation of lithium is specific for normal myeloid precursors or whether it would have similar effects on malignant cell growth. As a first step, the effect of lithium on the cell proliferation of a human myelogenous leukemia blast cell line, K562, was studied.

MATERIALS AND METHODS

Studies of the effect of lithium chloride on leukemic cell growth were performed using a myelogenous leukemic cell line, K562. The K562 cells were maintained in suspension culture in Waymouth/McCoy 5A (1:1) medium containing 10% heat inactivated fetal bovine serum. Cultures were maintained at 37°C in a humidified atmosphere of 95% air and 5% carbon dioxide. All studies of cells were carried out using untreated cells, and cells cultured in the presence of equivalent amounts of calcium chloride ($CaCl_2$), as controls for the effects of lithium chloride (LiCl).

For growth studies, cells were plated at a concentration of 1×10^5 cells/60 mm plate in 5 ml medium containing LiCl or $CaCl_2$ at the following concentrations: 0, 0.5, 1.0, 1.5, 2.0, 2.5, 3.0, 3.5, 4.0, 4.5 and 5.0 meq/liter. Six plates of control cells, and $CaCl_2$ and LiCl incubated cells were counted (Coulter Electronic Cell Counter) each day for four days at each salt concentration. Within the therapeutic drug range, 0.5 - 3.0 meq/liter, 20 plates were set up for each drug and time point.

Viability studies were run in parallel with the growth studies. The trypan blue exclusion method was used, and the percentage of live and dead cells obtained by counting cells in a hemocytometer. Studies of the effects of LiCl and $CaCl_2$ on the plating efficiency (colony forming ability) of K562 cells were carried out using a modified soft-agar technique. Cells were plated at 1×10^4 cells per 35 mm plate onto 1 ml of 0.3% agar in Waymouth/McCoy 5A medium containing 20% heat inactivated fetal bovine serum and incubated at 37°C for 24 hours to allow cell attachment. The cells were then overlayed with medium containing LiCl, $CaCl_2$, or no additions and incubated for eight days. Colony formation (≥ 50 cells) was determined under an inverted microscope and the number of colonies formed recorded. Plating efficiency was calculated using the formula:

$$\text{Plating Efficiency} = \frac{100 \times \text{mean number of colonies}}{\text{number of cells plated.}}$$

All data were subjected to statistical analyses, using analysis of variance and the Student t-test methods.

RESULTS

Within the therapeutic serum drug level range of 0.5 to 5.0 meq/liter lithium, the addition of lithium chloride, or an ionic equivalent (calcium chloride control drug) appeared to cause a mild stimulation of the growth of K562 cells in vitro. This was reflected in a small increase in the number of cells counted on days two and three after plating and a significant increase in maximal cell density on day four. This trend was apparent at drug doses of 0.5, 1.0, 1.5 and 2.0 meq/liter. This pattern is illustrated in Figures 1 and 2. Significant differences in maximal cell density were also found at doses higher than the normal therapeutic range. For example, there was an increased maximal cell density of cells grown in the presence of lithium compared to calcium at 3.0 meq/liter at the 0.02 significance level as tested by the Student's t-test.

There was no dose-response curve to lithium within the therapeutic range. However, when higher doses were used a dose-response could be seen for lithium at a much lower concentration (10 meq/liter) than for calcium as shown in Figure 3.

The growth of cells in the presence of added lithium and calcium was also monitored by viability assay using the trypan blue exclusion method. Viability in the presence of no added drug was normalized to 100% viability. By the use of this method it was again shown that at concentrations of lithium and calcium in the range from 2.0 - 4.0 meq/liter cell survival was slightly better than if no drug was added to the medium. When the level of drug added was increased there was a much greater loss of viability in the presence of added lithium than added calcium as shown in Figure 4.

Another more sensitive method of assaying cell behavior is plating efficiency. However, since the cell line K562 usually grows in suspension culture and only lightly attaches to the plastic culture flask surface this method could not be used. Therefore, an adaptation of the colony formation technique using soft agar was used. Cells were plated on 0.3% soft-agar using conditioned medium from K562 cell cultures and replacing the feeder layer with an overlay of agar-medium containing lithium and/or calcium salts and incubated for 8 days. Colony formation and calculation of plating efficiency was performed according to standard methods. An increased efficiency was seen with both calcium and lithium compared to the control, as shown in Table I. There appears to be a higher plating efficiency with lithium at 1 and 2 meq/liter compared to calcium but not at 3.0 meq/liter.

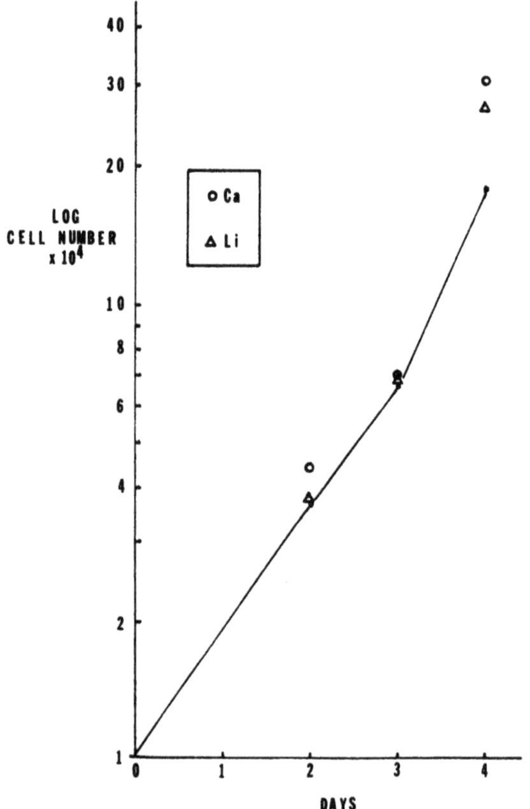

Figure 1. Growth of K562 cells seeded at 1 X 10^4 cells/plate in medium containing 20% FBS, with no additions (closed circles); 0.05 meq/liter $CaCl_2$ (open circles); and 0.5 meq/liter LiCl (open triangles).

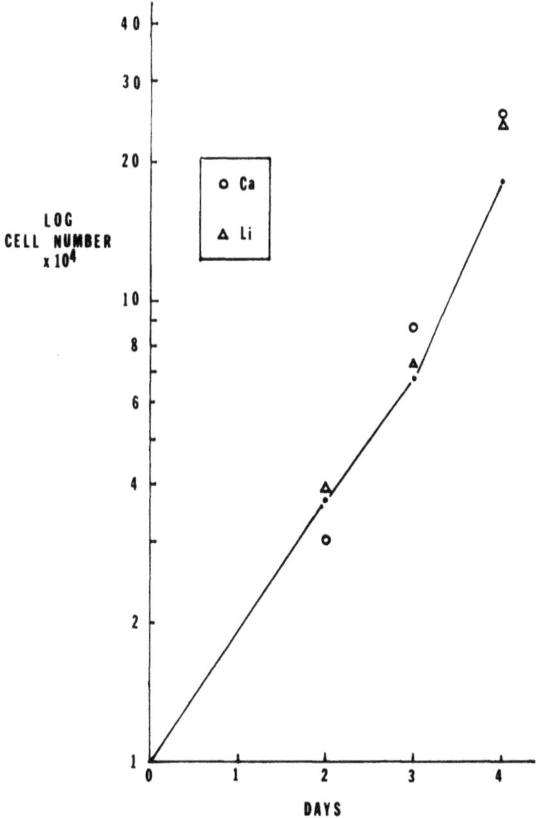

Figure 2. Growth of K562 cells seeded at 1 x 10^4 cells/plate in medium containing 20% FBS with no additions (closed circles); 1.0 meq/liter $CaCl_2$ (open circles) and 1.0 meq/liter LiCl (open triangles).

TABLE I

PERCENTAGE PLATING EFFICIENCY

(COLONY FORMATION ON SOFT AGAR ± 1 STANDARD DEVIATION)

Drug Dose (meq/liter)	Calcium Chloride	Lithium Chloride
0	29.20 ± 2.30	29.20 ± 2.30
1	30.12 ± 4.83	55.65 ± 6.10
2	27.70 ±4.45	42.77 ± 1.75
3	36.30 ± 3.14	37.00 ± 1.60

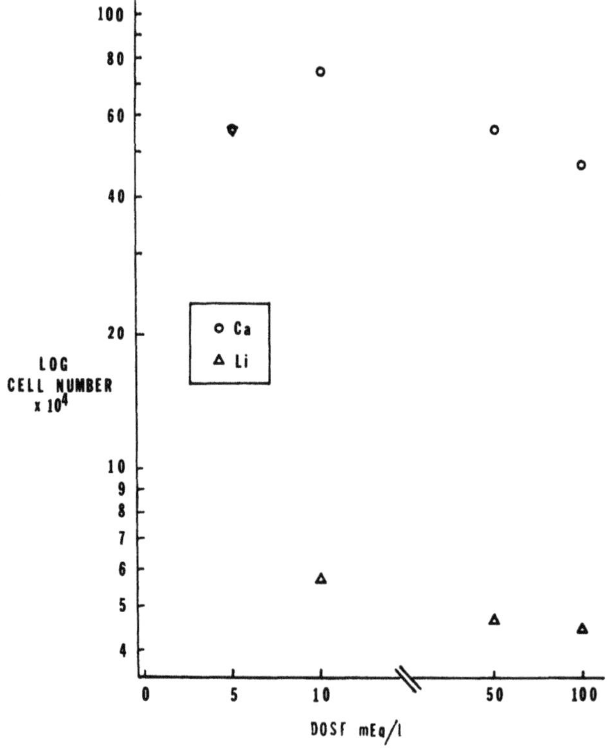

Figure 3. Growth of K562 cells seeded at 5×10^4 cells/plate in medium with the following additions: 0, 5, 10, 50 and 100 meq/liter of $CaCl_2$ (open circles) and LiCl (open triangles). Cell density on day 4 after plating is plotted against drug dose.

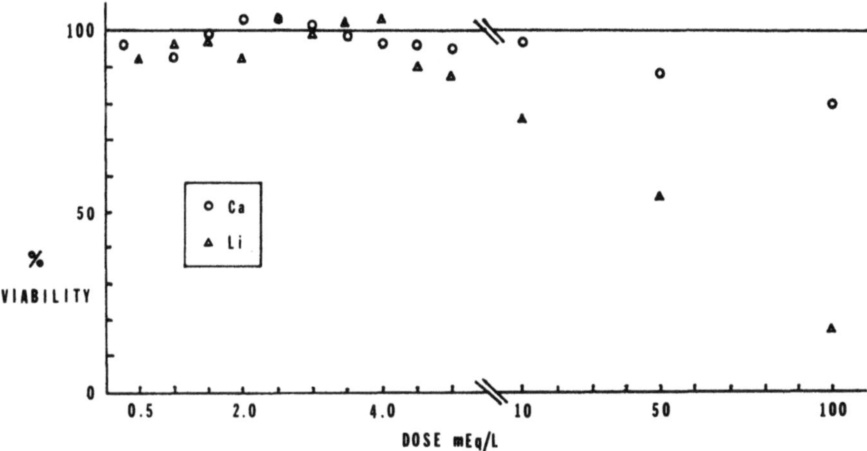

Figure 4. The percentage viability of cells (measured by trypan blue exclusion) is plotted against the dose of $CaCl_2$ (open circles) and LiCl (open triangles) in meq/liter. Viability of untreated cells was normalized to 100%

DISCUSSION

The granulocytic stimulation of lithium has great potential clinical benefit in patients with malignancy if the effect is specific and does not concomitantly increase the growth of the malignant cells. The studies of Bille et al. (1975) and of Malloy et al. (1978) showed the effects of lithium to include an increase in platelets. The mechanism of action of lithium on the myeloid elements seems to be by increasing the colony stimulating activity (CSA) so that the effect is at the level of the committed stem cell. Malignant cells, on the other hand, although usually involving some degree of cell line committment, have apparently different cell growth controlling factors than normal committed cells.

K562, the cell line chosen to determine if lithium could stimulate growth of a malignant cell line, is supposedly a malignant committed myeloid line. It retains the Philadelphia chromosome and has morphologic characteristics consistent with a myeloid blast cell. This cell line would appear to be close to a normal myeloid element and thereby most susceptible to the effect of lithium. There are factors which bring into question its lineage. The chromosome studies of Lozzio and Lozzio (1975) show it to contain both the Philadelphia chromosome and to be hypodiploid. Clinical studies in patients with chronic myelogenous leukemia (CML) in blast crises who have hypodiploid cells have a much better response to chemotherapy than such patients with other chromosome patterns (Rosenthal et al., 1977). Also, blast crises of CML with lymphoblasts respond well to drugs typically used in acute lymphatic leukemia. Cytochemical studies of this cell line with PAS, peroxidase, and Sudan Black show a pattern consistent with lymphoid characteristics despite the morphological appearance (Rosenstock, 1979). The positive effect on growth in this cell line at levels which may be reached intermittently in humans on oral lithium suggests that the effect of lithium may not be limited to committed normal myeloid cells. Malignant cells may also be stimulated in some way, and this effect may be by increasing individual cell growth or possibly by recruitment.

Further studies in vitro and especially in animals with different cell lines are necessary to explore the specificity of lithium on cell growth and to understand further the mechanism of cell growth in normal and malignant cells.

ACKNOWLEDGEMENT

The research presented in this manuscript was supported by Biomedical Research Support Grant 5-S07-RR05413.

REFERENCES

Barrett, A.J., Hugh-Jones, K., Newton, K. and Watson, J.G., 1977, Lithium therapy in aplastic anemia, The Lancet 2:202.

Bille, P.E., Jensen, M.K., Jensen, J.P. and Poulsen, J.C., 1975, Studies on the haematologic and cytogenetic effect of lithium, Acta Med. Scand. 198:281.

Lozzio, C.B. and Lozzio, B.B., 1975, Human chronic myelogenous leukemia cell-line with positive Philadelphia chromosome, Blood 45:321.

Malloy, N.L., Zauber, N.P., Chervenick, P., 1978, The effect of lithium on blood and marrow neutrophils, Blood 52:228, (Supplement 1).

Rosenstock, J.G., 1979, Unpublished observations.

Rosenthal, S., Canellos, G.P., Whang-Peng, J. and Gralnick, H.R., 1977, Blast crisis of chronic granulocytic leukemia, Am. J. Med. 63:542.

Shopsin, B., Friedmann, R. and Gershon, S., 1971, Lithium and leukocytosis, Clin. Pharmacol. Ther. 12:923.

Tisman, G. and Show-Jen, G.W., 1977, Lithium-induced granulocytosis, The Lancet 2:251.

Turner, A.R. and Allalunis, M.J., 1978, Mononuclear cell production of colony stimulating activity in humans taking oral lithium, Blood 52:234, (Supplement 1).

DRINKING WATER LITHIUM LEVELS FAIL TO PREDICT FOR THE INCIDENCES OF ACUTE OR CHRONIC GRANULOCYTIC LEUKEMIA

James L. Budd and Arthur H. Rossof

Pritzker School of Medicine of the University of Chicago and
Section of Medical Oncology, Department of Medicine
Rush Medical College, Chicago, Illinois

Frenkel and Herbert (1974) commented upon the inverse relationship between drinking water lithium ion (Li^+) content and the incidences of acute granulocytic leukemia (AML) in the Dallas-Ft. Worth standard metropolitan statistical area (SMSA) and in El Paso, Texas. They also noted a similar incidence of chronic granulocytic leukemia (CML) in the two areas, suggesting no relationship to drinking water Li^+ concentrations. We have further investigated these relationships by correlating the drinking water Li^+ concentrations with the incidence rates of AML and CML in 19 American cities, SMSAs, or states. For both AML and CML, we have determined no significant correlation ($p > 0.10$) between drinking water Li^+ content and the incidence data.

MATERIALS AND METHODS

Data on drinking water lithium levels were obtained from the U.S. Geological Survey Water Supply Paper No. 1812, "Public Water Supplies of the 100 Largest Cities in the United States, 1962" (Durfor and Becker, 1964). Certain assumptions were made by adjusting these data to relate them to the same geographical areas for which leukemia incidence data were available. These assumptions are explained in full in the legend to Table I.

Data on leukemia incidences in metropolitan New Orleans and the Seattle-Puget Sound 13 county area and of the states of Connecticut, Hawaii, Utah, and New Mexico were obtained from the background data for the Surveillance, Epidemiology, and End Results (SEER) Program report (Young, et al., 1978). These are incidence data for 1973-1976 and have been age-adjusted to the 1970 census. Incidence data for the Texas cities of Houston, Corpus Christi, San Antonio, and El Paso were background data for a recent publication (Macdonald and Heinze, 1978). These data were collected over the period 1962-1966 and were age adjusted to the 1970 census. Incidence data for the SMSAs of Pittsburgh, Birmingham, Dallas-Ft. Worth, Minneapolis-St. Paul, San Francisco-Oakland, Atlanta, and Detroit and for the States of Colorado and Iowa were obtained from the Third National Cancer Survey (TNCS) (Culter and Young, 1975) and were collected over 1969-1971. Raw data provided in the TNCS were corrected for those cases which were microscopically confirmed and incidences were calculated based on the 1970 census data as provided in the Survey publication. When the same areas were evaluated both in the SEER report and the TNCS, data from the latter were chosen for analysis in this study since they are more temporally-related to the data on water supply lithium levels. The data used in our analyses can be found in Table I.

In analyzing these data, we assumed that the incidences of AML and CML and the drinking water lithium levels were unchanged over the period under study. Since it was not possible to correct these data for migration into and out of these communities, it was assumed that the duration of exposure to a given environmental lithium level was sufficient to cause any possible effect on leukemia incidence. Linear regression analyses were calculated as described by Colton (1974).

RESULTS

Drinking water Li^+ levels and incidence rates of AML and CML in these 19 American communties are presented in Table I. Linear regression analysis for AML incidence as a function of drinking water Li^+ concentration gives a slope of -0.013 with p = 0.36 (See Figure 1). For CML, the slope is 0.000533 with p = 0.94 (See Figure 2).

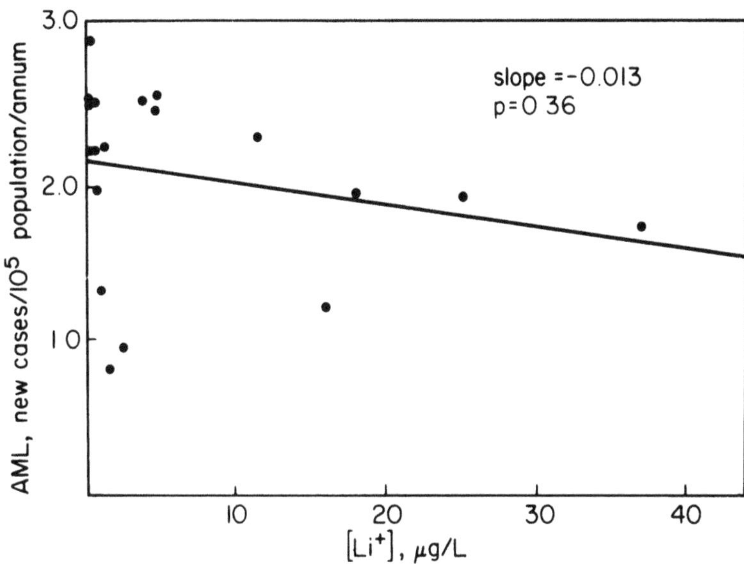

Figure 1. Incidences of acute myelogenous leukemia in 19 American communities plotted as a function of the drinking water lithium content.

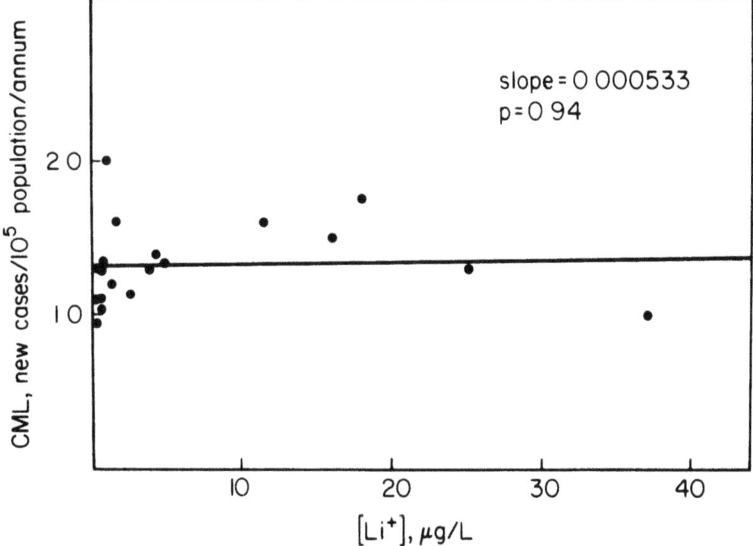

Figure 2. Incidences of chronic myelogenous leukemia in 19 American communities plotted as a function of the drinking water lithium content.

TABLE I

Location	Li^+, μg/L	Incidence Rates New Cases/10^5/Annum	
		AML	CML
Seattle-Puget Sound	0.1	2.5	1.1
Atlanta SMSA	0.1	2.18	0.94
Connecticut	0.3	2.5	1.3
Hawaii	0.3	2.9	1.1
Colorado	0.5	2.19	1.30
Detroit SMSA	0.7	1.93	1.34
Houston	0.9	1.3	2.0
Utah	1.2	2.2	1.2
San Francisco-Oakland SMSA	1.4	2.48	1.03
San Antonio	1.5	0.8	1.6
Birmingham SMSA	2.5	0.9	1.13
New Orleans	3.8	2.5	1.3
Dallas-Ft. Worth SMSA	4.6	2.47	1.34
Pittsburgh SMSA	4.8	2.53	1.33
Minneapolis-St. Paul SMSA	11.5	2.26	1.60
Corpus Christi	16.0	1.2	1.5
Iowa	18.0	1.91	1.76
New Mexico	25.0	1.9	1.3
El Paso	37.0	1.7	1.0

Table I. Drinking water lithium content and incidence rates for acute and chronic granulocytic leukemia for the 19 American communities under discussion.

The water supply lithium level of Seattle, WA represents the Seattle-Puget Sound area, while Atlanta, GA represents the Atlanta SMSA; Honolulu, HI represents Hawaii; Denver, CO represents Colorado; Detroit,

MI represents the Detroit SMSA; Salt Lake City, UT represents Utah; Birmingham, AL represents the Birmingham SMSA; Pittsburgh, PA represents the Pittsburgh SMSA; Des Moines, IO represents Iowa; and Albuquerque, NM represents New Mexico. The value for Connecticut (0.3 μg/L) represents the mean of the values for Bridgeport, CN (0.5), Hartford, CN (0.2), and New Haven, CN (0.1). The value for the San Francisco-Oakland SMSA (1.4) represents the mean of the values for San Francisco (0.6) and Oakland (2.1). The value for the Dallas-Ft. Worth SMSA (4.6) represents the mean of the values for Dallas (7.2) and Ft. Worth (2.0). The value for the Minneapolis-St. Paul SMSA (11.5) represents the mean of the values for Minneapolis (14.0) and St. Paul (8.9).

DISCUSSION

Our analyses of the data provided to us fail to confirm a significant positive or negative relationship between the drinking water Li^+ concentrations and the incidences of AML or CML in these 19 American communities. A number of assumptions were made in the analyses of these data which may or may not be entirely valid. One can speculate that environmental Li^+ exposure contributes to the regulation of normal granulopoiesis in man . There are, however, no direct data indicating that this is so and our analyses of these data concerning two forms of abnormal granulopoiesis (AML and CML) fail to indicate that such a relationship exists.

ACKNOWLEDGEMENTS

It is with deep appreciation that we acknowledge the generous assistance of Leland J. McCabe, Director, Field Studies Division, Health Effects Research Laboratory, United States Environmental Protection Agency, Cincinnati, Ohio; John W. Horm, Biometry Branch, National Cancer Institute, Bethesda, Maryland for the background data of the SEER Program report; and Dr. Eleanor J. Macdonald, Professor of Epidemiology, the University of Texas System Cancer Center, M.D. Anderson Hospital and Tumor Institute, Houston, Texas for data on the Texas cities of Houston, Corpus Christi, San Antonio, and El Paso. Dr. Richard J. Shekelle assisted with the statistical interpretations.

REFERENCES

Colton, T., 1974, Statistics in Medicine, Little, Brown, and Co., Boston.

Cutler, S.J. and Young, J.L., Jr. (Eds.), 1975, Third National Cancer Survey: Incidence Data, DHEW Publication No. (NIH) 75-787, National Cancer Institute Monograph 41.

Durfor, C.N. and Becker, E., 1964, Public Water Supplies of the 100 Largest Cities in the United States, 1962, U.S. Geological Survey Water Supply Paper 1812.

Frenkel, E.P. and Herbert, V., 1974, Frequency of granulocytic leukemia in populations drinking high -vs- low-lithium water, Clin. Res. 22:390A.

Macdonald, E.J. and Heinze, E.B., 1978, Epidemiology of Cancer in Texas: Incidence Analyzed by Type, Ethnic Group, and Geographic Location, Raven Press, New York.

Young, J.L., Jr., Asire, A.J., and Pollack, E.S. (Eds.), 1978, SEER Program: Cancer Incidence and Mortality in the United States, 1973-1976, DHEW Publication No. (NIH) 78-1837.

ADJUVANT-LIKE EFFECTS OF LITHIUM ON PERIPHERAL BLOOD MONONUCLEAR CELLS

William Borkowsky, Louis Shenkman, Scott Wadler,
Robert S. Holzman, and Baron Shopsin

Departments of Medicine and Neuropsychopharmacology
New York University Medical Center
New York, New York

Cyclic nucleotides appear to play a dynamic role in the modulation of immune responses. While an increase in lymphocyte cyclic-AMP (C-AMP) is required for the initiation of lymphocyte proliferation, a sustained elevation of cellular C-AMP levels results in a net inhibition of lymphocyte proliferation (Wang et al., 1978). Similarly, macrophage function is depressed in the presence of agents that increase cellular C-AMP (Schultz, 1978).

Although its exact mode of action on the central nervous system is not known, lithium has been shown to interfere with a variety of adenylate cyclase systems. Inhibition of adenylate cyclase has been observed in the thyroid, kidney, platelet, and other tissues (Singer et al., 1973; Murphy et al., 1973; Birnbaumer et al., 1969). In view of the inhibitory effects of C-AMP on immune function, we have investigated whether lithium, by inhibiting adenylate cyclase and lowering C-AMP levels, enhances the function of human peripheral blood mononuclear cells.

EFFECTS ON LYMPHOCYTE-SHEEP ERYTHROCYTE (SRBC) ROSETTE FORMATION

Lymphocytes isolated from normal human peripheral blood by Ficoll-Hypaque separation were allowed to form rosettes with washed sheep erythrocytes at room temperature and at 4°C. These rosettes are termed active, and total, respectively. Active rosettes represent the fraction of lymphocytes with high-affinity receptors for SRBC. These procedures were duplicated on identical lymphoid cells that had been incubated with various concentrations of lithium (Li).

Li at a concentration of 10^{-3}M increased the formation of active rosettes from 30.9 to 39.8% ($p < 0.01$ by paired T test). Higher concentrations of Li produced no additional increases in active rosettes. At a concentration of 10^{-3}M, Li increased the formation of total rosettes from 69.8 ± 3.0 to 72.0 ± 3.3%. At 5 x 10^{-3}M and 10^{-2}M, Li increased the percentage of total rosettes to 74.5 ± 3.3 and 74.7 ± 2.7%, respectively. Regression analyses showed a highly significant linear coefficient ($F(1,12) = 12.3$, $p < 0.005$).

EFFECTS ON MONOCYTE INGESTION OF LATEX BEADS

Phagocytosis of latex particles by adherent monocytes was studied by the method of Al-Ibrahim *et al.* (1976). Macrophage monolayers were cultured on glass coverslips for three days with Li in concentrations of 0 to 5 x 10^{-3}M. ^{99}Tc-labelled latex particles were added for 30 minutes. The cover slips were washed free of non-ingested particles and counted for 30 seconds in a gamma counter. Results were recorded as counts per milligram of protein.

Increasing the concentration of Li caused a progressive increase in macrophage phagocytosis (Figure 1). Analysis of variance showed a significant linear correlation coefficient ($F(1, 14) = 25.3$, $p < 0.005$) for the regression of phagocytosis on log Li concentrations.

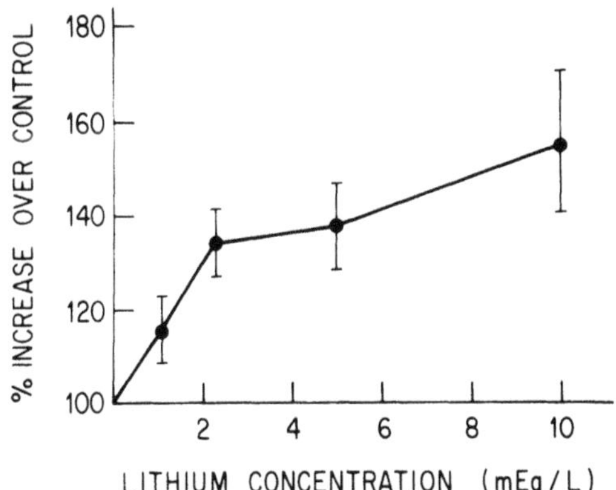

Figure 1. Effect of lithium on phagocytosis by macrophages, as assessed by the ingestion of ^{99}Tc-labeled latex particles.

EFFECTS ON LYMPHOCYTE PROLIFERATION TO HETEROLOGOUS LYMPHOID CELLS (TWO-WAY MIXED LYMPHOCYTE CULTURE (MLC)) AND SOLUBLE BACTERIAL ANTIGENS

MLC reactions were established in microculture plates by adding 0.1 ml of each of two HLA incompatible donor lymphocytes at a concentration of 750,000 mononuclear cells/ml to a well. Li solution or culture medium were added to create final Li concentrations from 0 to 5×10^{-3}M. Cultures were incubated for 6 days and (^{14}C)thymidine was added for an additional 18 hours. The cells were collected by an automatic harvester on glass fiber filters. The contents of each well were counted in a scintillation counter after the addition of a toluene scintillation liquid cocktail.

At a Li concentration of 5×10^{-3}M, thymidine incorporation was increased 52% over that seen in the absence of Li ($p < 0.05$). There was no significant increase at lower Li concentrations.

Lymphocyte proliferative responses to tuberculin (PPD), candida extract, and streptokinase-streptodornase (SKSD) were assessed by the method of Cohen et al. (1976). Lymphocyte donors were individuals with clearly demonstrated cell-mediated immune responses to these antigens as judged by skin test reactivity. When compared to control cultures, the addition of Li at concentrations of 2.5×10^{-3}M enhanced thymidine uptake by 11% (from 4600 ± 785 CPM to 5120 ± 790, mean ± S.E., $P < 0.01$ by paired T test).

EFFECTS OF LITHIUM ON LYMPHOCYTE PROLIFERATIVE RESPONSES TO MITOGENS

Lymphocytes were stimulated by optimal concentrations of phytohemagglutinin (PHA) in the presence and absence of Li. Although Li was not mitogenic itself, thymidine incorporation after PHA stimulation was significantly enhanced in the presence of Li (Figure 2). The kinetics of the enhancement revealed that the maximal effect of Li occurred after cultures had reached their peak of proliferation (i.e., after 72 hours of PHA stimulation). Thymidine incorporation was increased by 28% at Li concentrations of 1.25×10^{-3}M and by 40% at concentrations of 5×10^{-3}M ($p < 0.001$).

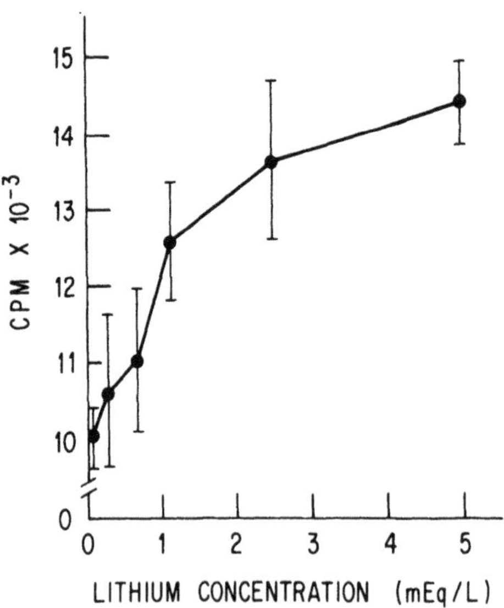

Figure 2. Effect of lithium on mitogenic response to PHA. The vertical axis depicts incorporation of ^{14}C-thymidine by PHA-stimulated lymphocytes.

Li also enhanced thymidine uptake by mononuclear cells stimulated by an optimally mitogenic concentration of concanavalin A (Con A, 15 μg/ml). At a concentration of 2.5×10^{-3} M of Li, there was a 51% increase in thymidine incorporation ($p < 0.01$).

In cultures containing submitogenic doses of Con A (0.1 μg/ml), Li decreased thymidine uptake by 29% (95 ± 41 without Li, 67 ± 57 with Li, mean ± SD). These results were also statistically significant at a p value of < 0.05.

EFFECTS OF LITHIUM ON LYMPHOCYTE RESPONSES TO PHA IN SYSTEMS SIMULATING ENHANCED SUPPRESSOR CELL ACTIVITY

The descriptions of prostaglandin-secreting macrophages in diseases associated with increased suppressor cell function prompted us to examine the effects of Li on PGE_1 inhibition of lymphocyte proliferation. PGE_1 at a concentration of 10^{-4}M significantly decreased the response to PHA. The addition of Li at a concentration of 1.25×10^{-3}M or greater completely reversed the inhibitory effect of PGE_1.

Other agents that increase white blood cell C-AMP have been reported to depress lymphocyte proliferation . Theophylline, at a concentration of 10^{-4}M, significantly decreased the incorporation of (^{14}C) thymidine from 7582 ± 1816 cpm (mean ± SD) to 3486 ± 399 cpm. The addition of Li at a concentration of 1.25×10^{-3}M partially reversed the inhibition by theophylline, with observed counts of 4429 ± 31 cpm ($p < 0.02$).

Incubation of cell cultures for 24 hours with Con A and subsequent addition of these mitomycin-treated cells to fresh autologous cells has been shown to decrease their DNA synthesis after stimulation with mitogens or antigens (Shou et al., 1976). Presumably, the decreased DNA synthesis is a reflection of enhanced suppressor cell activity induced by ConA.

We employed this system to measure the effects of Li in a suppressor-enriched system. Cell cultures were preincubated for 24 hours with or without Con A (50 μg/ml), and then exposed to mitomycin C (25 μg/ml) for

20 minutes at 37°C. The cells were washed with an α-methyl mannoside solution and added to equal aliquots of fresh lymphocytes stimulated with PHA, with or without Li. Cells precultured for 24 hours in the absence of Con A and subsequently treated as described above served as control cultures.

Con A-activated cells caused a decrease in thymidine incorporation by PHA-stimulated fresh cells. The suppression averaged 29%. When Li (2.5×10^{-3}M) was added to this suppressor-enriched culture, the suppression of thymidine incorporation was reversed.

EFFECTS OF LITHIUM ON LYMPHOCYTE RESPONSES TO CON A IN SYSTEMS PARTIALLY DEPLETED OF SUPPRESSOR CELLS

Preincubation of lymphocytes for 24 hours had been shown to increase DNA synthesis when Con A is subsequently added as a mitogenic stimulus, presumably because a population of labile suppressor cells is diminished by the preincubation (Dutton, 1972).

Cell cultures stimulated by Con A (15 μg/ml) at 0 to 24 hours were incubated for an additional 84 hours. Thymidine uptake was enhanced by 39% in the cells preincubated for 24 hours (suppressor-deficient system). When Li (2.5×10^{-3}M) was added to the suppressor-deficient system, an additional increase of 66% in thymidine uptake was noted (Figure 3). The additive effect of Li and the 24 hour preincubation resulted in a 130% increase of thymidine incorporation in Con A-stimulated lymphocytes.

EFFECTS OF LITHIUM ON IN VITRO RESPONSES TO MITOGENS IN LYMPHOCYTES FROM IMMUNOCOMPROMIZED INDIVIDUALS

Although the effects of Li on normal lymphocyte responses to mitogens was considerable (i.e. 40%-50% increases in (^{14}C) thymidine incorporation), we anticipated that the effects on abnormal lymphocytes would be even more marked.

Two individuals with clinical immunodeficiency, diminished number of T cells, and impaired lymphocyte responses to T cell mitogens were studied at various intervals of their disease. Their lymphocytes were stimulated by mitogens in the presence and absence of Li at a concentration of 2.5×10^{-3}M.

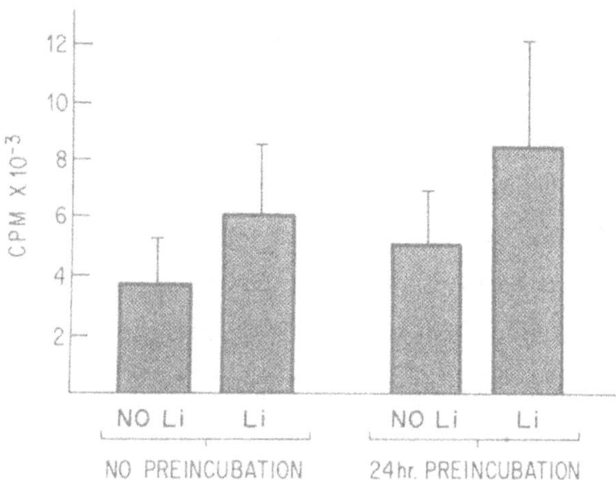

Figure 3. Effect of lithium on suppressor-deficient cultures. Con A (15µg/ml) was added at either 0 hours or after 24 hour pre-incubation. Cells were exposed to mitogen for 3.5 days and were labelled with ^{14}C-thymidine 16 hours before harvesting.

One individual demonstrated a 291% increase in response to Con A when Li was included in the lymphocyte culture (from 1844 ± 559 to 5370 ± 1409 cpm, mean ± S.E.). The second patient demonstrated a 217% increase in response to PHA with the addition of Li to the culture (2810 ± 836 to 6102 ± 1460). This latter patient was ultimately given a six-week trial of Li therapy. Prior to therapy, three determinations of T and B cell percentages and (^{14}C) thymidine incorporation to PHA were as follows: T cells: 41 ± 14% (mean ± S.D.); B cells: 41 ± 25%; thymidine uptake: 2849 ± 1024. The results of 8 determinations (mean ± S.D.) performed during Li therapy were as follows: T cells: 59 ± 6%; B cells: 11 ± 5%; thymidine uptake: 10,741 ± 3124. The highest serum Li concentration achieved in this patient was 0.7 mEq/L.

SUMMARY AND CONCLUSIONS

Lithium in concentrations readily achievable in humans affects human mononuclear cells in vitro and enhances the expression and various functions of these cells (Shenkman et al., 1978). Lithium increases macrophage phagocytosis of latex particles, active SRBC rosette formation, and normal lymphocyte proliferative responses to heterologous lymphocytes, antigens and mitogens. The latter effect is mediated by lithium's activity in both suppressor-enriched culture systems and in culture systems partially depleted of suppressor cell activity. Li has an even greater enhancing effect on the activity of lymphocytes derived from certain immunocompromised individuals. We postulate that Li's effects are a result of its known inhibitory action on adenylate cyclase systems and a consequent lowering of cellular C-AMP levels.

Activation of lymphoid cells is associated with a transient increase in C-AMP and a rapid return to normal levels within minutes (Wang et al., 1978). However, the addition of C-AMP analogues or progenitors to lymphocyte cultures is invariably accompanied by depression of lymphocyte transformation of T-cell expression (Hirschorn et al., 1970). It should be noted that these same inhibitory substances can be stimulatory at very low concentrations. This suggests that prolonged large increases in cell C-AMP levels inhibits lymphocyte responses (Wang et al., 1978), and that a substance capable of diminishing the duration and extent of the elevated C-AMP levels may enhance these responses.

Cell-cell interactions result in vectorial effects on responder lymphocytes. Thus, both "Helper" and "Suppressor" lymphocytes may exert effects on responder lymphocytes. Helper T cells have been shown to have an increased affinity for SRBC, while suppressor T cells have a decreased affinity for SRBC (West et al., 1976; Platsouchas et al., 1979). Agents which increase C-AMP levels cause suppressor T cells to dissociate from SRBC under optimal conditions for rosetting (Limatibul et al., 1978). Suppressor T cells may therefore have cell membranes that express enhanced mobility and diminished rosetting capabilities. Agents that increase C-AMP may also enhance membrane mobility, possibly by affecting the cell skeletal structure (i.e. microtubule dissociation).

Thus, Li's ability to increase active rosettes may be explained by its inhibition of adenylate cyclase with a resultant decrease in C-AMP levels, which in turn stabilizes cell surface membranes. If suppressor cell function is related to this postulated increase in cell membrane mobility, then perhaps Li is inhibiting suppressor cell function by decreasing cell membrane mobility.

Several additional observations support the view that Li acts to decrease suppressor cell function. First, Li counteracts the suppressive action of PGE_1 on lymphocyte proliferation. This observation is of particular interest in view of recent studies suggesting that specific receptors for prostaglandins of the E series are present in human peripheral blood mononuclear cells, and that these cells are probably T_γ cells (Bromberg et al., 1979). In addition, PGE_2-producing suppressor cells have been identified in some patients with Hodgkin's disease (Goodwin et al., 1977) and the presence of these cells may contribute to the depressed cellular immunity seen in these patients.

The ability of Li to counteract the effects of Con A-activated suppressor cells on lymphocyte response to PHA also suggests that Li is acting on the suppressor cell population. Finally, Li reverses the suppressive activity of serum from certain immunocompromised patients on the PHA response of normal lymphocytes. When serum from one of the immunodeficient patients reported here was added to normal lymphocyte populations, we observed a decrease in PHA response and an enhanced response to Con A. Since Gupta et al. (1978) have shown that suppressor cells respond preferentially to Con A, this suggests that this serum was increasing the activity of a suppressor cell population, with a resultant decrease in response to PHA. The addition of Li to these cultures restored to normal the response to PHA.

The observed enhancement of lymphocyte proliferation caused by Li in cultures partially depleted of suppressor cells indicates that Li may be affecting helper cells as well as suppressor cells.

Finally, the results of Li therapy in an immunocompromised individual suggest that Li may have a greater ability to enhance immune function in individuals with deranged immunoregulatory mechanisms than in normals. The normalization of B cell numbers as well as T cells implies that Li may also affect the regulation and expression of immunoglobulin-bearing cells.

ACKNOWLEDGEMENT

Louis Shenkman, M.D. is a recipient of a Career Scientist Award from the Irma T. Hirschl Trust.

REFERENCES

Al-Ibrahim, M.S., Chandra, R., Kishore, R., Valentine, F.T., and Lawrence, H.S., 1976, A micromethod for evaluating the phagocytic activity of human macrophages by ingestion of radio-labelled polystyrene particles, J. Immunol. Meth. 10:207.

Birnbaumer, L., Pohl, S.L., and Rodell, M., 1969, Adenyl cyclase in fat cells, J. Biol. Chem. 244:3468.

Bromberg, S., Goodwin, J.S., Peake, G.T., and Messner, R.P., 1979, Receptors for prostaglandin E on human peripheral blood mononuclear cells, Clin. Res. 27:321A.

Cohen, L., Holzman, R.S., Valentine, F.T., and Lawrence, H.S., 1976, Requirement of precommitted cells as targets for the augmentation of lymphocyte proliferation by leucocyte dialysates, J. Exp. Med. 143:791.

Dutton, R.W., 1972, Inhibitory and stimulatory effects of concanavalin A on the response of mouse spleen cell suspensions to antigen, I. Characterization of the inhibitory cell activity, J. Exp. Med. 136:1445.

Goodwin, J.S., Messner, R.P., Bankhurst, A.D., Peake, G.T., Saiki, J.H., and Williams, Jr., R.C., 1977, Prostaglandin-producing suppressor cells in Hodgkin's Disease, New Engl. J. Med. 297:963.

Gupta, S. and Good, R.A., 1978. Human T cell subsets in health and disease, in "Human Lymphocyte Differentiation: Its Application to Cancer," Inserim Symposium No. 8, (B. Serrou and C. Rosenfeld, Editors), p. 367, Elsevier/North Holland Biomedical Press.

Hirschhorn, R., Grossman, J. and Weissmann, G., 1970, Effect of cyclic 3', 5' - adenosine monophosphate and theophylline on lymphocyte transformation, Proc. Soc. Exp. Biol. Med. 133:1361.

Limatibul, S., Shore, A., Dosch, H-M. and Gelfand, E.W., 1978, Theophylline modulation of E-rosette formation: An indicator of T-cell maturation, Clin. Exp. Immunol. 33:503.

Murphy, D.L., Donnelly, B.S., and Moskowitz, J., 1973, Inhibition by lithium of prostaglandin E, and norepinephrine effects on cyclic adenosine monophosphate production in human platelets, Clin. Pharmacol. Ther. 14:810.

Platsoucas, C.D., Good, R.A., and Gupta, S., 1979, Separation of human T lymphocyte subpopulations by density gradient electrophoresis, Proc. Natl. Acad. Sci. 76, 1972.

Shenkman, L., Borkowsky, W., Holzman, R.S., and Shopsin, B., 1978, Enhancement of lymphocyte and macrophage function *in vitro* by lithium chloride, Clin. Immunol. Immunopathol. 10:187.

Shou, L., Schwartz, S., and Good, R., 1976, Suppressor cell activity after Concanavalin A treatment of lymphocytes from normal donors, J. Exper. Med. 143:1100.

Singer, I. and Rotenberg, D., 1973, Mechanisms of lithium action, New Engl. J. Med. 289:254.

Wang, T., Sheppard, J.R., and Foker, J.E., 1978, Rise and fall of cyclic AMP required for onset of lymphocyte DNA synthesis, Science, 201:155.

West, W.H., Payne, S.M., Weese, J.L., and Herberman, R.B., 1976, E-rosette forming affinity and the F_c receptor, J. Immunol. 119:548.

CHARACTERIZATION OF LITHIUM EFFECTS ON TWO ASPECTS OF T-CELL FUNCTION

E.W. Gelfand, R. Cheung, D. Hastings, and H-M. Dosch

Division of Immunology
Research Institute
Hospital for Sick Children
Toronto, Canada

There is increasing evidence that positive and negative feedback control mechanisms regulate the immune response. At the molecular level, candidates for these regulatory effects are the cyclic nucleotides. Although most of the studies demonstrating a role for these compounds have involved non-lymphoid tissues, cyclic nucleotides also appear to be important mediators in the regulation of a variety of specific lymphocyte functions. These functions include triggering of differentiation, expression of discrete receptor activities, lymphocyte proliferation, cytotoxicity, antibody production and the release of lymphokines (Strom *et al.*, 1977). We have examined the role of drugs known to involve cyclic nucleotide synthesis or degradation, in modulating the expression of different lymphocyte responses, and have investigated the potential of lithium as a putative blocker of membrane adenylate cyclase, to counter these effects. In this paper we will describe our studies of lithium effects on two aspects of T-cell function, namely the ability to express the receptor for sheep red blood cells (SRBC) and the proliferative response to a number of mitogens. In the accompanying paper, the effect of lithium on the expression of suppressor cell activity *in vitro* and *in vivo* will be discussed.

E-ROSETTE FORMATION

It is known that E-rosette formation by human T cells is inhibited by drugs that result in increased levels of cyclic AMP (Chisari and Edgington, 1974; Galant and Remo, 1975; Grieco et al., 1976). We have previously characterized the effects of one of these agents, theophylline, on E-rosette formation (Limatibul et al., 1978) and have extended these findings to show that, salbutamol, isoproterenol, and dibutyryl cyclic AMP also lead to a dose dependent inhibition of rosette formation (Gelfand et al., 1979).

As shown in Table I at a maximal inhibitory dose of each of the drugs, there was a 50-60% inhibition of E-rosette formation. If lithium was added 30 minutes prior to the addition of the drug there was virtually a complete reversal of the inhibitory effect in all cases except for dibutyryl cyclic AMP.

TABLE I

EFFECT OF LITHIUM ON E-ROSETTE FORMATION

	% Inhibition E-Rosette Formation* Lithium (5mM)	
	-	+
Control	0	0
Theophylline (5mM)	53	4
Salbutamol (100 μM)	52	2
Isoproterenol (100 μM)	50	0
Dibutyryl cAMP (100 μM)	57	55

*Means of three experiments

The time kinetics of these drug interactions are illustrated in Figure 1. In Figure 1A, we see that following 30 minute incubation of 5 mM theophylline at 37°C, a plateau is reached so that there is little additional inhibition with 120 minutes preincubation with the drug. Preincubation with lithium for as little as 5 minutes prior to the addition of theophylline is sufficient to abrogate the inhibitory activity. In contrast, once theophylline is added, lithium cannot reverse this effect. Similar results are shown for salbutamol (Figure 1B) and isoproterenol (Isuprel) (Figure 1C). In contrast, on no occasion could lithium prevent the dibutyryl cyclic AMP effect, even if added 60 minutes prior to the drug (Figure 1D).

This effect of lithium (like the effects of the drugs) was 37°C dependent. As shown in Table II, preincubation with lithium at 4°C did not result in abrogation of the theophylline-induced inhibition of E-rosette formation.

Additional studies were carried out to determine if lithium could prevent the drug induced inhibition of rosette formation by agents acting in different ways than those studied above. In these studies (Table III) we used isobutylmethylxanthine (IBMX), a calcium-independent inhibitor of phosphodiesterase activity, cholera toxin, a potent and direct stimulator of adenylate cyclase, the calcium ionophore A23187, and adenosine. Adenosine is a potent activator of adenylate cyclase in brain (Sattin and Rall, 1970), cultured human cell lines (Clark _et al._, 1974), bone cells (Peck _et al._, 1974) and lymphocytes (Wolberg _et al._, 1975). Lithium chloride or lithium carbonate were equally capable of reversing the activity of theophylline and IBMX. The reversal with IBMX was generally slightly less than with theophylline itself. Cholera toxin resulted in a dose dependent inhibition of E-rosette formation and this inhibition was reversible by lithium. At higher concentrations of the toxin, this reversal was incomplete. Lithium similarly was effective in reversing the adenosine-mediated inhibition of rosette formation but was incapable of reversing the ionophore-induced inhibition. These studies thus confirm that lithium is capable of interfering with the effects of drugs known to lead to an increase in intracellular levels of cyclic AMP, through adenylate cyclase

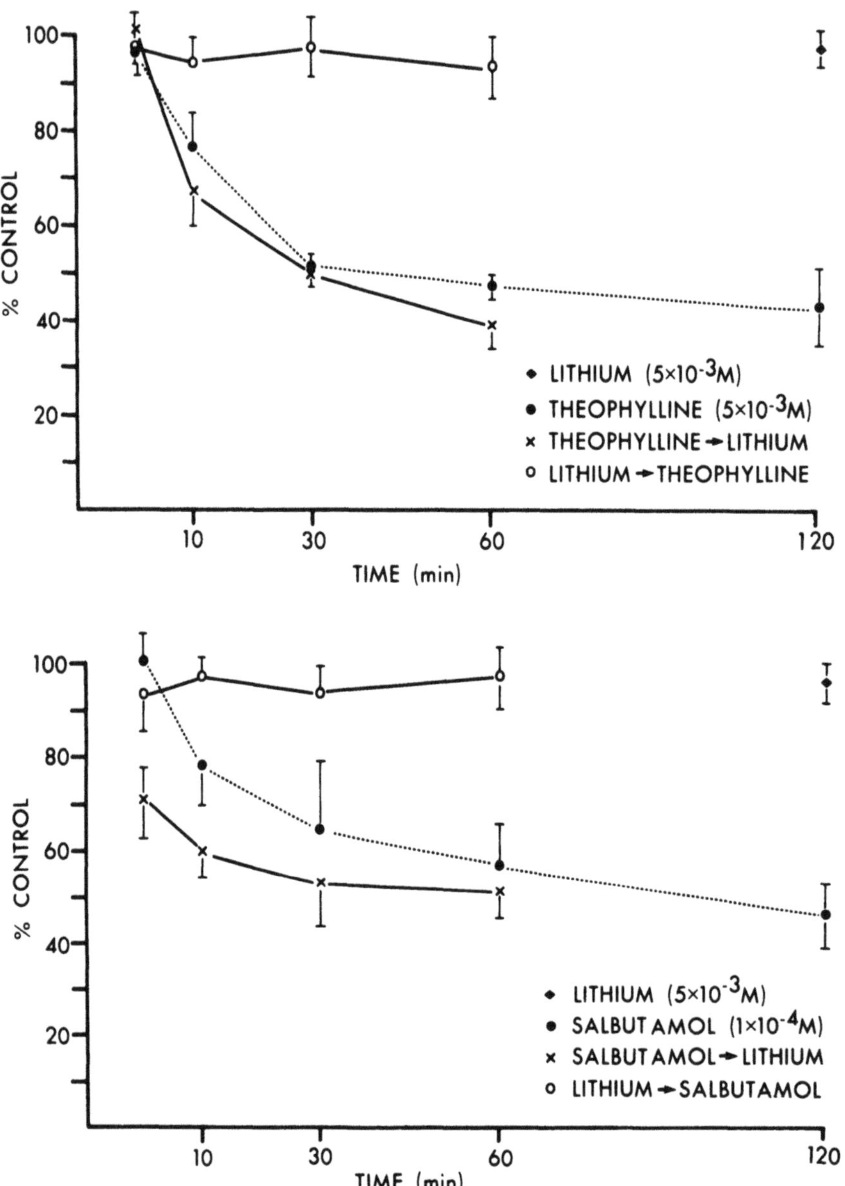

Figure 1. Lithium modulation of drug effects on E-rosette formation. A: Theophylline; B: Salbutamol; C: Isuprel; D: Dibutyryl cyclic AMP. The closed diamonds indicate incubation with lithium for 120 min. The closed circles indicate incubation with the drug for the indicated period prior to

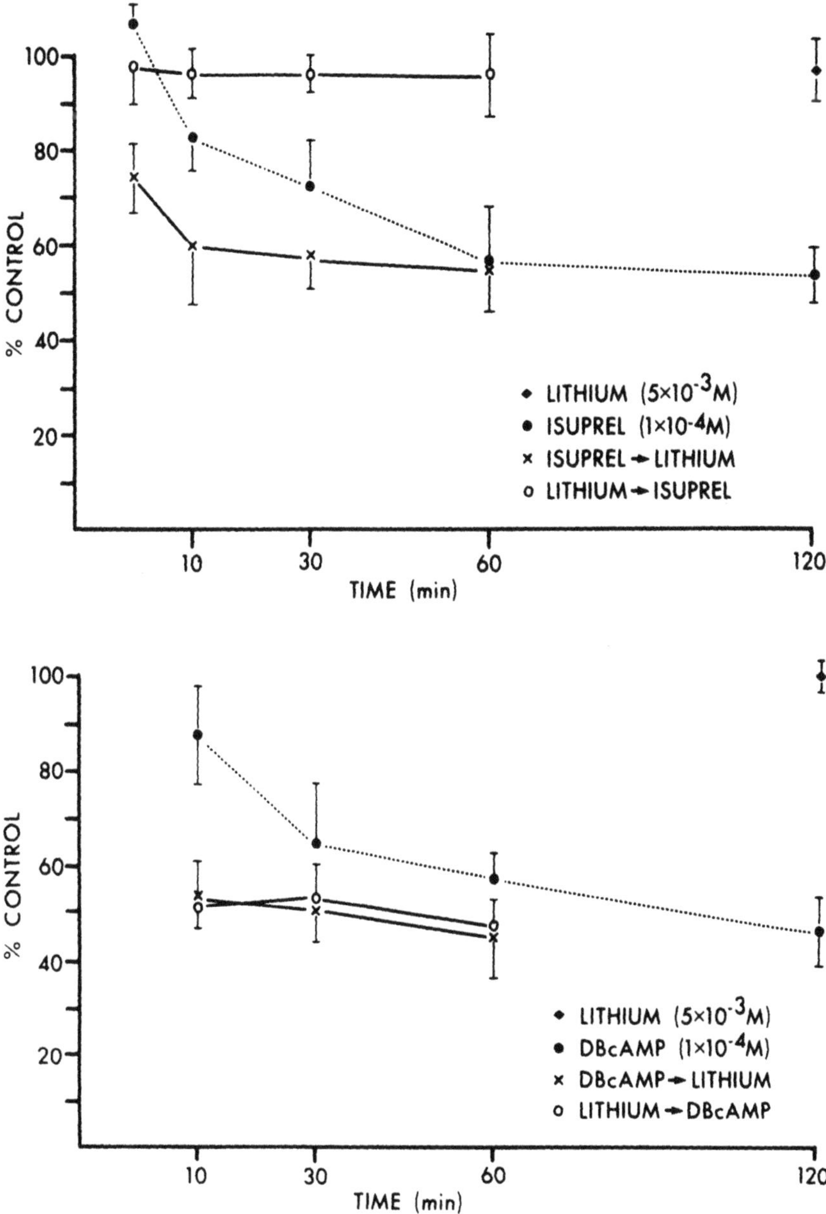

the addition of SRBC. X's indicate incubation with the drug for the indicated period of time followed by a 60 min incubation with lithium prior to the addition of SRBC. The open circles indicate incubation with lithium for the indicated period of time followed by a 60 min incubation with the drug prior to the addition of SRBC.

stimulation directly (cholera toxin, adenosine), by β-agonists (salbutamol, isoproterenol), or phosphodiesterase inhibition (theophylline, IBMX). Lithium could not reverse the inhibitory effects of dibutyryl cyclic AMP or the calcium ionophore A23187 which likely acts through adenylate cyclase-independent pathways. The lithium effects therefore appear to be somewhat specific to drugs involved in the synthesis or degradation of the cyclic nucleotides.

TABLE II

TEMPERATURE DEPENDENCE OF LITHIUM EFFECT ON E-ROSETTE FORMATION

	% Inhibition E-Rosette Formation*
Lithium (3mM) (37°C)	1
Theophylline (3mM) (37°C)	48
Lithium (4°C) → Theophylline (4°C)**	10
Lithium (4°C) → Theophylline (37°C)	41
Lithium (37°C) → Theophylline (37°C)	6

* Means of two experiments

** Incubations with lithium were for 5 minutes followed by the addition of theophylline and a further incubation period of 45 minutes prior to the addition of SRBC.

TABLE III

DRUG-INDUCED INHIBITION OF E-ROSETTE FORMATION

		% Inhibition E-Rosette Formation*		
		-	LiCl	Li_2CO_3
Theophylline (3mM)		47	0	0
IBMX (30 &M)		48	11	11
Cholera toxin	(20 ng/ml)	38	0	
	(200 ng/ml)	50	13	
	(2000 ng/ml)	59	17	
A23187	(0.05 µg/ml)	44	40	
Adenosine	(0.1 µM)	47	5	

*Means of three experiments.

An interesting aspect of the studies with adenosine was the comparison of lithium to theophylline in modulating the adenosine-induced inhibition. Classically, theophylline is thought to act via inhibition of phosphodiesterase, promoting cyclic AMP accumulation. It is now recognized that theophylline is an adenosine antagonist as well, with inhibition of adenosine-induced accumulation of cyclic AMP demonstrated in brain, erythrocytes, cultured cell lines, blood vessels (Clark and Seney, 1976; Wahl and Kuschinsky, 1976), lymphocytes (Schwartz et al., 1978) and mast cells (Marquardt et al., 1978). Adenosine resulted in a dose dependent inhibition of E-rosette formation (Table IV). Indeed at higher concentrations of adenosine the effect was less apparent. Low concentrations of theophylline (10^{-6}M), which themselves were unable to affect E-rosette formation (Limatibul et al., 1978), were capable of preventing the adenosine-mediated inhibition. This unique effect of theophylline to block the effect of adenosine was mirrored by lithium. Since it has been suggested that adenosine activates a particular pool of adenylate cyclase, at least within the membrane of turkey erythrocytes (Tolkovsky and Levitzki, 1978), our studies indicate that lithium as well as theophylline, can interfere with this activation.

TABLE IV
EFFECT OF ADENOSINE ON E-ROSETTE FORMATION

		% Inhibition E-Rosette Formation*		
		-	LiCl	Theophylline(10^{-6}M)
Adenosine	0.1 μM	49	0	0
	0.01 μM	16	0	0
	0.001 μM	12	0	0

*Means of three experiments

EFFECTS ON LYMPHOCYTE PROLIFERATION

Numerous studies have attempted to correlate or define a relationship between cyclic AMP levels and cell proliferation (Strom et al., 1977). It has generally been held that cyclic AMP can act as an inhibitor of cell division since agents which result in increased intracellular levels of cyclic AMP inhibit the multiplication of a variety of cultured cells (Johnson and Pastan, 1971; Sheppard, 1971). Following interaction with phytohemagglutinin (PHA) or concanavalin A, adenylate cyclase is activated and there appears to be a concomitant rise in intracellular cyclic AMP (Smith et al., 1971; Wang et al., 1978). Since one proposed mecnanism for lithium action is through inhibition of membrane adenylate cyclase (Singer and Rotenberg, 1973), we investigated the effect of lithium in PHA-induced proliferation of T-lymphocytes.

Addition of lithium at the same time, or up to 1 hour prior to the addition of PHA, resulted in a dose-dependent augmentation of ^{3}H-thymidine uptake. One such experiment is illustrated in Table V where optimal enhancement (approximately 60%) was observed with 5 mM lithium. Despite some variation between individuals and from one experiment to another, between 1-5 mM lithium regularly enhanced the PHA response with levels of enhancement ranging from 15-80%. Concentrations of lithium greater than 10 mM were inhibitory. The degree of enhancement often appeared greater at suboptimal concentrations of PHA. This effect of lithium was virtually eliminated if the addition of PHA was delayed to 4 hours or if PHA was added prior to lithium.

Lithium also consistently resulted in an increased response to other T-cell mitogens. In the experiments illustrated in Table VI, a 16-30% increase in response to PHA, concanavalin A, pokeweed and Staphylococcus aureus protein A was observed. Enhancement of the response to the B-cell mitogen, S. aureus (formalinized Cowan I Strain) was less apparent.

TABLE V

EFFECT OF LITHIUM ON PHA-INDUCED PROLIFERATION

Lithium Concentration (x 10^{-3}M)	^{3}H-Thymidine Uptake (cpm)*
-	68,400 ± 15,700
0.5	81,300 ± 17,100
1	88,500 ± 10,900
5	110,600 ± 41,700
10	83,400 ± 29,000
20	38,300 ± 10,900

*Means ± S.D. of two separate experiments.

Further studies considering potential differences of lithium on T versus B cell proliferative responses are currently underway. The addition of theophylline to the incubation mixture resulted in a dose dependent inhibition of proliferation (Figure 2). In the presence of lithium, there was a partial reversal of the theophylline-induced suppression of the response and the degree of reversal was dependent on the dose of theophylline. In the presence of theophylline however, we did not observe a lithium-induced augmentation of the PHA response.

TABLE VI

EFFECT OF LITHIUM ON MITOGEN-INDUCED PROLIFERATION

Mitogen	Lithium (5 mM)	cpm*	% Increase
Phytohemagglutinin	+	112.0	21
	-	92.4	
Concanavalin A	+	92.9	30
	-	71.5	
Pokeweed	+	28.8	21
	-	23.8	
S. aureus, Protein A	+	126.9	16
	-	109.1	
S. aureus, formalinized	+	31.5	8
	-	29.9	

*Mean counts per minute ^{3}H-thymidine uptake (x 10^{-3}) of triplicate cultures.

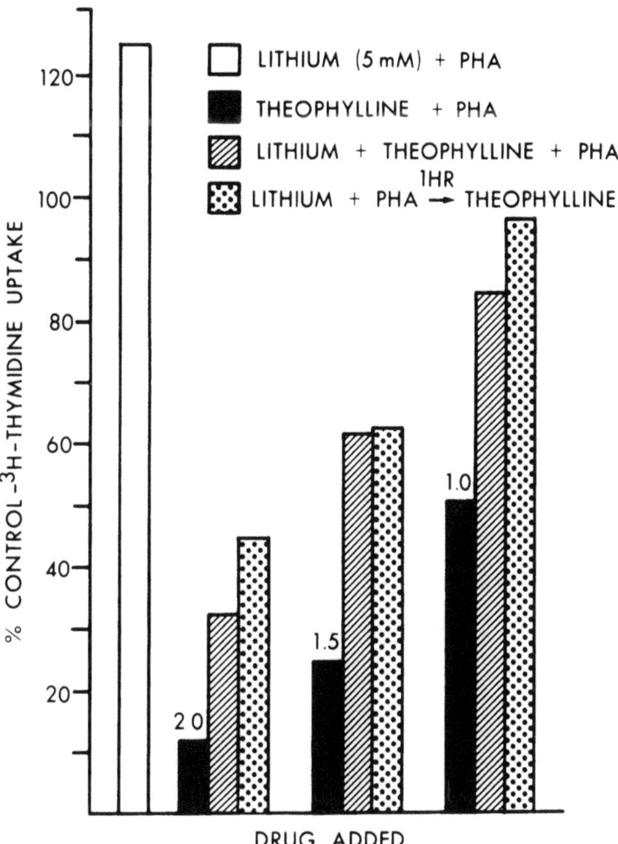

Figure 2. Modulation of the PHA response. Numbers above the solid bars refer to the concentration (mM) of theophylline added.

MECHANISM OF LITHIUM ACTION

Lithium has important effects in many different organ systems. In several of these systems it appears that lithium may interfere with cyclic AMP-mediated processes particularly those which are regulated by polypeptide hormones (Singer and Rotenberg, 1973). Thus, lithium has a profound effect on the secretion of hormones such as thyroid-stimulating hormone and vasopression. The biochemical mechanism(s) of action of lithium on human lymphocyte functions remain to be determined and it is uncertain whether all effects can be explained by a common event. Many of the effects in this and the companion paper appear to be in agreement with an effect at the level of adenylate cyclase blockade. Certainly the effects on lectin-induced proliferation, IgM secretion and interference with the expression of suppressor cell activity can not be mimicked by other monovalent cations, further supporting this hypothesis. However, in several systems monovalent cations can influence certain cellular events in parallel to lithium. For example, in a system measuring epinephrine-stimulated adenylate cyclase of glial cells, lithium enhanced the epinephrine effect (Schimmer, 1971). Sodium and potassium had similar effects with an order of potency Li > Na > K. In studies of ionic permeability of nerve membranes, it is now known that the sodium channel of the active nerve membrane is not exclusively permeable for sodium ions and that other ions can also move through this channel (Meves, 1970). The sequence of permeability proposed for the sodium channel of the active nerve membrane is Li > Na > K > Rb > Cs.

Since the sharing of physical and chemical properties with the biologically important Na^+ and K^+ may account for some of the biologic properties of lithium (Singer and Rotenberg, 1973), particularly in assays where rapid effects may be assessed, we studied the effects of monovalent and divalant cations on E-rosette formation. Surprisingly, we could show an effect using other monovalent cations on theophylline-induced inhibition of E-rosette formation. As shown in Table VII, preincubation (30 minutes) with lithium, sodium, and potassium could interfere with the theophylline-mediated inhibition of rosette formation. Cesium was much less effective and calcium and choline were ineffective. Thus, in this assay as well, there was a suggestion for the order of potency of Li > Na > K > Cs.

The efficacy of sodium in preventing many of the drug-induced effects is compared to lithium in Table VIII. Preincubation with 5 mM sodium chloride could prevent the theophylline or IBMX-induced inhibition as well as lithium, but was much less effective with salbutamol or adenosine. Both cations were ineffective with dibutyryl cyclic AMP or the calcium ionophore, A23187.

TABLE VII

EFFECT OF CATIONS ON THEOPHYLLINE-MEDIATED INHIBITION OF E-ROSETTE FORMATION

	% Inhibition E-Rosette Formation
Theophylline + 0	47
LiCl	12
NaCl	13
KCl	16
CsCl	36
$CaCl_2$	53
Choline	52

All reagents were used at a concentration of 5 mM in phosphate buffered saline. Results represent the means of two separate experiments.

TABLE VIII

COMPARISON OF LITHIUM AND SODIUM IN PREVENTING DRUG-INDUCED INHIBITION OF E-ROSETTE FORMATION

	% Inhibition E-Rosette Formation*		
	-	LiCl	NaCl
Theophylline	56	7	12
IBMX	50	0	3
Salbutamol	49	3	23
DBcAMP	43	47	49
Ionophore	50	52	49
Adenosine	53	0	25

*Means of two experiments

These findings, particularly with the xanthine derivatives, suggested that exceedingly small changes in osmolarity could prevent these drug induced effects. This was further examined by carrying out the E-rosette studies in the presence of increasing amounts of added water (Table IX). The addition of increasing amounts of water to the standard phosphate buffered saline (PBS) resulted in a progressive diminution in the ability of LiCl or NaCl to interfere with the theophylline-induced effect. With 500 &l added water (a 5% change in osmolarity), neither lithium nor sodium were effective. Thus small changes in osmolarity appeared to modulate many of the changes observed in our studies of E-rosette formation. The nature of these changes are currently being studied in an attempt to relate them to the changes observed in the assays of lymphocyte function.

TABLE IX

EFFECT OF SMALL CHANGES IN OSMOLARITY

	% E-Rosettes* 10 ml PBS			
	+ 100 μl H_2O	+ 200 μl H_2O	+ 300 μl H_2O	+ 500 μl H_2O
--	55			
Theophylline	29			
LiCl + Theophylline	54	48	33	27
NaCl + Theophylline	50	50	30	29

*Means of two experiments

PBS: Phosphate buffered saline

TABLE X

TIME DEPENDENCY OF THE CATION EFFECTS

	% E-Rosettes*				
Time (min)	0	15	60	120	150
NaCl	50	54	53	33	27
LiCl	52	56	52	41	29

Untreated = 52%

Theophylline = 27%

*Means of two experiments

These changes, induced by the monovalent cations and which may be related to simple shifts in osmolarity, were reversible with time. As shown in Table X, preincubation with either NaCl or LiCl for periods of time beyond 60 minutes prior to the addition of theophylline, tended to interfere with the capacity of the cations to prevent the theophylline-induced inhibition of rosette formation. These results may indicate that the cells have the capacity, with time, to adapt or readjust to the changes resulting from the addition of small amounts of salt. There was no effect of the addition of water on other assays of lymphocyte function including cell proliferation or the plaque-forming cell response.

SUMMARY

Cell surface receptors receive, transduce and relay a variety of environmental signals. These phenomena, which have been extensively characterized in non-lymphoid cells, also appear to play a crucial role in dictating the degree of lymphocyte responsiveness. The nature of these regulatory events is only beginning to be unraveled but the adenylate cyclase-cyclic AMP axis appears to be one of the important controlling systems. Lithium appears to be as important a modulator of lymphocyte responsiveness as previously shown for a variety of other cells and the mechanism of action, in general, is consistent with its role as a putative blocker of adenylate cyclase activation. Indeed, lithium may exert its role as a regulator of lymphocyte responsiveness by acting on specific lymphocyte subpopulations. Direct proof for this is still wanting and consideration of its capacity for action as an imperfect substitute for normal extra- or intracellular cations or on the physiochemical state of the plasma membrane is necessary. Nevertheless, these studies indicate the validity of using lithium for assessing the role of the lymphocyte adenylate cyclase-cyclic AMP system in the generation and expression of regulatory signals leading to modulation of the immune system.

ACKNOWLEDGEMENTS

This work was supported by grants from the Medical Research Council of Canada (MT4875), and the National Foundation, March of Dimes (6-190).

REFERENCES

Chisaro, F.V. and Edgington, T.S., 1974, Human T lymphocytes "E" rosette function, I. A progress modulated by intracellular cyclic AMP, J. Exp. Med. 140:1122.

Clark, R.B. and Seney, M.N., 1976, Regulation of adenylate cyclase from cultured human cell lines by adenosine, J. Biol. Chem., 251:4239.

Clark, R.B., Gross, R., Su, Y.F., and Perkins, J.P., 1974, Regulation of adenosine 3':5'-monophosphate content in human astrocytoma cells by adenosine and the adenine nucleotides, J. Biol. Chem., 249:5296.

Galant, S.P. and Remo, R.A., 1975, β-Adrenergic inhibition of human T lymphocyte rosettes, J. Immunol., 114:512.

Gelfand, E.W., Dosch, H-M., Hastings, D., and Shore, A., 1979, Lithium: A modulator of cyclic AMP-dependent events in lymphocytes, Science, 203:365.

Grieco, M.H., Siegel, I., and Goel, Z., 1976, Modulation of human T lymphocyte rosette formation by autonomic agonists and cyclic nucleotides, J. Allerg. Clin. Immunol., 58:149.

Johnson, G.S. and Pastan, I.H., 1971, Change in growth and morphology of fibroblasts by prostaglandins, J. Nat. Cancer Inst., 47:1357.

Limatibul, S., Shore, A., Dosch, H-M., and Gelfand, E.W., 1978, Theophylline modulation of E-rosette formation: An indicator of T-cell maturation, Clin. Exp. Immunol., 33:503.

Marquardt, D.L., Parker, C.W., and Sullivan, T.J., 1978, Potentiation of mast cell mediator release by adenosine, J. Immunol., 120:871.

Meves, H., 1970, The ionic permeability of nerve membranes, in "Permeability and Function of Biological Membranes," (L. Bolis, A. Katchalski, R.D. Keynes, W.R. Loewenstein, and B.A. Pethica, eds.), Elsevier, Amsterdam.

Peck, W.A., Carpenter, J., and Messinger, K., 1974, Cyclic 3',5'-adenosine monophosphate in isolated bone cells. II. Responses to adenosine and parathyroid hormone, Endocrinology, 94:148.

Sattin, A. and Rall, T.W., 1970, The effects of adenosine and adenine nucleotides on the cyclic adenosine 3'-5'-phosphate content of guinea pig cerebral cortex slices, Mol. Pharmacol., 6:13.

Schimmer, B.P., 1971, Effects of catecholamines and monovalent cations on adenylate cyclase activity in cultured glial tumor cells, Bioch. Biophys. Acta., 252:567.

Schwartz, A.L., Stern, R.C., and Polmar, S.H., 1978, Demonstration of an adenosine receptor on human lymphocytes in vitro and its possible role in the adenosine deaminase-deficient form of severe combined immunodeficiency, Clin. Immunol. Immunopath., 9:499.

Sheppard, J.R., 1971, Restoration of contact-inhibited growth to transformed cells by dibutyryl adenosine 3':5'-cyclic monophosphate, Proc. Nat. Acad. Sci., 68:1316.

Singer, I. and Rotenberg, D., 1973, Mechanisms of lithium action, New Eng. J. Med., 289:254.

Smith, J.W., Steiner, A.L., Newberry, W.M., and Parker, C.W., 1971, Cyclic adenosine 3',5'-monophosphate in human lymphocytes, Alterations after phytohemagglutinin stimulation, J. Clin. Invest., 50:432.

Strom, T.B., Lundin, A.P., and Carpenter, C.B., 1977, The role of cyclic nucleotides in lymphocyte activation and function, Progr. Clin. Immunol., 3:115.

Tolkovsky, A.M. and Levitzki, A., 1978, Coupling of a single adenylate cyclase to two receptors: Adenosine and catecholamine, Biochemistry, 17:3811.

Wahl, M. and Kuschinsky, W., 1976, The dilatory action of adenosine on pial arteries of cats and its inhibition by theophylline, Pflueger's Arch., 362:55.

Wang, T., Sheppard, J.R., and Foker, J.E., 1978, Rise and fall of cyclic AMP required for onset of lymphocyte DNA synthesis, Science, 201:155.

Wolberg, G., Zimmerman, T.P., Hiemstra, K., Winston, M., and Chu, L.C., Adenosine inhibition of lymphocyte-mediated cytolysis: Possible role of cyclic adenosine monophosphate, Science, 187:957.

ANTI-SUPPRESSOR CELL EFFECTS OF LITHIUM *IN VITRO* AND *IN VIVO*

Hans-Michael Dosch, David Matheson,
Ruud K.B. Schuurman, and Erwin W. Gelfand

Division of Immunology
Research Institute
Hospital for Sick Children
Toronto, Ontario M5G 1X8
Canada

Studies of cellular immunity have recently begun to unravel a highly complex network of regulatory events in which a particular effector function is shown to represent the net result of multiple cell interactions which are modulated by antigenic experience, genetic restrictions, polyclonal effects, and, probably, nutritional and hormonal factors. Because of its complexity and ability to accomodate external and internal stimuli in an adaptive learning fashion, the immune network has been compared to the central nervous system (Jerne, 1974).

We have concentrated on the human immune system, using normal lymphocytes and tissues from patients with immune deficiency (Gelfand *et al.*, 1974). Similar to the central nervous system, diminished or absent immune responsiveness may either reflect the absence of a required cell-type or function, or alternatively, may be due to regulative events with a negative net outcome, i.e. the suppression of response. In view of the growing list of diseases where faulty immune regulation has been invoked

(Gelfand and Dosch, 1979; Waldmann et al., 1979), the understanding of the regulatory circuits involved and their cellular and molecular requirements is prerequisite for rational attempts at manipulation of these immunoregulatory abnormalities.

Antigen specific, hemolytic plaque forming cell (PFC) responses have been utilized to study different categories of human regulatory T-cells in vitro (reviewed in Dosch and Gelfand, 1979a): A) Suppressor cell activity generated in PFC cultures at supraoptimal concentrations of antigens (Dosch et al., 1979). These are suppressor cells which interfere with the development of an immune response in an antigen specific fashion. B) Spontaneous suppressor T-cells, directly interfering with immunoglobulin secretion in previously generated PFC (end point suppression) (Dosch and Gelfand, 1978). These were detected in freshly drawn peripheral blood lymphocytes (PBL) from several patients with antibody deficiency syndromes (Gelfand and Dosch, 1979).

In both experimental systems, cell-cell interactions were defined and in both cases suppressor activity was mediated by the small theophylline-sensitive T-lymphocyte subset (Limatibul et al., 1979a).

We have begun to characterize the interacting cell populations and some of their functional, antigenic and biochemical requirements. In some of these studies we made use of the knowledge that the adenylate cyclase/cyclic AMP system plays an important role in the translation or transmission of regulatory signals between interacting cells, including those of the immune system (Teh and Paetkau, 1974; Cook et al., 1975). Utilizing β-agonists and lithium as probes, we found that both the antigen-induced activities of regulatory T-cells in culture and the spontaneous suppression of immunoglobulin secretion mediated by lymphocytes from certain patients appear to involve an activation of the adenylate cyclase/cyclic AMP system. In the latter case, the ability of lithium to interfere with spontaneous suppressor cell activity has now resulted in the initiation of a phase I clinical trial in appropriate patients.

EXPERIMENTAL APPROACH

Specific in vitro PFC Responses

All procedures have been described in detail (Dosch, et al., 1977; Dosch and Gelfand, 1978; Dosch and Gelfand, 1979a; Dosch et al., 1979). Cultures of 3 x 10^6 Ficoll-Hypaque separated mononuclear cells in 10 ml serum-supplemented RPMI-1640 received an optimal concentration of antigen (e.g. 0.1 μg ovalbumin (OA)) at the beginning of culture. Following 5-7 days of incubation, cells were washed and aliquots were assayed for direct hemolytic plaques on poly-L-lysine coupled monolayers of antigen-coated erythrocytes in microtest-II-plates (Dosch and Gelfand, 1977).

Antigen Induced Suppressor Activity (AISA)

Mononuclear cells from various tissues or lymphocyte subpopulations purified by rosette depletion techniques (Shore et al., 1978; Dosch et al., 1979; Schuurman et al., 1979a) were cultured in the presence of supraoptimal antigen concentrations (e.g. 100 μg OA) whereas control cultures received optimal amounts (Dosch and Gelfand, 1977; Dosch and Gelfand, 1979a). Following 5-6 days of incubation the cells were thoroughly washed and the numbers of specific PFC generated were compared to optimally stimulated cultures. Under these conditions decreased responses have been shown to reflect antigen induced T-suppressor cell activity (Shore et al., 1978). In some experiments purified lymphocyte preparations were incubated with the high antigen dose for only 20 hours ("primed"), washed and added to optimally stimulated target cultures with similar results (Dosch et al., 1979).

Spontaneous Suppressor Cell Activity (SSA)

PFC, generated at optimal antigen concentrations were harvested on day 5 or 6 of culture, washed and assayed as described. Aliquots of these cells, containing a constant, known number of PFC (e.g. 80 per individual assay) were then used in the spontaneous suppressor cell (SSA) assay (Dosch and Gelfand, 1978). Increasing numbers (1-100 x 10^3) of fresh PBL, obtained from patients with antibody deficiency or from normal controls were mixed with these PFC prior to their assay for PFC activity. In this report SSA is expressed as the number of PFC in these mixtures which remained active (Gelfand and Dosch, 1979).

Patients Studied

Five patients with congenital agammaglobulinemia (Aγ) and 17 with common variable immunodeficiency (CVID) were studied. The majority of these patients have been described (Dosch et al., 1977; Dosch and Gelfand, 1978; Gelfand and Dosch, 1979). All patients with Aγ lacked circulating immunoglobulin bearing B-lymphocytes and plasma cells in lymphoid tissue. In contrast, CVID patients were heterogeneous with respect to the presence or absence of B-lymphocytes and serum immunoglobulin but all showed a deficiency of specific antibody formation. All patients were studied while receiving gammaglobulin replacement therapy and in the absence of acute infection.

RESULTS AND DISCUSSION

Antigen Induced Suppressor Cell Activity (AISA)

We have previously observed that the specific in vitro PFC response of human lymphocytes is largely dependent on the antigen concentration present in culture (Dosch and Gelfand, 1977). Thus, high concentrations of SRBC were found to abrogate the development of SRBC-specific PFC and high concentrations of soluble antigens, such as ovalbumin (OA), interfered with the generation of optimal responses to these antigens (Dosch et al., 1977; Dosch and Gelfand, 1979). This effect was found to be specific for the inducing antigen and was later shown to reflect the presence of suppressor cells which were activated in an antigen dose dependent fashion early during culture (Shore et al., 1978; Dosch et al., 1979). The cellular origin of AISA has been characterized in cell separation studies where aliquots of the purified populations were primed with 100 μg OA for 20 hours until added to target cultures of 3×10^6 autologous PBL (Dosch et al., 1979). AISA is mediated by a non-adherent, E-rosette forming and theophylline-sensitive (T-sens) T-lymphocyte subpopulation (see below, Table IV).

AISA appears to reflect a fairly mature T-cell function. When different normal tissues were studied, suppressor activity could easily be demonstrated in PBL and peripheral lymphoid tissues. Cell dilution experiments suggested that PBL are especially rich in antigen recruitable suppressor cell precursors. In contrast, bone marrow proved to be a poor source of these cells and virtually none were found among thymocytes. In an attempt to obtain insight into the biochemical pathways involved in the generation and expression of AISA, we utilized theophylline and lithium. These agents were chosen since both have been found to affect the same human T-cell subset which mediates AISA, presumeably via modulation of the T-cell adenylate cyclase/cyclic AMP system (Gelfand et al., 1979c). As described in our preceding report in this volume (Gelfand et al., 1979a), a clearcut antagonism was delineated between theophylline and lithium with respect to both surface receptor modulation on theophylline-sensitive T-lymphocytes and mitogen induced T-cell proliferation.

Theophylline and/or lithium (chloride or carbonate) were added to cultures of PBL or tonsil cells together with a high antigen concentration (100 μg OA) for the generation of AISA (Table I). In the experiment shown the optimal anti-OA PFC response (1890 ± 250 PFC/culture) was found at an antigen dose of 0.3 μg OA and, as expected, at 100 μg OA significant suppression was observed (380 ± 50 PFC/culture). To our surprise both lithium and theophylline interfered with this antigen-induced suppression permitting the generation of near optimal responses when either lithium or theophylline was present. Furthermore, in cultures containing both drugs, their effects seemed additive and certainly not antagonistic. This abrogation of high dose antigen-induced suppression could reflect the failure of development and/or expression of suppressor cell activity itself or the protection of differentiating PFC precursor B-lymphocytes from suppressor cells. The effects of lithium and theophylline were dose dependent. At concentrations of ≥ 1 mM lithium and ≥ 1-3 mM theophylline, cell survival and PFC responses were often found to decline. No consistent antagonism for this conceivably toxic effect could be delineated between lithium and theophylline.

The mechanism underlying the additive effect of lithium and theophylline on AISA is unclear but the results suggest that the adenylate cyclase/cyclic AMP system may play a role during the induction or expression of AISA. Attempts to demonstrate significant alterations in culture of intracellular cyclic AMP levels have not been successful so far. However, this does not rule out such an effect in a small cell population such as antigen-triggered suppressor cells (Dosch et al., 1979). This view is reinforced by the preliminary finding that low concentrations of salbutamol and dibutyryl cAMP have the same effects as theophylline.

TABLE I

PHARMACOLOGIC MODULATION OF AISA*

	Theophylline (3×10^{-4}M)	
Lithium	–	+
------	380 ± 50	1170 ± 110
10 μM	810 ± 70	1790 ± 90
100 μM	1970 ± 160	2650 ± 180
3.0 mM	590 ± 370	640 ± 460

* PFC response/culture ($\bar{x}$ ± 1 S.D.)

Table I. AISA was induced in cultures of 3×10^6 tonsil cells with a high antigen dose (100 μg OA). Lithium and/or theophylline were added just prior to the addition of antigen. Results are expressed as PFC response/culture ($\bar{x}$ ± 1 S.D.). The optimal control response was 1890 ± 250 PFC per culture containing 0.3 μg OA.

The target cells manifesting the lithium and/or theophylline effects are unknown and studies are underway to establish whether kinetic differences between the action of the two agents can be delineated. Furthermore, it should be noted that for the effects on receptor modulation the lithium/theophylline antagonism appears to be rather short lived and disappears after several hours of incubation (Gelfand _et al._, 1979a; Gelfand _et al._, 1979c). This could apply similarly to T-cell mitogen-induced proliferation where the induction of cell triggering occurs very rapidly, within minutes of interaction between mitogen and T-lymphocyte. If the effects of both agents are mediated through elevated intracellular levels of cyclic AMP in susceptible lymphocyte populations, then one possible result of this elevation may be interference with cell division via inhibition of ribonucleotide reductase (Gelfand _et al._, 1979b); with their requirement for rapid cycles of cell division early in culture (Dosch _et al._, 1979), antigen triggered T-sens may be very susceptible to such a mechanism.

Spontaneous Suppressor Cell Activity (SSA)

In vitro PFC responses have been studied in patients with a variety of primary immune deficiency disorders (Gelfand and Dosch, 1979; Dosch and Gelfand, 1979a). One surprising finding was the consistent generation of lower but nonetheless significant PFC responses in certain patients with antibody deficiency, including agammaglobulinemia (Dosch _et al._, 1977). Since the development of PFC in patients could be prevented by altering culture conditions and addition of T-cell mitogens, attempts were made to circumvent tissue culture.

A short-term assay was developed for the detection of spontaneous suppressor cell activity (SSA) in fresh patient PBL which exploits the following observation: plaque forming activity of generated PFC is abrogated when they were mixed with appropriate fresh patient (but not normal) PBL just prior to the hemolytic plaque assay (Dosch and Gelfand, 1978). Extensive studies have been performed to characterize the mode of action, cellular and functional requirements of SSA (Dosch and Gelfand,

1978). The data indicated a) that SSA is mediated by a small, theophylline-sensitive T-cell subset; b) that it demonstrated a requirement for direct cell-cell contact at 37°C; c) that suppression was reversible (and thus not directly cytotoxic); and d) suppression appeared non-specific, since PFC from different donors and specific for different antigens were suppressed equally. However, suppression appeared restricted to B-cells since other secretory phenomena, such as histamine release, were unaffected.

TABLE II

PHARMACOLOGICAL ENHANCEMENT OF SSA

Fresh PBL added	PFC/well			
-----	82 ± 4.9	68 ± 4.4	76 ± 4.0	26 ± 4.4
Normal	81 ± 5.0	70 ± 3.9	75 ± 4.3	24 ± 3.1
Aγ	39 ± 3.9	11 ± 2.1	10 ± 0.9	<2
Aγ	44 ± 3.7	9 ± 1.2	11 ± 1.1	<2
CVID	42 ± 4.3	10 ± 1.0	9 ± 0.7	<2
Salbutamol (M)	----	3×10^{-7}	----	3×10^{-7}
Theophylline (M)	----	----	3×10^{-5}	3×10^{-5}

Table II. Normal OA specific PFC ($82 \pm 4.9/2.2 \times 10^4$ cultured cells) were mixed with fresh PBL from a normal donor or patients with Aγ or CVID in the presence or absence of the drugs indicated. A number of fresh PBL was chosen where patient cells suppressed approximately half of the PFC ($1\text{-}4 \times 10^4$/well).

The expression of SSA was studied with pharmacological probes known to modulate the adenylate cyclase/cyclic AMP system. In Table II, fresh PBL from three SSA-positive patients with Aγ or CVID were mixed with anti-OA PFC which had been generated during 5 days in culture as described above. A concentration of patient PBL was chosen where approximately half of the PFC were suppressed. Fresh normal PBL served as controls. As shown, the addition to these cell mixtures of low concentrations of salbutamol or theophylline resulted in enhancement of suppressor cell activity. When both drugs were added, their effects were synergistic. Salbutamol, particularly in the presence of theophylline, interfered with hemolytic plaque formation even in the absence of patient cells, i.e. of SSA. This inhibition occurred at the level of PFC since control experiments demonstrated that the complement-mediated lysis of erythrocytes used in the plaque assay were unaffected by drugs. Theophylline alone had no consistent effect on plaque formation alone whereas it induced a significant enhancement of SSA.

Lithium completely abrogated SSA without any detectable effect on plaque formation itself (Table III). This effect was dose dependent and maximal at a concentration of 0.1 - 1.0 mM. Furthermore, when lithium was tested together with salbutamol and theophylline, it abrogated both the direct inhibitory drug effects in SSA-free controls and the drug-induced enhancement of SSA.

These data indicated an active regulatory role of the adenylate cyclase/cyclic AMP system for IgM secretion by PFC as well as for the expression of SSA by fresh patient PBL. These conclusions were confirmed in experiments where the analogue dibutyryl-3', 5'-cyclic AMP (DBcAMP) was tested. As shown (Figure 1), DBcAMP had a direct inhibitory effect on PFC activity (in the absence of SSA). As well, it enhanced SSA of patient PBL. In contrast to theophylline or salbutamol, this activity was not blocked in the presence of lithium, suggesting that lithium did not interfere with the effect of the cyclic nucleotide once generated or added.

The drug-induced enhancement of SSA may reflect an increase either in efficiency of suppressor cells or in susceptibility of PFC. Similarily, lithium may protect target PFC not only from drug-induced inhibition, but, in addition, from SSA or, alternatively, it may directly block the activity of suppressor cells. Thus, although the drug effects appear clear, the target cells of drugs and lithium are as unclear as their role in the studies of AISA. As summarized in Table IV, AISA and SSA may involve different

TABLE III

PHARMACOLOGICAL MODULATION OF SSA: EFFECT OF LITHIUM

Fresh PBL added	PFC/well					
-----	82 ± 4.9	84 ± 4.1	83 ± 3.7	80 ± 3.3	26 ± 4.4	76 ± 5.2
Normal	81 ± 5.0	82 ± 3.5	85 ± 5.2	84 ± 3.9	24 ± 3.1	78 ± 4.7
Aγ	39 ± 3.9	80 ± 4.7	73 ± 4.3	43 ± 3.6	<2	74 ± 5.1
Aγ	44 ± 3.7	79 ± 3.0	78 ± 5.0	49 ± 5.7	<2	69 ± 3.8
CVID	42 ± 4.3	79 ± 4.4	72 ± 4.8	43 ± 5.2	<2	68 ± 4.9
LiCl (M)	----	1×10^{-3}	1×10^{-4}	1×10^{-5}	----	1×10^{-3}
Salbutamol (M)	----	----	----	----	3×10^{-7}	3×10^{-7}
Theophylline (M)	----	----	----	----	3×10^{-5}	3×10^{-5}

Table III. Normal OA specific PFC ($82 \pm 4.9/2.2 \times 10^4$ cultured cells) were mixed with fresh PBL from a normal donor or patients with Aγ or CVID in the presence or absence of the drugs indicated. A number of fresh PBL was chosen where patient cells suppressed approximately half of the PFC ($1\text{-}4 \times 10^4$/well).

events and/or cell populations. Our studies emphasize the complexity of the regulatory events investigated. In addition, they delineate the potential that such agents may provide as probes for unraveling complex cell interactions in normals and patients with immunological disorders.

TABLE IV

COMPARISON OF AISA AND SSA

	Cell Separation Studies			Functional Studies	
	AISA	SSA		AISA	SSA
PBL	+	+	Normal Cells	+	-
AC	-	-	Aγ/CVID	+	+*
non AC	+	+	Culture		
E^+	+	+	Specificity	+	-
E^-	-	-	Cell-cell contact	-	+
T-sens	+	+	Theophylline		
T-res	-	-	Lithium		

* 2/3 of patients tested

Table IV. Cellular requirements and properties of AISA and SSA are compared utilizing results of cell separation experiments and functional studies. Detailed descriptions are referred to in the text. Abbreviations: PBL, peripheral blood lymphocytes; AC, plastic adherent mononuclear cells from PBL; non AC, adherent cell depleted PBL; E^+, purified E-rosette forming lymphocytes; E^-, E-rosette depleted (non T-) cells; T-sens, theophylline sensitive T-cells; T-res, theophylline resistant T-cells.

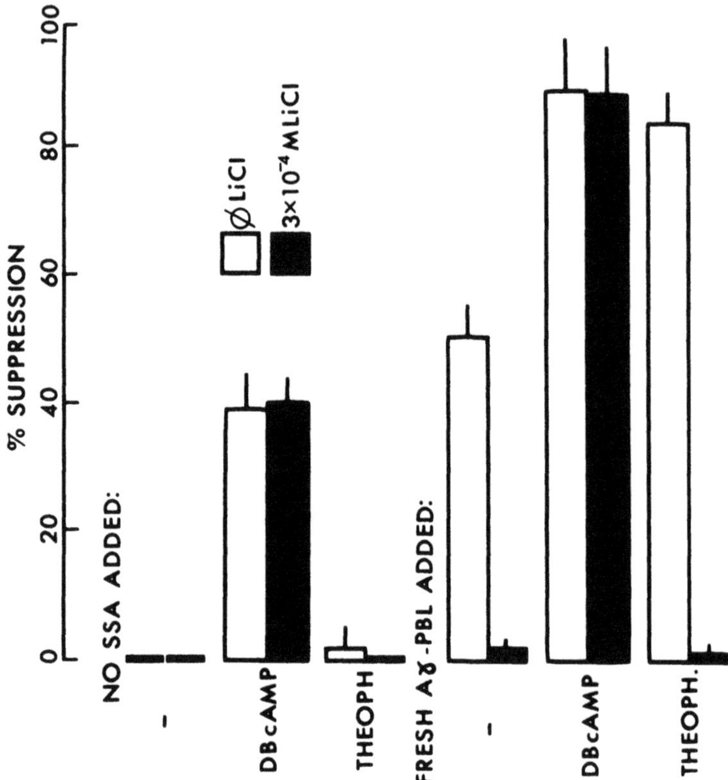

Figure 1. Differential effect of lithium on the drug-induced enhancement of SSA. Dibutyryl-3', 5'-cAMP (DBcAMP, 1×10^{-7}M) or theophylline (1×10^{-4}M) were added to PFC assays in the presence or absence of SSA (fresh PBL from a patient with Aγ). Lithium (3×10^{-4}M) abrogates theophylline effects and SSA itself but fails to alter DBcAMP effects.

Lithium Therapy in Patients with SSA

SSA was consistently found in more than 2,000 assays over a 30-month follow-up study of the positive patients (Dosch and Gelfand, 1978). On all occasions tested, lithium effectively inhibited SSA. About 60% of our patients with Aγ and CVID belonged to this group, but the number is small and preliminary studies on patients from other centres suggest that, overall, a somewhat larger proportion of patients with antibody deficiency may be expected in the PFC- and SSA-negative group (Gelfand and Dosch, 1979).

On the basis of our findings, a phase-I clinical trial was initiated in an attempt to institute B-cell maturation and function *in vivo*. Preliminary observations in patient MT, a 15 year old male with the X-linked form of congenital Aγ are summarized in Table V. Prior to lithium therapy, no surface immunoglobulin (sIg) positive lymphocytes or plasma cells had been found on numerous occasions in peripheral blood, bone marrow or a lymph node biopsy. T-lymphocytes were normal in number and for a variety of functions. In contrast, there was no proliferative response to the B-cell mitogen STA (formalinized *Staph. aureus*) whereas the proliferative response to the T-cell mitogen, soluble Protein A (SpA), was unimpaired (Schuurman *et al.*, 1979b).

TABLE V

EFFECT OF LITHIUM ADMINISTRATION

Date	Serum Level Lithium meq/L	SpA	STA	sIgM	SSA
		cpm		%	
Mar 7	0	99,000	600	0	+++
Mar 14	0.21	94,000	2,400	0.1	+
Mar 21	0.34	85,000	3,700	0.3	(±)
Mar 28	0.36	91,000	5,000	2.9	-
Apr 4	0.18	102,000	5,900	5.4	-
May 9	0.20	92,000	4,800	4.7	-

Table V. A 15 year old male patient with the X-linked form of congenital Aγ (Bruton type) and positive SSA in his fresh peripheral blood was treated with oral lithium carbonate. Serum lithium levels are indicated. Results of proliferative responses to a T-cell mitogen (SpA) and a B-cell mitogen (STA), are compared to the proportions of sIgM positive cells and the detection of spontaneous suppressor cell activity (SSA) in PBL.

Lithium therapy was initiated with a low dose (150 mg/d) aiming for serum levels of $\leq$ 0.5 meq/liter since in vitro effects were still optimal at only 0.1 mM (Table III). After two weeks of therapy low numbers of sIg positive B-cells appeared in peripheral blood together with a proliferative response to STA. In parallel a significant fall in SSA was noted, which continued until SSA was no longer detectable. By this time, close to normal numbers of sIg bearing B-lymphocytes were found, mostly expressing sIgM and sIgD. Significant changes in serum levels of IgM, IgE or IgA have not been observed so far. Since the patient remains on gammaglobulin replacement therapy, IgG levels may be less reliable indicators but no unusual elevations were noted and we have only just begun active immunization.

Although these observations are encouraging, the ultimate goal, i.e. the development of antibody production in vivo, has not been achieved so far. However, the time requirements for this development and the effect of the concomittant gammaglobulin replacement therapy are unknown. Our earlier conclusion, that even in congenital Aγ, certain (SSA-positive) patients may possess populations of precursor B-lymphocytes, able to complete at least certain stages of differentiation, has been confirmed in this patient. One further patient with this form of agammaglobulinemia, entered recently into the lithium trial, has shown similar results.

If the rationale derived from in vitro studies of SSA and drug/lithium effects is correct, then these preliminary observations may reinforce the concept that abnormal T-suppressor lymphocytes (SSA) could play a perpetuating role in certain antibody deficiency syndromes (Dosch et al., 1977; Gelfand and Dosch, 1979). The efficacy of anti-suppressor cell therapy with litnium and the inherent functionality of B-lymphoid cells will require further study. However, these findings do suggest that lithium or similar agents are useful probes for the study of immunoregulatory circuits and provide promising approaches in clinical therapy for the selective modulation of adverse immune reactivities.

ACKNOWLEDGEMENTS

This work was supported by the Medical Research Council of Canada (MT-4875) and the National Foundation, March of Dimes.

REFERENCES

Cook, R.G., Stavitsky, A.B., Schoenberg, M.D., 1975, Regulation of the in vitro early anamnestic antibody response by exogenous cholera enterotoxin and cyclic AMP, J. Immunol. 114:426.

Dosch, H-M. and Gelfand, E.W., 1977, Generation of human plaque-forming cells in culture: tissue distribution, antigenic and cellular requirements, J. Immunol. 118:302.

Dosch, H-M. and Gelfand, E.W., 1978, Functional differentiation of B-lymphocytes in agammaglobulinemia. III. Characterization of spontaneous suppressor cell activity, J. Immunol. 121:2097.

Dosch, H-M. and Gelfand, E.W., 1979a, Specific in vitro IgM response of human B-cells: A complex regulatory network modulated by antigen, Immunol. Rev. 45:242.

Dosch, H-M. and Gelfand, E.W., 1979b, Antigen-induced regulation of the PFC response in man, in "In vitro Induction and Measurements of Antibody Synthesis in Man" (A.S. Fauci, R.E. Ballieux, eds.), pp. 121, Academic Press, New York.

Dosch, H-M., Percy, M.E., and Gelfand, E.W., 1977, Functional differentiation of B-lymphocytes in congenital agammaglobulinemia. I. Generation of hemolytic plaque forming cells, J. Immunol. 119:1959.

Dosch, H-M., Shore, A., and Gelfand, E.W., 1979, Regulation of the specific PFC-response in man: Restraint of B-cell responsiveness, Eur. J. Immunol., in press.

Gelfand, E.W., Biggar, W.D., and Orange, R.P., 1974, Immunological deficiency: Evaluation, diagnosis and therapy, Ped. Clin. N. Amer. 21:745.

Gelfand, E.W., Cheung, R., Hastings, D., and Dosch, H-M., 1979a, Characterization of lithium effects on two aspects of T-cell function, (This volume).

Gelfand, E.W. and Dosch, H-M., 1979, In vitro function heterogeneity of cellular and humoral immune deficiency states, in "In vitro Induction and Measurements of Antibody Synthesis in Man" (A.S. Fauci, R.E. Ballieux, eds.), pp 309, Academic Press, New York.

Gelfand, E.W., Lee, J.J.W., and Dosch, H-M., 1979b, Selective toxicity of purine deoxynucleosides for human lymphocyte growth and function, Proc. Natl. Acad. Sci. USA. 76:1998.

Gelfand, E.W., Dosch, H-M., Hastings, D., and Shore, A., 1979c, Lithium: A modulator of cyclic AMP-dependent events in lymphocytes?, Science 203:365.

Jerne, N.K., 1974, Towards a network theory of the immune system, Ann. Immunol. 125c:373.

Limatibul, S., Shore, A.H., Dosch, H-M, and Gelfand, E.W., 1978, Theophylline modulation of E-rosette formation: An indicator of T-cell maturation, Clin. Exp. Immunol. 33:503.

Schuurman, R.K.B., Gelfand, E.W., Matheson, D., Zimmerman, B., and Dosch, H-M., 1979a, Identification of Ia on a subpopulation of human T-lymphocytes which stimulate in a mixed lymphocyte reaction, J. Immunol. Submitted.

Schuurman, R.K.B., Dosch, H-M., and Gelfand, E.W., 1979b, Polyclonal activation of human lymphocytes in vitro. I. Characterization of a B-cell mitogen in normals and immunodeficient patients, J. Immunol, Submitted.

Shore, A., Dosch, H-M., and Gelfand, E.W., 1978, Induction and separation of antigen-dependent T-helper and T-suppressor cells in man, Nature 274:586.

Teh, H-S. and Paetkau, V., 1974, Biphasic effect of cyclic AMP on an immune response, Nature 250:505.

Waldmann, A., Broder, S., Blaese, R.M., Durm, M., Goldman, C., and Muul, L., 1979, The role of suppressor cells in human disease, in "The Biological Basis for Immunodeficiency Disease" (E.W. Gelfand, H-M. Dosch, eds.), In press, Raven Press, New York.

LITHIUM AND IMMUNE FUNCTION IN MAN

F. Anthony Greco

Division of Oncology
Department of Medicine
Vanderbilt University Medical Center
Nashville, Tennessee 37232

Lithium has diverse biologic effect on many organ systems. The effects of lithium on the central nervous system, thyroid gland, kidney, heart, gastrointestinal tract, and bone marrow have been investigated (Singer and Rotenburg, 1973; Rothstein et al., 1978). Lithium appears to exert some physiologic actions by interfering with cyclic AMP mediated processes which are regulated by polypeptide hormones (Smith et al., 1977).

Since cyclic AMP mediated events are involved in the regulation of human lymphocyte activation during the response to antigen (Parker, 1976), one could speculate that lithium might effect immune function in man. In addition, immuno-stimulatory activity of lithium was demonstrated by in vitro testing of human lymphocytes and macrophages and lithium augmented thymidine incorporation of phytohemagglutinin-stimulated lymphocytes, mixed lymphocyte culture responses and phagocytosis of latex particles by macrophages (Shenkman et al., 1976). In mice, lithium enhanced resistance to a transplanted tumor (Shenkman et al., 1976). The present study was designed to assess the immune function of patients and normal volunteers receiving lithium

PATIENTS

Eight subjects were studied in this evaluation. Five manic depressive patients and three normal volunteers, who were not taking any other medication except lithium carbonate, had serial evaluations of their immune function. The dose of lithium carbonate was 300 mg by mouth three times a day for three weeks in the volunteers. The patients started at this dose but most were escalated to 600 mg three times daily. The patients had immune evaluation before and during lithium administration and the volunteers before, during, and after lithium.

METHODS

Delayed hypersensitivity skin testing was done with standard recall antigens: purified protein derivative (PPD) (0.1 cc - Intermediate strength), mumps (0.1 cc), and streptokinase-streptodornase (SKSD) (10 units). These antigens were injected intradermally and read at 48 hours for millimeters of induration. Five millimeters of induration was considered a positive skin test. The primary antigen, keyhole limpet hemocyanin (KLH) was used to assess primary immune response (Paul et al., 1974). The immunizing dose of KLH was given intramuscularly at a dose of 2.5 mg and the delayed hypersensitivity response measured by skin testing with 0.1 mg of antigen intradermally as described above for the recall antigens. Antibody response to KLH was also measured.

For the in vitro assays, 15 ml of whole blood was separated by Ficoll-Hypaque gradient to obtain a mononuclear cell preparation. The T cell rosette assay utilized was the total "T" rosette assay as previously described (West et al., 1976). One-tenth ml of lymphocyte suspension (5 x 10^6/ml) was mixed well with 0.2 ml fetal calf serum and then with 0.2 ml of sheep red blood cells (SRBC) (5 x 10^7/ml). The tubes were incubated at 37° for 5 minutes, then centrifuged at 200 X G for five minutes. The resulting lymphocyte/SRBC suspension was incubated at 4^oC overnight. The cells were gently resuspended by hand and counted in a hemocytometer chamber to obtain the percentage of rosette forming cells. The adherence of at least three sheep blood cells to a lymphocyte was required to define a rosette forming cell. All tests were run in triplicate.

Lymphocyte blastogenesis was performed using the mononuclear cell preparation obtained as described above. Blastogenesis was done in our microculture assay as previously described (Dean et al., 1975a; Dean et al., 1975b). Phytohemagglutinin (PHA) was selected as the mitogen for this study. Our results were reported in the form of relative proliferative index (RPI), a value comparing the net patient's counts per minute (CPM) with the average CPM of three normals tested the same day (Dean et al., 1977). The RPI is less variable than the stimulation index which may vary widely according to the baseline CPM. Variation among individuals from day to day is standardized by the RPI. The RPI is defined as:

$$\text{RPI} = \frac{\begin{array}{c}\text{CPM of patient lymphocytes}\\ \text{in the presence of stimulant (E)}\end{array} - \begin{array}{c}\text{CPM of patient}\\ \text{lymphocytes alone (C)}\end{array}}{\text{Mean E - C of normal controls included in the same assay}}$$

Our previous studies have indicated that an RPI in the range of 0.5 to 1.5 is within the normal range of 95% of the normal population.

In the normal volunteers the skin testing, peripheral blood T rosette levels, in vitro lymphocyte transformation and KLH immunization were done three weeks prior to the beginning of the administration of lithium carbonate. Serial reevaluations, including KLH antibody titers, and quantitation of immunoglobulins IgG and IgM were done after one and three weeks of lithium administration and one month after stopping lithium. In the five manic depressive patients, initial evaluation was done one week before beginning lithium carbonate, and thereafter every two to three weeks while on lithium for a total of three tests in most patients.

RESULTS

There was no difference in the percentage of T rosettes or the degree of lymphocyte transformation concomitant with the administration of lithium carbonate (Table I). There was no difference in the serial skin testing during this study and the percentage of T rosette forming cells remained relatively stable during the administration of lithium. Response to PHA did not appear to be affected by the administration of lithium and the response to KLH was consistent with that seen previously in normal volunteers in the absence of lithium (Table II) (Paul et al., 1974). No quantitative changes in the immunoglobulins of IgG or IgM were noted.

TABLE I

IMMUNOLOGICAL TESTS

Patients	% T Rosettes*			Lymphocyte Blastogenesis**		
	Before Li_2CO_3	1 week Li_2CO_3	3 weeks Li_2CO_3	Before Li_2CO_3	1 week Li_2CO_3	3 weeks Li_2CO_3
1	75	73	77	—	—	—
2	68	65	64	—	—	—
3	70	72	69	1.14	0.95	1.13
4	69	72	66	1.17	1.14	1.20
5	—	73	70	0.88	0.96	0.90
Normal Volunteers**						
1	83	84	81	2.04	2.24	1.79
2	81	86	78	1.10	1.81	1.00
3	79	76	77	1.72	1.86	1.56

* % Rosette at $4^{o}C$

** Lymphocyte blastogenesis to PHA expressed as RPI (See Text)

*** Normals were off Li_2CO_3 at 3 week test point

TABLE II

EFFECTS OF LITHIUM ON ANTIBODY FORMATION

	KLH TITER		
Patients	Before Li_2CO_3	During Li_2CO_3	After Li_2CO_3
1	1:4	1:256	-----
2	1:16	1:256	-----
3	1:32	1:256	-----
4	----	-----	-----
5	1:64	1:2048	-----
Normals			
1	1:64	1:1024	1:2048
2	1:8	1:1048	1:2048
3	1:8	1:8192	1:4096

DISCUSSION

Our results failed to show any evidence of immunological abnormality as measured by these assays in manic depressive and normal subjects after short-term administration of lithium carbonate. These results in man do not support the *in vitro* data suggesting that lithium is an immunostimulant. There was no effect three weeks after discontinuation of lithium in the three normal volunteers nor any effect in the patients who continued the drug.

These results are of interest because lithium is currently being utilized in several clinical trials attempting to take advantage of its diverse biologic activity. Lithium is being used to treat patients with the syndrome of inappropriate anti-diuretic hormone secretion (White and Fetner, 1975; Baker *et al*., 1977) and research continues in patients with hyperthyroidism (Temple *et al*., 1972). Lithium stimulates human neutrophil production (Rothstein *et al*., 1978) and lithium is being investigated in patients with granulocytopenia (Greco and Brereton, 1977; Stein et al., 1977). Since lithium carbonate is being used in a wider clinical setting, including those patients with granulocytopenia and on cancer chemotherapy, the lack of immunological depression may favor its use in these trials. There are recent data suggesting lithium in vitro increases mitogen-induced lymphocyte proliferation and inhibits suppressor T cell activity by modulating cyclic AMP-dependent events in lymphocytes (Gelfand et al., 1979). Lithium in vivo does not appear to increase mitogen-induced lymphocyte proliferation. Regulation of suppressor cell expression in individuals receiving lithium was not addressed by this study and has not been eliminated as a possibility. The present study demonstrates no short-term immunological depression in man following the administration of lithium

REFERENCES

Baker, R.S., Hurley, R.M., Feldman, W., 1977, Treatment of recurrent syndrome of inappropriate secretion of antidiuretic hormone with lithium, J. Ped. 90:480.

Dean, J.H., Silva, J.S., McCoy, J.L., Leonard, C.M., Middleton, M., Cannon, G.B., and Herbman, R.B., 1975a, Lymphocyte blastogenesis induced by 3M KCl extracts of allogenic breast carcinoma and lymphoid cells, J. Natl. Cancer Inst. 54:1295.

Dean, J.H., Silva, J.S., McCoy, J.L., Chan, S.P., Baker, J.J., Leonard, C., and Herbman, R.B., 1975b, In vitro human reactivity to staphylococcal phage lysate, J. Immunol. 115:1060.

Dean, J.H., Connor, R., Herbman, R.B., Silva, J., McCoy, J.L., Oldham, R.K., 1977, The relative proliferation index as a more sensitive parameter for evaluating lymphoproliferative responses of cancer patients to mitogens and alloantigens, Int. J. Cancer 20:359.

Gelfand, E.W., Dosch, H.M., Hastings, D., Shore, A., 1979, Lithium: A modulator of cyclic AMP-dependent events in lymphocytes, Science 203:365.

Greco, F.A., and Brereton, H., 1977, Effect of lithium carbonate on the neutropenia caused by chemotherapy: A preliminary clinical trial, Oncology 34:153.

Parker, C.W., 1976, Control of lymphocyte function, New Eng. J. Med. 295:1180.

Paul, S., Kenny, A.B., Hitzig, W.H., 1974, Immune response to keyhole-limpet hemocyanin in the human, Inter. Arch. Aller. Appl. Immunol. 47:155.

Rothstein, G., Clarkson, D.R., Larsen, W., Grosser, B.I., Athens, J.W., 1978, Effect of lithium on neutrophil mass and production, New Eng. J. Med. 298:178.

Shenkman, L., Borkowsky, W., Holzman, R.S., Shopsin, B., 1976, Lithium chloride, an immunologic adjuvant, Clin. Res. 27:634A.

Singer, E., and Rotenberg, D., 1973, Mechanisms of lithium action, New Eng. J. Med. 289:254.

Smith, J.W., Steiner, A.L., Newberry, W.M., Parker, C.W., 1971, Cyclic adenosine 3', 5' - monophosphate in human lymphocytes. Alterations after phytohemagglutinin stimulation, J. Clin. Invest. 50:432.

Stein, R.S., Beaman, C., Ali, M.Y., Hanson, R., Jenkins, D.D., Jume'an, H.G., 1977, Lithium attenuation of chemotherapy-induced neutropenia, New Eng. J. Med. 179:430.

Temple, R., Berman, M., Robbins, J., and Wolfe, J., 1972, The use of lithium in the treatment of thyroxtoxicosis, J. Clin. Invest. 51:2746.

West, W., Sienknecht, C.W., Townes, A.S., Herberman, R.B., 1976, Performance of a rosette assay between lymphocytes and sheep erythrocytes at elevated temperatures to study patients with cancer and other diseases, J. Clin. Immunol. Immunopath. 5:60.

White, M.G., and Fetner, C.D., 1975, Treatment of the syndrome of inappropriate secretion of antidiuretic hormone with lithium carbonate, New Eng. J. Med. 292:390.

INDEX

GPSR Compliance
The European Union's (EU) General Product Safety Regulation (GPSR) is a set of rules that requires consumer products to be safe and our obligations to ensure this.

If you have any concerns about our products, you can contact us on

ProductSafety@springernature.com

In case Publisher is established outside the EU, the EU authorized representative is:

Springer Nature Customer Service Center GmbH
Europaplatz 3
69115 Heidelberg, Germany

www.ingramcontent.com/pod-product-compliance
Ingram Content Group UK Ltd.
Pitfield, Milton Keynes, MK11 3LW, UK
UKHW051127260726
13967UKWH00010B/2911
* 9 7 8 1 4 7 5 7 0 2 6 0 6 *